Health Informatics

This series is directed to healthcare professionals leading the transformation of healthcare by using information and knowledge. For over 20 years, Health Informatics has offered a broad range of titles: some address specific professions such as nursing, medicine, and health administration; others cover special areas of practice such as trauma and radiology; still other books in the series focus on interdisciplinary issues, such as the computer based patient record, electronic health records, and networked healthcare systems. Editors and authors, eminent experts in their fields, offer their accounts of innovations in health informatics. Increasingly, these accounts go beyond hardware and software to address the role of information in influencing the transformation of healthcare delivery systems around the world. The series also increasingly focuses on the users of the information and systems: the organizational, behavioral, and societal changes that accompany the diffusion of information technology in health services environments.

Developments in healthcare delivery are constant; in recent years, bioinformatics has emerged as a new field in health informatics to support emerging and ongoing developments in molecular biology. At the same time, further evolution of the field of health informatics is reflected in the introduction of concepts at the macro or health systems delivery level with major national initiatives related to electronic health records (EHR), data standards, and public health informatics.

These changes will continue to shape health services in the twenty-first century. By making full and creative use of the technology to tame data and to transform information, Health Informatics will foster the development and use of new knowledge in healthcare.

Paolo Maria Matricardi • Stephanie Dramburg

Digital Allergology

From Theory to Practice

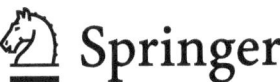 Springer

Paolo Maria Matricardi 🔟
Department of Pediatric Respiratory Medicine
Immunology and Critical Care Medicine
Charité–Universitätsmedizin Berlin,
a corporate member of Freie Universität
Berlin and Humboldt–Universität zu Berlin
Berlin, Germany

Institute of Allergology
Charité—Universitätsmedizin Berlin
Corporate Member of Freie Universität Berlin
and Humboldt-Universität zu Berlin
Berlin, Germany

Fraunhofer Institute for Translational
Medicine and Pharmacology ITMP
Allergology and Immunology
Berlin, Germany

Stephanie Dramburg 🔟
Department of Pediatric Respiratory Medicine
Immunology and Critical Care Medicine
Charité–Universitätsmedizin Berlin,
a corporate member of Freie Universität
Berlin and Humboldt–Universität zu Berlin
Berlin, Germany

ISSN 1431-1917   ISSN 2197-3741   (electronic)
Health Informatics
ISBN 978-3-031-71020-9   ISBN 978-3-031-71021-6   (eBook)
https://doi.org/10.1007/978-3-031-71021-6

This book is dedicated to the memory of Marcus Maurer, a most brilliant mind, charismatic scientist, enthusiastic mentor, and generous colleague.
The editors.

Foreword

Digital health is revolutionizing allergology, with the increasing adoption of mobile devices and applications in allergy practices. The European Academy of Allergy and Clinical Immunology (EAACI) has taken a leading role in developing guidelines and position papers on digital health in allergology. This emerging field is transforming the management of allergic conditions by harnessing technologies such as mobile apps, telemedicine, and electronic health records. One of the main advantages is personalized care, where digital tools enable tailored diagnostic and therapeutic approaches. This improves patient stratification and treatment outcomes, allowing for precision medicine in allergology. For instance, digital platforms can analyze individual patient data to create customized treatment plans and follow up of treatments and side effects in a personalized fashion.

Digital health is transforming allergology, with mobile devices and apps becoming increasingly prevalent in allergy practices. The European Academy of Allergy and Clinical Immunology (EAACI) has been at the forefront of developing guidelines and position papers on digital health in allergology. A 2017 EAACI Task Force meeting in Berlin, leading to a position paper on digital health in allergy was a front leader in the area. This book, *Digital Health for Allergology: From Theory to Practice*, provides a comprehensive overview of mHealth in allergy across various diseases.

Remote monitoring is an important significant benefit of digital health. Apps like MASK-Air and AllergyMonitor help patients track their symptoms and exposure to allergens, facilitating self-management and informed decision-making. Real-time tracking of environmental factors can be enabled in these tools that affect allergies, providing important data for the analysis of long-term trends. Telemedicine is another area where digital health excels. Video consultations enhance patient-doctor communication, particularly during regular follow-ups for treatments such as allergen immunotherapy. This increases accessibility to specialist care, especially in remote areas, and reduces travel time and costs for patients.

However, with these advancements comes the need for a major problem, namely better data protection and regulation. There is a pressing requirement for robust data protection measures, certification programs for digital health tools, and appropriate reimbursement systems. Ensuring compliance with evolving healthcare regulations is also crucial. Digital health solutions significantly enhance patient engagement by encouraging active participation in health management. They improve health literacy through educational content and facilitate better communication between patients and healthcare providers. Additionally, digital platforms boost treatment adherence by providing reminders and tracking tools, which can visually demonstrate treatment progress and motivate patients.

The integration of big data and AI further supports clinical decision-making by analyzing large-scale data to identify patterns and trends. AI algorithms can predict allergy flare-ups based on various factors, offering valuable insights for healthcare providers. Wearable technology also plays a role by integrating with smartwatches and other devices for continuous monitoring. These tools track vital signs and environmental factors in real-time, providing early warning systems for potential allergic reactions. Moreover, digital therapeutics offer cognitive behavioral therapy for managing anxiety related to allergies. They provide guided relaxation techniques to help manage symptoms and incorporate gamification elements to encourage consistent self-care practices. Digital health solutions may also streamline and improve clinical trials by facilitating patient recruitment and data collection for research. They enable remote participation in clinical trials, increasing diversity and providing more comprehensive and continuous data for study analysis. Finally, digital health enhances interdisciplinary care coordination by improving communication between different specialists involved in allergy care. It facilitates seamless sharing of patient data across healthcare teams, enhancing continuity of care for patients with multiple allergic conditions.

To implement digital health solutions for allergic diseases, several significant challenges will have to be endured. The main challenges in implementing digital health solutions for allergic diseases can be listed as follows. Data Privacy and Security: Keeping patient information safe and secure is a big challenge. Interoperability and Standardization: Different healthcare systems don't always work well together, making it hard to share data between them. There's a need for a common language so that different platforms can communicate easily. Clinical Validation and Regulatory Approval: Digital health tools need to be proven safe and effective, just like any other medical treatment. Getting approval from regulatory bodies can be complex and should be based on clear rules. User Adoption and Digital Literacy: Some healthcare providers and patients might not be comfortable using new technology. An important hurdle is to make sure everyone can use easily these tools. Cost and Reimbursement: Developing digital health solutions can be expensive, and it's not always clear how these costs will be covered by insurance or healthcare systems. Data Quality and Reliability: Making sure the information collected is accurate and useful is important. This includes managing a lot of data and using them effectively. Integration into Clinical Workflow: Digital tools need to fit smoothly into how healthcare providers already work. This means avoiding too much extra work and balancing interaction with digital tools for personal care. There is no chance to overloading the healthcare systems by digital tools.

Overall, digital health in allergology not only enhances patient engagement, adherence to treatment plans, and quality of life for those with allergic conditions, but also revolutionizes the way allergic diseases are diagnosed, monitored, and treated. It empowers both patients and healthcare providers with tools that were previously unavailable, leading to more efficient management of allergic diseases. However, an extensive collaboration is required between healthcare providers, technology developers, policymakers, and patients to address key challenges to create effective and sustainable digital health solutions. These challenges need to be addressed so that digital health solutions can be effective and helpful for people with allergies. Addressing these challenges requires collaboration between healthcare providers, technology developers, policymakers, and patients to create effective and sustainable digital health solutions for allergic diseases.

I sincerely congratulate the authors for this very useful and easily readable book.

Davos, Switzerland   Cezmi Akdis
April 2025

Preface

Worldwide, a billion people experience an allergic reaction at least once in their life.

Pollen, mites, animal epithelia, fungi, any sort of food, insect venom, drugs and occupational agents, innocuous for most humans, can be dangerous to those who develop an allergic reaction to them. Luckily, the biotechnology revolution remarkably improved diagnostic precision and new therapeutic options emerge steadily. However, the gap between a declining number of allergists offering highly specialized care and an increasing number of patients with complex allergic diseases is widening. Given this scenario, even the best solutions for diagnostics and therapy reach only a tiny minority of the vast population of allergic patients.

Digital health is defined by the World Health Organization (WHO) as "a field of knowledge and practice associated with the development and use of digital technologies to improve health". The comprehensive WHO definition also addresses the universe of smart devices and connected equipment, as well as related areas, such as artificial intelligence, big data, block chain, interoperability of health data systems, the internet of things, and telemedicine. Based on this great diversity of flexible opportunities, digital health is considered to have immense potential when it comes to reducing the above-mentioned gap between a growing need for and declining offer of personalized healthcare in all areas of medicine, including allergology.

"Digital Allergology: From Theory to Practice" is a first attempt to define the new area of Digital Allergology and collate theoretical background with reports of pragmatic experiences in one single book. Being Digital Allergology still in its infancy, this book is neither a textbook, nor a systematic report of every project related to digital health and allergology in the world. It is rather aimed at initiating the scientific community into this new, yet rapidly moving field, where opinion leaders and researchers share their knowledge and visions. Another aim of ours is to promote further research in this area by inspiring scientists, clinicians, engineers, public health experts, and many other stakeholders to join efforts for new developments in this highly multi-disciplinary field.

The first section of the book includes an introductory overview of all chapters, as well as comprehensive summaries of definitions, general concepts, and the regulatory framework of digital tools in healthcare. Building up on this general knowledge, a second section compiles reports on how digital health technologies have been recently implemented for the most prevalent allergic diseases, including allergic rhino-conjunctivitis, with a focus on pollen allergies, asthma, pre-school wheezing, chronic urticaria, atopic dermatitis, and drug allergies. A third section then focuses on tools and methodologies like wearables, sensors, clinical decision support systems, databanks, expert systems, machine learning approaches and finally social media. Finally, the book is concluded by three chapters offering a detailed depiction of the implementation of digital allergy care in three prototype countries, namely Germany, Spain, and Australia.

After 12 months of intense and exciting work, the Editors wish to express their warm gratitude to all the outstanding experts who enthusiastically accepted their invitation to contribute to this common enterprise. A special acknowledgement to the Springer book editorial team for their continuous, scrupulous and patient support. Last but not least, we also thank in advance all readers for sharing their impressions, comments, criticism and suggestions with us. Our wish is that "Digital Allergology", now just a newborn, will quickly become a vital, strong adolescent, so that very soon new books will be published to disseminate knowledge and help decisionmakers in healthcare systems to provide digitally aided care to their allergic citizens.

Berlin, Germany   Paolo Maria Matricardi
Berlin, Germany   Stephanie Dramburg
May 2024

Contents

xiii

Chapter 1
Digital Allergology: State of the Art, 2024

Paolo Maria Matricardi (ID) **and Oliver Pfaar** (ID)

Contents

This book chapter is an extended summary of the content of other 21 chapters of the Book "Digital Allergology: From Theory to Practice". Matricardi PM, Dramburg S. (Editors). 2024. Springer.

P. M. Matricardi (✉)
Department of Pediatric Respiratory Medicine, Immunology and Critical Care Medicine, Charité–Universitätsmedizin Berlin, a corporate member of Freie Universität Berlin and Humboldt–Universität zu Berlin, Berlin, Germany

Institute of Allergology, Charité—Universitätsmedizin Berlin, Corporate Member of Freie Universität Berlin and Humboldt-Universität zu Berlin, Berlin, Germany

Fraunhofer Institute for Translational Medicine and Pharmacology ITMP, Allergology and Immunology, Berlin, Germany
e-mail: paolo.matricardi@charite.de

O. Pfaar
Department of Otorhinolaryngology, Head and Neck Surgery, Section of Rhinology and Allergy, University Hospital Marburg, Philipps-Universität Marburg, Marburg, Germany
e-mail: oliver@pfaar.org

P. M. Matricardi, S. Dramburg, *Digital Allergology*, Health Informatics, https://doi.org/10.1007/978-3-031-71021-6_1

Abstract The enormous expansion of digital health will increasingly impact allergy practice and its scientific background. This development is so substantial that it generated a new area of interest, defined "Digital Allergology" and was first described with a position paper of the European Academy of Allergy and Clinical Immunology (EAACI). After describing pioneering initiatives, this introductory chapter continues as an extended summary of the book "Digital Allergology: from theory to practice." The state of the art of digital allergology is described in terms of definitions and regulatory issues, e-Diaries for allergic rhinitis, allergic asthma, and wheezing disorders, chronic urticaria and atopic dermatitis, as well as drug allergies. Sections are also dedicated to wearables and social media, omics science, big data, and artificial intelligence. A description of how digital technologies are implemented in real life scenarios in large countries is also given, with a focus on Spain, Germany, and Australia.

Abbreviations

A&AA	Allergy and Anaphylaxis Australia
ADFS	Allergen Database for Food Safety
ADHA	Australian Digital Health Agency
AI	Artificial Intelligence
AIT	Allergen Immunotherapy
AR	Allergic Rhinitis
ASCIA	Australasian Society of Clinical Immunology and Allergy
ASD	Allergy Study Directory
ANN	Artificial Neural Networks
ARIA	Allergic Rhinitis and its Impact on Asthma
ANZCTR	Australian and New Zealand Clinical Trials registry
AusCAR	Australasian Registry of Severe Cutaneous Adverse Reactions
CARAT	Control of Allergic Rhinitis and Asthma Test
CDSS	Clinical Decision Support Systems
COMPARE	Comprehensive Protein Allergen Resource
CRUSE	Chronic Urticaria Self-evaluation
CURE	Chronic Urticaria Registry
EAACI	European Academy of Allergy and Clinical Immunology
ePROMs	Electronic Patient-Reported Outcomes
DHS	Digital Health Strategy
GDPR	General Data Protection Regulation
HCP	Health Care Providers
HER	Electronic Health Records
IUS	International Union of Immunological Societies
iNAAN	International Network of Antibiotic Allergy Nations
LCA	Latent Class Analysis
ML	Machine Learning

MDA	Multi-dimensional Analyses
MDR	Medical Device Regulation
mHealth	mobile Health
NACE	National Allergy Centre of Excellence
NHS	National Health Survey
PCC	Person-Centered Care
SCORAD	SCORing Atopic Dermatitis
TF	Task Force
UCARE	Urticaria Centers of Reference and Excellence
UCARE 4 U	Chronic Urticaria Comprehensive Patient Care
WHO	World Health Organization

1.1   Introduction to Digital Health in Allergology and to an EAACI Position Paper

Principles of digital mobile Health have increasingly been identified for optimizing therapeutic care in all areas of medicine [1]. Consequently, the Organization for Economic Coordination and Development (OECD) has recently underlined the impact and potential of using, e.g., mHealth digital tools and health information system approaches for the optimized management of chronic diseases aiming to alert key strategic priorities to policy makers [2]. A first attempt to summarize digital health knowledge and experiences in allergology was completed by the European Academy of Allergy and Clinical Immunology (EAACI) as an expert Task Force (TF) project. As the largest specialist society in the field of allergy, the EAACI has elaborated and still develops many guidelines, position papers, and consensus reports in a variety of topics aimed to provide evidence-based recommendations for clinical care in allergology.

The EAACI-TF "Digital Health" met in Berlin in April 2017, and the fruitful debate between experts gave rise to a position paper published the following year in the journal *Allergy* [3]. At that time, mobile communication devices, including smartphones, tablet computers, and sensors, were already widely used in allergy practices and by allergic patients with several different targets, but neither validation studies nor guidelines were available to support doctors and patients in their proper use. Nevertheless, it was clear that mobile devices were going to support and, in some cases, hopefully improve allergy-related health services, to facilitate the flow of data and information, reinforce patient self-management, disease surveillance and monitoring, and improve adherence to disease management guidelines in allergy diagnosis, prevention, and therapy. By endorsing the general orientation promoted by the World Health Organization's (WHO) initiative "Be He@lthy, Be Mobile," the Task Force discussed in depth the quality, usability, efficiency, advantages, limitations, and risks of several categories of mobile devices for allergic patients and their caregivers. Starting with an analysis of the, at that time recently introduced, GDPR ("General Data Protection Regulation") and of other Medical

Directives of the European Community, the Task Force evaluated the scopes, design, patient's participation, medical and scientific content, efficiency and impact, credibility and accountability, and privacy of several mHealth products. Conclusions of that document focused also on the need to continuously update position papers and didactic material to minimize the gap between specific training of the healthcare professionals and the rapidly evolving world of digital health, producing innovation at a very quick pace [3].

In the light of the importance of person-centered care (PCC), especially in the field of allergy, e.g., by optimizing therapeutic strategies, EAACI supported subsequent TF-projects together with the global Allergic Rhinitis and its Impact on Asthma (ARIA)-initiative [4]. A most recent position paper focuses on the potential role of mHealth apps as "digital biomarkers" for improving PCC in allergen immunotherapy (AIT) [5]. EAACI experts highlighted the current applicability of apps, their advantages in the clinical and study-related setting and current limitations, and elaborated recommendations for further development and impact in the field [5].

This introductory chapter aims to meet the challenge posed by the EAACI Position Papers and presents a state of the art regarding the theoretical background and the practical application of digital health technologies in allergy care, based on a recent article collection under the title "Digital Health for Allergology: from theory to practice" [6]. The collection combines contributions from 58 experts and provides a state of the art overview on the field of mHealth in allergy in 22 chapters, ranging from definitions and regulatory issues, digital health innovation for several allergic diseases, including allergic rhinitis, asthma and preschool wheezing disorders, chronic urticaria, atopic dermatitis and drug allergies, databanks, artificial intelligence, and their use in clinical decision support systems (CDSS), wearables, social media, telemedicine, and current examples of digital allergology implementation in three countries: Spain, Germany, and Australia [6].

1.2   Definition and Regulatory Issues

"Digital Health" has acquired a long list of definitions and encompasses several different scientific and informatic technological areas. This list includes also e-Health, telehealth, telemedicine, telemonitoring, mHealth, social media, artificial intelligence, machine learning, deep learning, big data, omic science, and others. In her chapter [7], Esther Metting provides definitions not only for most of these words, but also informs about the complex interplay among these knowledge areas. She describes how in the last few decades, home computers and internet are progressively liberating medical offices, clinical records, and medical science itself from paper. A model based on paper archives with a priviliged access limited to the doctors and scientists, is transforming into a paper-free, digitalized network offering every stakeholder easy access to medical science and information to individual patients, demolishing barriers of knowledge, and facilitating a more active and aware participation of the patients in their own disease management process. The communication between patients and their health-care providers, once limited by space and time, is becoming more efficient through digitalization, allowing remote assistance (telemedicine) and asynchronous exchange of information and advice (telemonitoring). If properly used, patient training through digital meetings, consultations, and platforms is strongly supporting adherence to treatment instructions and guidelines, while reducing stress, time, and costs due to transportation. Overall, this digital revolution in medicine will allow the progressive integration of most recent and effective technologies, reduce costs, and make innovative healthcare affordable and accessible for all.

Artificial intelligence is a great opportunity, and its unpreceded power is a challenge for humanity. Big players in the world are developing more and more powerful AI systems to exponentially gain global influence in most areas of life, from economy to war systems, from research and innovation to population control. Meanwhile, the European Union is elaborating more and more complex regulations, in the hope that a juristic approach to this matter will protect Europeans' freedom, sinking economy, and privileged lifestyle. AI is closely related to digital health issues and deals also with personal health data, i.e., the most sensitive ones. In his comprehensive chapter on legal and regulatory challenges for digital health technologies [8], Sebastian Dramburg first introduces this discipline and then describes in detail, with a European perspective, many topics concerning DH systems certification, liability issues, data protection and security aspects, and legal and ethical challenges concerning digital health and artificial intelligence [8]. Mobile health applications are medical devices and must follow, in Europe, the Medical Device Regulation (MDR) in the attempt to guarantee safety, functionality, and public trust of medical devices [9]. This is obtained with complex registration systems including a thorough evaluation of adherence to regulatory requirements. Legislation is also identifying liability for damages or fines and harm of reputation for failure to comply with the European regulations, violation of intellectual property rights, defamation, or unlawful activities [8]. Data protection and safety are fundamental and complex areas for healthcare providers and their institutions. The General Data Protection Regulation (GDPR) [10] is the European legislative response to the needs of European citizens. GDPR regulates fundamental principles of ethical data handling and security, focusing on purpose limitation, data minimisation, standard contractual clauses, and binding corporate rules [8]. GDPR is still marginally considering the novel legal implications posed by AI on the production and use of medical devices and applications. For example, it is not immediately clear who is responsible in case of malfunctioning of an AI-based medical device (programmer, manufacturer, supplier or distributor, operator or user). An initiative has been recently taken by the EU Commission to face this additional challenge [8].

1.3 E-Diaries for Allergic Rhinitis

Perhaps the most popular digital tool for allergic diseases is the so-called e-Diary for allergic rhinitis (AR). Pollen is a major trigger of symptoms in most patients with AR, whose symptoms tend to be seasonal. Monitoring the concentration of pollen grains in the air is therefore important for diagnosis, prediction, and prevention of seasonal allergic rhinitis. Pollen monitoring is also instrumental in evaluating the impact of drug therapy and allergen immunotherapy during the pollen season. Daily monitoring of pollen grain concentration in the atmosphere is almost as old as the concept of pollinosis. A first pollen trap producing data to draw trajectories of grass pollen counts was produced and used by Sir Charles Blackley already in the second half of the nineteenth century [11]. The use of computer-based clinical diaries, registering trajectories of symptoms is dating back to the 1970s of the twentieth century [12]. However, this diagnostic tool has never been popular until recently when digital apps for smartphones and tablets made almost real-time information on the concentration of pollen in the atmosphere available to patients with pollen allergy [13].

First, in a chapter on automated pollen monitoring and exposure prediction for pollen allergic patients [14], Mariel Suarez-Suarez et al. illustrate how pollen capture and registration systems are becoming automatic thanks to reading devices based on deep learning. Pollen monitoring stations are spread in some areas only, such as Europe [15], where they are organized in networks. Pollen data are disseminated through networks organizing pollen stations and made available through the media, websites, and smartphone apps [16]. However, many apps are providing pollen forecast information in the absence of any scientific validation or certification of their monitoring and prediction systems. However, networks based on automated pollen stations, molecular measures of pollen allergenicity and co-exposure to microbial products or pollutants, and new AI algorithms will probably overcome this problem [16]. Most pollen stations are based on manual methods, with a delay in delivery of the data. By contrast, automatic pollen monitors can provide (near)-real-time data, relevant for diagnosing, monitoring, and forecasting symptoms triggered by exposure to the culprit pollen [17]. Several automated pollen monitors are commercially available, and comparative studies (including also some traditional Hirst-type traps) have shown that different devices produce heterogeneous results [18]. The chapter also presents the "allergic nose as pollen biosensor" concept [19], proposing that data provided by monosensitized index patients, when acquired through e-Diaries and with a citizen science approach, may reflect pollen concentrations and trends in the future [20–22] or may work as a valuable proxy of it in geographic areas where no pollen station is available [19]. On the other hand, also social media posts on allergy symptoms may help measuring pollen exposure, as observed in several cohorts [23, 24].

A widely popular e-Diary dedicated to the patient with pollen allergy has been produced and used since 2009 by the Austrian pollen information service of the Medical University of Vienna. In their chapter [25], Uwe Berger et al. summarize over a decade of experience and scientific studies based on their App. With "Pollen," users can follow daily not only the current trends, but also the short-term forecasts of the concentration of most relevant allergenic pollen grains all over their country. Patients can also enter personal symptom data, thus allowing the app to produce their own symptom report. This report can be used by patients and healthcare providers to visualize clinically significant correlations between personal symptoms and certain pollen types. Finally, the system can guide patients in their prevention strategies, aimed in general at avoiding exposure during critical days in specific areas characterized by very high pollen exposure. The field experience with the "Pollen" app is accompanied by a series of solid scientific studies, dedicated to design or use allergic rhinitis symptom scores [26], define pollen seasons [27], comparatively analyze pollen levels, allergen content, phenological data [28–30], and outdoor air pollution [31]. Similar mHealth applications have been implemented in daily practice in Germany (Husteblume) [32] or are planned to be implemented in other European countries (EU project PASYFO) [25]; moreover, "Pollen" is now integrating new features (Ragweed Finder) aimed at monitoring, through a citizen science approach, the rapid expansion of ragweed and ragweed allergy in some European geographic areas [25].

Also in 2009 started the long-lasting experience of AllergyMonitor®, an e-Diary for smartphones and tablets. In their chapter [33], Salvatore Tripodi et al. highlight major characteristics of the APP and its peculiar back-office enabling doctors to adapt the App's front-end according to the needs of their patient [34]. Moreover, patients can record their medication, immunotherapy intake and possible side effects, so the app also allows to monitor the adherence to treatment. As in the case of "Pollen," results can be viewed by both the patient and the health caregiver and reports for specific pre-selected monitoring periods are produced. AllergyMonitor® has been the basis for a series of scientific studies on pollen allergy diagnosis [35], allergen immunotherapy prescription [36], adherence and compliance to e-Diary compilation [37], medication [38], sublingual immunotherapy [39], disease severity score investigation [40], and epidemiological surveys [41].

1.4   Digital Health for Wheezing Disorders and Allergic Asthma

One of the respiratory and allergic diseases with the most advanced use of mobile medical devices and smartphone Apps is asthma. In their chapter [42], João Fonseca et al. review how digital solutions, including Apps, electronic patient-reported outcomes (ePROMs), clinical decision support systems (CDSS), and real-world data (e.g., asthma registries) contribute to improving unmet needs on asthma surveillance, diagnosis, and management [43]. The combined use of infodemiology data, including Google Trends and social media data [44], and of electronic health records (EHR) [45] will help improving digital surveillance-supporting tools in asthma and alert services forecasting exacerbations [42]. Mostly based on daily collection of patient's symptoms and medication data, disease severity scores for asthma have been developed, useful to measure and monitor its severity, identify disease clusters, and control patterns [46]. Digital health interventions with short message service (SMS)-based dose reminders [47], telemedicine intervention [48], and mobile apps [49] seem to be accepted [50] and efficient [51–54] in improving asthma management. An impressive series of digitalized medical devices, including smart inhalers, digital spirometers, digital oximeters, physical activity trackers, and air quality sensors, communicate with apps and complete the information provided directly by the patient [42]. Even the smartphone microphone is used to record and reproduce sounds produced by breathing and coughing, thus objectively monitoring the patient's monitoring status [42]. This information can be combined with ePROMS data collected with asthma apps, which generate disease severity scores—like the recent eDASTHMA [55] measuring short-term asthma control and the well-established Control of Allergic Rhinitis and Asthma Test (CARAT) [42] and measuring long-term asthma control. These tools are being integrated in CDSS for asthma diagnosis, monitoring and management, an area of investigation requiring further development and still understudied [56–58]. The chapter also reviews how registries for severe asthma, a valuable example of which is active in Portugal [59] can be interconnected with apps, thus allowing a broader view of the disease trends at population level, and facilitating classification and stratification studies [42]. Last, all the above-mentioned tools are going to be combined in a platform aiming at a complex digital health integrated asthma care pathway, targeted for diagnosis, surveillance, personalization and stratification, management, and shared decision medicine [42]. In another chapter on the same topic [60], Cefaloni et al. add further knowledge around digital applications, smarthalers, and asthma apps. Among other devices also mentioned in the above-listed chapters, the chapter focuses on digital devices monitoring exhaled nitric oxide, a key marker of eosinophilic airway inflammation [61], on regulatory and registration aspects conditioning this area of medicine, and on initiatives integrating digital data with remote care [60].

The development of digital health tools for wheezing disorders at preschool age, perhaps the most frequent and relevant pathology in pediatrics in high income countries, reflects the peculiar characteristic of this condition, quite different from asthma in adulthood. In their chapter [62], Do et al. summarize available information on Digital Health technologies for young children with wheeze and their potential role in the disease management of these pediatric conditions. Different categories of digital health interventions have been reviewed, including the use of deep learning-trained automatic wheeze-detectors, telemedicine strategies, wheeze monitoring apps, asthma gamification tools, and multicomponent digital interventions [62]. A special focus is dedicated to smart devices aimed at detection of pathological airway sounds in preschool children. These devices aim at helping parents in discriminating wheezing from other sounds, better modulate anti-symptomatic therapy, reduce family stress and needless doctor's consultations, and facilitate early diagnosis by at home monitoring [62]. Other sections are dedicated to smart nebulizers and smarthalers, alerting the doctor of patients' poor adherence to regular medication [62], smart devices promoting physical activity at home [63], multifunctional remote examination devices, recording and transmitting lung sounds [64], and pediatric mobile health clinic, drastically reducing the no-show-rate [65]. Asthma education also takes advantage from the digital world through gamification, which is obtained by software aimed at young children, combining informative sessions with games testing the acquired knowledge concerning disease and its self-management [66]. Last, an example of a multicomponent platform is discussed, which combines smartwatch applications with a commercially available wireless dust-sensor and a smart spirometer to forecast with confidence asthma exacerbation risk [67].

1.5   Digital Health for Chronic Urticaria, Atopic Dermatitis, and Drug Allergies

Among chronic allergic diseases, chronic urticaria and angioedema belong to those with highest impact on the patients' quality of life. In their chapter [68], Maurer et al. report on several digital tools and platforms targeted to improvement of patient and physician education, to monitoring disease activity, symptoms control, and response to treatment. They review the nature and first results obtained by apps for chronic urticaria self-evaluation (CRUSE), patient–physician communication, chronic urticaria comprehensive patient care (UCARE 4 U), and by a Chronic Urticaria Registry (CURE). Activation of the patient with chronic urticaria is promoted through digital care pathways adopting digital technologies aimed at shared decision-making intervention [69, 70]. A network of Urticaria Centers of Reference and Excellence (UCARE) provides lists of experts acting locally, many of which also offer teleconsultation and provide digital questionnaires rapidly evaluated for diagnosis and disease severity evaluation. In parallel, online webinars and publications with real-world evidence produced by the patient's registries (CURE, CARE) help doctors' education [71], also thanks to a UCARE LevelUp program based on regular webinars, podcasts, websites, journal clubs, grand rounds, and newsletter. With the recently launched CRUSE app, patients can monitor their disease activity and control, based on several disease severity indexes while being educated to a more successful outcome [68]. Importantly, the chapter informs "that through digital patient-physician communication, education, and disease monitoring, CU patients and their treating physicians share a common sense of empowerment" [68]. Moreover, digital tools save time and allow a more equal flow of information and a balanced interaction among patients and their caregivers [68]. It is also noted that the expansion of digital health in chronic urticaria will generate large databanks from geographically different areas, which will allow the use of data analytics and machine learning algorithms, thus further expanding the potential of the network in generating new knowledge and tailored treatment [68].

Another highly frequent and highly fastidious allergic disease of the skin is atopic dermatitis. A first mature software for calculation of the SCORing Atopic

Dermatitis (SCORAD) was already scientifically validated in 2002 [72]. Nevertheless, digital health tools for the management of patients with atopic dermatitis are not as advanced as those for chronic urticaria described above. In their chapter, Sebastian Sitaru et al. describe digital tools for AD patients as web searches, social media platforms, wearables, mobile apps, 3D full body scanners, and optical coherence tomography [72]. Unfortunately, the general quality of AD-related information online is considered rather low and often misleading. There is still insufficient data validating the clinical use of apps in AD. Similarly, although a plethora of Apps for AD is available in app stores, clinical validation of their use is scarce or missing [73]. Wearables, such as scratch measurement by wrist-worn non-invasive sensors [74], or trackers of the disease activity have been produced and require further clinical investigation [72]. As in other dermatological diseases, 2D and 3D image data are nowadays read, analyzed, and interpreted by automatic systems adopting deep learning procedures [75]. While studies suggest that it will be possible to predict persistence of AD beyond infancy with AI procedures, the implementation of this and similar approach in clinical practice is still only foreseen [76].

Digital health is also changing the approach to drug allergy diagnosis, monitoring, and management. In their chapter [77], Shuayb Elkhalifa et al. show how digital health improves patient safety, healthcare efficiency, accurate data management, interoperability, and continuity of care for patients with drug allergies. Electronic Health Records (EHRs) include nowadays comprehensive drug allergy profiles for patients, so that vital allergy information is promptly available to any doctor having access to the patient's EHR. At individual level, this allows alert messages to pop-up and prevent prescription of drugs that are dangerous for the patient, while at community level this allows monitoring trends of drug allergies and even identifying new, unpredicted drug allergies. On the one hand, oversimplification in codification is still a problem; on the other hand, not all doctors are educated to deal with similar information, therefore new systems should be accompanied by a parallel educational program to be properly used by all involved parties. Another problem lays with the poor standard definitions, overreporting and underreporting of drug allergies, which is adding confusion to the interpretation of the acquired information. Mobile applications give patients alerts and reminders if they enter drug allergies, and they also inform on drug interactions. Some apps are dedicated to drug allergy de-labeling, a very important issue for patients [78]. They help doctors correctly diagnose allergy to penicillin, and, conversely, help them in de-labeling, if they have received a wrong diagnosis. They may include clinical decision support systems not only for allergists, but also for non-allergist doctors [78].

1.6 Wearables and Social Media

Wearable technology will revolutionize healthcare services by empowering remote patient monitoring and expand a new form of medicine based more on objective patient's data than on reported and subjective impressions. In their chapter [79],

Justin Greiwe et al. start with describing Apple Watch, whose promises as a reliable health device were disattended by some hardware problems. In a few years, however, a vast and differentiated production of wearables opened the avenue to both active and passive data collection in many areas of medicine. The chapter reviews wearables for asthma, primary immunodeficiency, and atopic dermatitis. In asthmatic patients, wereables have been used to monitor sleep in adult women [80] and in children [81], physical activity [79], and breathing patterns [82, 83]. Other digital devices, measuring VO2 max or other lung function parameters, have been produced and investigated, but their reliability and efficiency is questioned and further high-quality studies are needed [79]. Wearables have been also used in immunodeficiencies, for immunoglobulin infusion (Wearable Infusor, IFI) [84], in atopic dermatitis, to measure scratching movements [85], and in food allergy, for food allergen detection [86]. Next-generation wearables, smaller, smarter, integrated with clothing or jewelry are rapidly being developed and released, and their targets and impact will be broader and broader, while their accuracy, usability, and concrete use will have to be demonstrated [79].

Social media platforms are being increasingly utilized to support allergy patients in diverse forms. In their two chapters [87, 88], Florin-Dan Popescu and Stephanie Dramburg present the historical background and basic functions of the most relevant social media and discuss how they can improve allergic disease management by addressing health education, patient's awareness, patient engagement as well as patient's support, monitoring of disease, and public health initiatives [89–91]. Allergy organizations and advocacy groups are linked with patients, receive and send information, educational material and support, not only through Facebook but also with many other social channels. Moreover, many doctors and health services also promote their activities through Facebook. Groups of patient support use social networks to exchange experiences, resources, and information on their diseases [89]. In parallel, allergies and asthma are commonly discussed on "X" by clinicians, patients and their organizations. Hashtags related to allergy topics guide users in finding information of their own interest [92]. Many Instagram accounts focus on allergies, and users can find information about so-called allergy-friendly foods and about products and lifestyle tips for allergic patients. Visual information is also circulated through Instagram and other social media by allergy associations, advocacy groups, health care providers (HCPs), companies, and allergy journals. An unsolved major problem, common to all social media, is that discrimination of true from false or inaccurate information can be very difficult for social media users, and the advantages of this development are balanced by this intrinsic risk [93]. Similarly, YouTube [94] and Tik-Tok [95] can become a source of valuable medical information for allergy patients, but the dangers of obtaining nonscientific, misleading, or even harmful information are not negligible [96]. To meet this challenge, allergists must increase their engagement in online networking and tackle medical misinformation related to allergy practice; they should also educate their patients in selecting proper sources of information in social media and consider the specialist as their reference counterpart [97].

1.7 Omics Science, Big Data, and Artificial Intelligence

Health electronic record forms and disease register generate databases concerning the patients. Allergic diseases and allergic symptoms are, by definition, caused and triggered by patient's exposure to allergens acquired from the external environment. In his chapter [98], Ronald Van Ree starts with mentioning the first, official World Health Organization (WHO) and International Union of Immunological Societies (IUIS) Allergen Nomenclature Subcommittee database [99] and describes existing allergen databases, their characteristics, and the way they can serve for scientific and clinical purposes. Allergen Online (AOL) [100], Allergen Database for Food Safety (ADFS) [101, 102], and Comprehensive Protein Allergen Resource (COMPARE) [103] contain basic information useful to compare primary sequences, predict or explain allergenicity, and investigate risk assessment. The first category of databanks feed training datasets of machine learning systems aimed at extracting from the primary sequence of the allergenic protein probabilistic information of de-novo allergenicity or cross-reactivity with already characterized allergens [98]. This is particularly useful for the food industry, whose goal in this area is to prevent, with a bioinformatic approach, the generation or use of molecules with high food allergenic potential [98]. Algorithms developed by bioinformaticians (e/g/ EVALLER) [104], aller-Stat [105], and others are improving in their efficiency, but 100% accuracy in prediction, given the complexity of allergenicity, cannot be reached so the criteria used by regulatory authorities for evaluation and selection are debated [98]. All Fam [106], the Structural Database of Allergenic Proteins (SDAP) [107], the Immune Epitope database (IEDB) [108], and the AllerBase database [109] focus more on allergen structure and investigate the inter-relationship of allergen molecules within structurally and functionally homogeneous families, as defined by the Protein Family database (Pfam) [110]. Last, ALLERGOME [111] is a very complex web-based platform providing broader information on allergens' taxonomical, biochemical, structural, functional, immunological, clinical, and epidemiological data. Allergome reaches a broader and differentiated stakeholder audience, spanning from molecular biologists to biochemists, from clinicians to epidemiologists, from regulators to laboratory doctors, and is instrumental to get a comprehensive State of the Art knowledge not only on the allergen molecules themselves, but also on the current use they serve in different areas of allergology [98].

Nowadays big databases are analyzed with methodologies of artificial intelligence, particularly machine learning (ML). In their chapter [112], Adnan Custovic and colleagues summarize the most recent development of the use of machine learning for the management of allergies and asthma in childhood. Unsupervised ML, such as clustering, is targeted to identify patterns or clusters in the database that may be totally hidden to the human eye or to the most sophisticated, but traditional statistical methods [113]. Supervised ML, such as classical regression models, support vector machines, and deep learning based on artificial neural networks (ANN), is targeted to predict output variables from input variables [113]. Given this distinction, ML has been used in attempts to generate prediction models for childhood asthma [114], latent class analysis (LCA) has been targeted to understand wheezing phenotypes [115], and new homogeneous and stable wheeze phenotypes have been discovered using multi-dimensional analyses (MDAs) [116]. Similarly, ML has been applied to the analysis of big datasets of allergic IgE sensitization generated by serological testing with allergen microarrays [112]. In this case, unsupervised analyses have been used to test whether sensitization trajectories are associated with different temporal patterns of wheezing, eczema, or allergic multimorbidity [112]. ML also suggested the existence of several different clusters of IgE sensitization and allowed discovering one of them, characterized by multiple, early IgE response to a broad set of allergenic molecules, as strongly associated with asthma diagnosis [117, 118]. Similarly, microarray data examined with ML disclosed that early, but not late-onset grass pollen sensitization was associated with allergic asthma [119]. Network analysis was applied to investigate interactions and connectivity patterns between IgE and molecules within a CRD array and relate them to a diagnosis of asthma [120]. Remarkable consistencies in the connectivity structure among IgE responses emerged from studies in populations from different countries, which may open avenues to novel diagnostic algorithms [112].

CDSSs are «information systems designed to improve clinical decision making». In their chapter [121], Paolo Maria Matricardi and Jean Bousquet review the benefits, challenges, and barriers to the use of CDSS in clinical allergology. CDSSs are extremely heterogeneous digital diagnostic tools, with algorithms, targets, timing, integration with existing systems, users, and other characteristics defining their category [121]. While their number, diffusion, and users are increasing in allergology, their effectiveness, limitations, and appropriateness are hotly debated [121]. MASK-Air® [122] and @IT-2020 [123] are two examples of electronic CDSS for allergic rhinitis supported by scientific publications, the first is targeted to support the day-by-day disease self-management and drug modulation [122], the second aims at supporting etiological diagnosis and identification of the culprit allergen in seasonal allergic rhinitis [36, 123]. Many other CDSS are mentioned, concerning (a) targeting early identification of severe asthma [124], asthma self-management improvement [125–128], proper use of SABA [127]; (b) monitoring and self-management of chronic urticaria [129]; (c) preventing drug allergies [130]. Some of these CDSSs are also presented in different chapters of this book. While some CDSSs are based on Bayesian algorithms, other adopt AI approaches (mostly ML). A long list of limitations of CDSS is discussed, and trials have shown only in some cases clinical usefulness and impact. However, this area of investigation is rapidly developing and, in general, the more CDSSs are used, the larger is the dataset they can analyze, and the more accurate they become [121].

1.8 Digital Allergology in Countries: Spain, Germany, Australia

The implementation of digital allergology in the real world is not only a free initiative of patients and doctors, but also part of the policy and plans of many governments and national health systems. The European next-generation plan incorporates digital health as one of its priorities, aiming at reducing costs and improving quality and equalness in assistance.

In their chapter [131], Antolin-Amerigo et al. describe how digital allergology is being implemented in Spain. The digital transformation of the public administration has received strong attention in Spain, and a Digital Health Strategy (DHS), articulated in 10 axes, is also involving the health sector. Within this framework, the new Spanish Strategy for Science, Technology, and Innovation, 2021–2027 is opening avenues to innovation in several aspects, including reimbursement structures, mobile health developments, telemedicine, remote care access, and integration of digital health tools in daily practice. Galicia, the Basque Country, Cataluña, and Andalusia have established tele-dermatology services, with Galicia playing a pioneer role also in conducting teleconsultations for pneumology [132]. COVID-19 heavily affected Spain in 2020, and most allergy practices implemented in a few weeks' telemedicine consultations [133], with reports registering high patient satisfaction [134]. Telemedicine for asthma and allergic rhinitis works well in Spain, and many asthmatic patients use digital devices to monitor their lung function and share their own data online with healthcare providers, thus facilitating early detection of asthma exacerbations and timely intervention [131]. Improved accessibility to care, remote monitoring, cost-effective intervention, enhanced allergy education, better disease management, rapid response during emergencies, flexibility and convenience, and timely medical advice are considered the main benefits that telemedicine is producing in Spain within the allergy practice [131]. Many Allergy apps have been developed in Spain or translated in Spanish, at least seven of which covering the area of pollen control, five dedicated to food allergy and anaphylaxis, and others to asthma, mastocytosis, atopic dermatitis, hereditary angioedema, and urticaria [131]. However, research in this area is still sporadic.

COVID-19 has had a great impact on the development of telemedicine initiatives also in Germany. In their chapter [135], Ludger Klimek et al. report that the rapid adoption of telemedicine and remote ambulatory healthcare during the COVID-19 pandemic has accelerated the use of digital health applications in allergology. This chapter explores the implementation and potential of digital technologies in allergen immunotherapy (AIT) in Germany and highlights the advantages and challenges they present. In addition, it provides an overview of e-health and its various terms, such as digital health, mHealth, and healthtech, and their role in the convergence of the internet and medicine in Germany. The potential cost savings and benefits of mobile applications in healthcare are explored, along with the concept of blended care. The chapter also emphasizes the need to leverage the positive experiences and lessons learned from the pandemic to improve patient care in the future.

The unmet needs related to prevention, diagnosis, and treatment of allergic diseases are challenges in many world countries. In her comprehensive, detailed, and very informative chapter [136], Janet Davies describes challenges, successes, and defeats of digital health strategies and tools in Australia in general, and in the field of Allergology in particular. This large country has established a sophisticated digital health ecosystem, with focus on electronic health records, mobile health applications, and potential for large data analytics in context characterized by cyber security and proper privacy legislation [137, 138] and dedicated national institutions, such as the Australian Digital Health Agency (ADHA) [136]. Notwithstanding, data are skewed to inpatients with more severe allergies, as patients with milder disease are not directly captured in national datasets [136]. Allergy or adverse reactions and their triggers can be reported by patients or their clinicians within each Australian citizen's "MyHealth Record" [139, 140], but the scope and completeness of compilation of these tools are still quite limited [141]. To meet this challenge, national scientific societies, such as the Australasian Society of Clinical Immunology and Allergy (ASCIA), and patient associations, such as the Allergy and Anaphylaxis Australia (A&AA) joined the National Allergy Council in an effort of educating patients, general practitioners, and nurses on the proper use of the existing digital health tools, including the patient's MyHealth record, also in the area of allergy [142, 143]. On this basis, nationwide datasets including information on allergic diseases are emerging and becoming available within the Allergy Study Directory (ASD) [144], The National Health Survey [145], and the Australian and New Zealand Clinical Trials registry (ANZCTR) [146]. In parallel, among 56 Investigator initiated studies for allergy and anaphylaxis registered by the National Allergy Centre of Excellence (NACE) [147], two are registries using digital health tools for drug allergies, i.e., the Australasian Registry of Severe Cutaneous Adverse Reactions (AusCAR) [148] and the International Network of Antibiotic Allergy Nations (iNAAN) de-labeling study (ANZCTR) [149]. Digital tools are also used in studies on food, insect, and respiratory allergies, the latter focusing on digital asthma inhaler [150], a citizen science Grass Gazers project on sources of airborne pollen [151], and an app to track allergic respiratory symptoms [152]. Other IIS and registries producing broad epidemiological information on allergic diseases and adopting digital tools in Australia are not captured by the NACE ASD. These studies are based on data generated by the National Health Survey (NHS) conducted in 2022 by the Australian Bureau of Statistics [145]. Given the national scenario, a major challenge for the future of Digital Allergology in Australia is understanding the associated digital health landscape [153] and how initiatives from government agencies and non-governmental initiative may interact in the future to influence, enable, and accelerate advancement of digital health capabilities for allergic patients.

1.9 Outlook in the Future

The enormous expansion of digital health will increasingly impact allergy practice and its scientific background. While some areas, such as allergic rhinitis, asthma, chronic urticaria, and others (food allergies, venom allergies, drug allergies) are less penetrated by digital technologies. However, it is easy to predict that allergists, PHC doctors, and the allergic patients themselves will be increasingly using digital technologies in allergic disease management. Considering that laws and regulations will presumably minimally affect this trend, and that countries have barriers in properly integrating these new technologies in their national health systems, the balance between advantages and disadvantages of this digital revolution in allergology will be mostly based on proper divulgation of sound scientific information and education of all the stakeholders.

Acknowledgments A special thanks to all the Co-Authors of the Book "Digital Allergology: From Theory to Practice". Matricardi PM, Dramburg S. (Editors). 2024. Springer, whose chapters are the basis for this summary chapter.

Lastname	Firstname	Email
Alvarez-Perea	Alberto	alberto@alvarezperea.com
Antolín-Amérigo	Darío	dario.antolin@gmail.com
Bastl	Katharina	katharina.bastl@meduniwien.ac.at
Bastl	Maximillian	maximilian.bastl@meduniwien.ac.at
Becker	Sven	Sven.Becker@med.uni-tuebingen.de
Berger	Uwe	uwe.berger@pollenresearch.com
Berger	Markus	markus.berger@pollenresearch.com
Bousquet	Jean	jean.bousquet@orange.fr
Bouwes	Wieke Ellen	w.e.bouwes@umcg.nl
Buters	Jeroen	buters@tum.de
Casper	Ingrid	Ingrid.Casper@allergiezentrum.org
Cerecedo	Inmaculada	cerecei@ClevelandClinicAbuDhabi.ae
Cherrez-Ojeda	Ivan	ivancherrez@gmail.com
Custovic	Adnan	a.custovic@imperial.ac.uk
Custovic	Darije	darije.custovic@imperial.ac.uk
Davies	Janet M	j36.davies@qut.edu.au
Di Stasio	Mario	mario-distasio@virgilio.it
Dirr	Lukas	lukas.dirr@meduniwien.ac.at
Do	Hoang Yen	hoang-yen.do@charite.de
Dramburg	Sebastian	dramburg@gmail.com
Dramburg	Stephanie	stephanie.dramburg@charite.de
Elbashir	Haggar MI	haggar@doctors.net.uk
Elkhalifa	Shuayb	shuayb@doctors.net.uk
Feleszko	Wojciech	wojciech.feleszko@wum.edu.pl
Fonseca	Joao A	fonseca.ja@gmail.com
Fontanella	Sara	s.fontanella@imperial.ac.uk
Francesca	Cefaloni	francesca.cefaloni@unicatt.it
García-Gutiérrez	Irene	irene.g.g.m.f@gmail.com
Garriga-Baraut	Teresa	teresagarriga@gmail.com
Gonzalez-Alonso	Monica	monica.gonzalez-alonso@tum.de
Greiwe	Justin	jcgreiwe@gmail.com
Jácome	Cristina	cristinajacome.ft@gmail.com
Kianfar	Roya	Roya.Kianfar@allergiezentrum.org
Klimek	Ludger	Ludger.Klimek@allergiezentrum.org
Kolkhir	Pavel	pavel.kolkhir@charite.de
Matricardi	Paolo Maria	paolo.matricardi@charite.de

Lastname	Firstname	Email
Matteo	Bonini	matteo.bonini@uniroma1.it
Maurer	Marcus	marcus.maurer@charite.de
Metting	Esther	e.i.metting@rug.nl
Nanda	Anil	anilnanda@yahoo.com
Nyenhuis	Sharmilee	snyenhuis@bsd.uchicago.edu
Passantino	Luca	passantinoluca01@gmail.com
Pelosi	Simone	stratopelo@gmail.com
Pereira	Ana Margarida	ambrpereira@gmail.com
Pfaar	Oliver	oliver@pfaar.org
Popescu	Florin Dan	florindanpopescu@allergist.com
Ramanauskaite	Aiste	aiste.ramanauskaite@charite.de
Röseler	Stefani	sroeseler@ukaachen.de
Salvo	Fulvio	salvof@clevelandclinicabudhabi.ae
Schareina	Astrid	a.schareina@praxisschareina-lind.de
Sitaru	Sebastian	sebastian.sitaru@tum.de
Sousa-Pinto	Bernardo	bernardosousapinto@protonmail.com
Suarez-Suarez	Mariel	mariel.suarez@tum.de
Tripodi	Salvatore	salvatore.tripodi@gmail.com
Uso	Walter	HNOWalter@t-online.de
van Ree	Ronald	r.vanree@amsterdamumc.nl
Wrede	Holger	wrede@gmx.de
Zink	Alexander	alexander.zink@tum.de

Disclosure of Potential Conflict of Interest   Dr. Matricardi reports research support from Omron Healthcare, Euroimmun, Hycor, MAD-X, Thermo Fisher Scientific, TPS software production, personal fees from Anallergo, Omron Healthcare, Hycor, speaker's fees from Euroimmun, Hycor, MAD-X, Thermo Fisher Scientific, Allergopharma, ALK-Abellò, Angelini, Bencard Allergie, HAL, Stallergenes, all outside the submitted work.

Dr. Pfaar reports grants and/or personal fees and/or travel support from ALK-Abelló, Allergopharma, Stallergenes Greer, HAL Allergy Holding B.V./HAL Allergie GmbH, Bencard Allergie GmbH/Allergy Therapeutics, Laboratorios LETI/LETI Pharma, GlaxoSmithKline, ROXALL Medizin, Novartis, Sanofi-Aventis and Sanofi-Genzyme, Med Update Europe GmbH, streamedup! GmbH, Pohl-Boskamp, Inmunotek S.L., John Wiley and Sons/AS, Paul-Martini-Stiftung (PMS), Regeneron Pharmaceuticals Inc., RG Aerztefortbildung, Institut für Disease Management, Springer GmbH, AstraZeneca, IQVIA Commercial, Ingress Health, Wort&Bild Verlag, Verlag ME, Procter&Gamble, ALTAMIRA, Meinhardt Congress GmbH, Deutsche Forschungsgemeinschaft, Thieme, Deutsche AllergieLiga e.V., AeDA, Alfried-Krupp Krankenhaus, Red Maple Trials Inc., Königlich Dänisches Generalkonsulat, Medizinische Hochschule Hannover, ECM Expro&Conference Management, Technical University Dresden, Lilly, Japanese Society of Allergy, Forum für Medizinische Fortbildung, Dustri-Verlag, Pneumolive, ASIT Biotech, LOFARMA, Almirall, Paul-Ehrlich-Institut, all outside the submitted work; and he is member of EAACI Excom, member of ext. board of directors DGAKI; coordinator, main- or co-author of different position papers and guidelines in rhinology, allergology and allergen immunotherapy; he is associate editor (AE) of Allergy and Clinical Translational Allergy.

References

1. Granstrom E, Wannheden C, Brommels M, Hvitfeldt H, Nystrom ME. Digital tools as promoters for person-centered care practices in chronic care? Healthcare professionals' experiences from rheumatology care. BMC Health Serv Res. 2020;20(1):1108.
2. OECD. Integrating care to prevent and manage chronic diseases: best practices in public health. OECD Publishing; 2023.
3. Matricardi PM, Dramburg S, Alvarez-Perea A, Antolín-Amérigo D, Apfelbacher C, Atanaskovic-Markovic M, et al. The role of mobile health technologies in allergy care: An EAACI position paper. Allergy. 2020;75(2):259–72. https://doi.org/10.1111/all.13953.
4. Bousquet J, Pfaar O, Togias A, et al. 2019 ARIA Care pathways for allergen immunotherapy. Allergy. 2019;74(11):2087–102.
5. Pfaar O, Sousa-Pinto B, Papadopoulos NG, et al. Digitally-enabled, person-centred care (PCC) in allergen immunotherapy: an ARIA-EAACI position paper. Allergy. 2024; in press
6. Matricardi PM, Dramburg S, editors. Digital allergology: from theory to practice. Springer; 2024.
7. Metting E. Digital health: general concepts and terminology. In: Matricardi PM, Dramburg S, editors. Digital allergology: from theory to practice. Springer; 2024.
8. Dramburg S. Legal and regulatory challenges for digital health technologies. In: Matricardi PM, Dramburg S, editors. Digital allergology: from theory to practice. Springer; 2024.
9. www.enforcementtracker.com: Europe-wide overview of fines imposed by data protection authorities for corresponding violations; 2024.
10. https://eur-lex.europa.eu/eli/reg/2016/679/oj; 2024.
11. Kay AB. Landmarks in allergy during the 19th century. Chem Immunol Allergy. 2014;100:21–6. https://doi.org/10.1159/000358477.
12. Tippett LO, Zeleznick LD, Knowles WE. The use of computer based diaries for the assessment of subjective symptomatology. Methods Inf Med. 1975;14(2):62–8.
13. Sousa-Pinto B, Pfaar O, Bousquet J. Real-life evidence in allergen immunotherapy: moving forward with mHealth apps. Allergol Select. 2023;7:47–56. https://doi.org/10.5414/ALX02343E.
14. Suarez-Suarez M, Alonso M, Matricardi PM, Dramburg S, Buters J. Automated pollen monitoring and exposure prediction for pollen allergic patients. In: Matricardi PM, Dramburg S, editors. Digital allergology: from theory to practice. Springer; 2024.
15. Buters JTM, Antunes C, Galveias A, Bergmann KC, Thibaudon M, Galán C, et al. Pollen and spore monitoring in the world. Clin Transl Allergy. 2018;8:9. https://doi.org/10.1186/s13601-018-0197-8.
16. Suarez-Suarez M, Maya-Manzano JM, Clot B, Graber M-J, Sallin C, Tummon F, Buters J. Accuracy of a hand-held resistance-free flowmeters for flow adjustments of Hirst-Type pollen traps. Aerobiologia. 2023;39:143–8.
17. Tummon F, Arboledas LA, Bonini M, Guinot B, Hicke M, Jacob C, Kendrovski V, McCairns W, Petermann E, Peuch V-H, Pfaar O, Sicard M, Sikoparija B, Clot B. The need for Pan-European automatic pollen and fungal spore monitoring: a stakeholder workshop position paper. Clin Transl Allergy. 2021b;11:e12015. https://doi.org/10.1002/clt2.12015.
18. Maya-Manzano JM, Tummon F, Abt R, Allan N, Bunderson L, Clot B, Crouzy B, Daunys G, Erb S, Gonzalez-Alonso M, Graf E, Grewling L, Haus J, Kadantsev E, Kawashima S, Martinez-Bracero M, Matavulj P, Mills S, Niederberger E, Lieberherr G, Lucas RW, O'Connor DJ, Oteros J, Palamarchuk J, Pope FD, Rojo J, Šauliené I, Schäfer S, Schmidt-Weber CB, Schnitzler M, Šikoparija B, Skjøth CA, Sofiev M, Stemmler T, Triviño M, Zeder Y, Buters J. Towards European automatic bioaerosol monitoring: comparison of 9 automatic pollen observational instruments with classic Hirst-type traps. Sci Total Environ. 2023;866:161220. https://doi.org/10.1016/j.scitotenv.2022.161220.

19. Matricardi PM, Hoffmann T, Dramburg S. The "allergic nose as a pollen detector" concept: e-Diaries to predict pollen trends. Pediatr Allergy Immunol. 2023;34:e13966. https://doi.org/10.1111/pai.13966.
20. Bastl K, Kmenta M, Geller-Bernstein C, Berger U, Jäger S. Can we improve pollen season definitions by using the symptom load index in addition to pollen counts? Environ Pollut. 2015;204:109–16. https://doi.org/10.1016/j.envpol.2015.04.016.
21. Bastl K, Berger U, Kmenta M. Evaluation of Pollen apps forecasts: the need for quality control in an ehealth service. J Med Internet Res. 2017;19:e7426. https://doi.org/10.2196/jmir.7426.
22. Damialis A, Häring F, Gökkaya M, Rauer D, Reiger M, Bezold S, Bounas-Pyrros N, Eyerich K, Todorova A, Hammel G, Gilles S, Traidl-Hoffmann C. Human exposure to airborne pollen and relationships with symptoms and immune responses: Indoors versus outdoors, circadian patterns and meteorological effects in alpine and urban environments. Sci Total Environ. 2019;653:190–9. https://doi.org/10.1016/j.scitotenv.2018.10.366.
23. Sitaru S, Wecker H, Buters J, Biedermann T, Zink A. Social media to monitor prevalent diseases: Hay fever and Twitter activity in Germany. Allergy. 2023;78:2777–80. https://doi.org/10.1111/all.15787.
24. Wakamiya S, Matsune S, Okubo K, Aramaki E. Causal relationships among pollen counts, tweet numbers, and patient numbers for seasonal allergic rhinitis surveillance: retrospective analysis. J Med Internet Res. 2019;21:e10450. https://doi.org/10.2196/10450.
25. Berger M, Bastl K, Bastl M, Dir L, Berger U. Digital Health for patients with Pollen Allergy: the Pollen App experience and beyond. In: Matricardi PM, Dramburg S, editors. Digital allergology: from theory to practice. Springer; 2024.
26. Bastl K, Bastl M, Bergmann KC, Berger M, Berger U. Translating the burden of pollen allergy into numbers using electronically generated symptom data from the patient's hayfever diary in Austria and Germany: 10-year observational study. J Med Internet Res. 2020;22(2)
27. Bastl K, Kmenta M, Berger UE. Defining Pollen seasons: background and recommendations. Curr Allergy Asthma Rep. 2018;18(12)
28. Bastl K, Kmenta M, Berger M, Berger U. The connection of pollen concentrations and crowd-sourced symptom data: new insights from daily and seasonal symptom load index data from 2013 to 2017 in Vienna. World Allergy Org J. 2018;11(1):24. https://doi.org/10.1186/s40413-018-0203-6.
29. Bastl K, Kmenta M, Pessi AMAM, Prank M, Saarto A, Sofiev M, et al. First comparison of symptom data with allergen content (Bet v 1 and Phl p 5 measurements) and pollen data from four European regions during 2009–2011. Sci Total Environ. 2016;548–549:229–35.
30. Kmenta M, Bastl K, Kramer MF, Hewings SJ, Mwange J, Zetter R, et al. The grass pollen season 2014 in Vienna: a pilot study combining phenology, aerobiology and symptom data. Sci Total Environ. 2016;566–567:1614–20. https://doi.org/10.1016/j.scitotenv.2016.06.059.
31. Berger M, Bastl K, Bastl M, Dirr L, Hutter HPP, Moshammer H, et al. Impact of air pollution on symptom severity during the birch, grass and ragweed pollen period in Vienna, Austria: importance of O3 in 2010–2018. Environ Pollut. 2020;263:1–9. Available from: https://linkinghub.elsevier.com/retrieve/pii/S0269749119373038
32. Sousa-Pinto B, Anto A, Berger M, Dramburg S, Pfaar O, Klimek L, et al. Real-world data using mHealth apps in rhinitis, rhinosinusitis and their multimorbidities. Clin Transl Allergy. 2022;12(11)
33. Tripodi S, Matricardi PM. Digital solutions for pollen allergy and allergen immunotherapy: the AllergyMonitor® experience. In: Matricardi PM, Dramburg S, editors. Digital allergology: from theory to practice. Springer; 2024.
34. Tripodi S, Giannone A, Sfika I, et al. Digital technologies for an improved management of respiratory allergic diseases: 10 years of clinical studies using an online platform for patients and physicians. Ital J Pediatr. 2020;46(1):105. https://doi.org/10.1186/s13052-020-00870-z.

35. Bianchi A, Tsilochristou O, Gabrielli F, Tripodi S, Matricardi PM. The smartphone: a novel diagnostic tool in pollen allergy? J Investig Allergol Clin Immunol. 2016;26:204–7.
36. Arasi S, Castelli S, Di Fraia M, et al. @IT2020: an innovative algorithm for allergen immunotherapy prescription in seasonal allergic rhinitis. Clin Exp Allergy. 2021;51:821–8. https://doi.org/10.1111/cea.13867.
37. Di Fraia M, Tripodi S, Arasi S, et al. Adherence to prescribed E-diary recording by patients with seasonal allergic rhinitis in the @IT-2020 project: observational study. J Med Internet Res. 2019;22(3):e16642.
38. Pizzulli A, Perna S, Florack J, Pizzulli A, Giordani P, Tripodi S, et al. The impact of tele-monitoring on adherence to nasal corticosteroid treatment in children with seasonal allergic rhinoconjunctivitis. Clin Exp Allergy. 2014;44:1246–54.
39. Tripodi S, Comberiati P, Di Rienzo BA. A web-based tool for improving adherence to sublingual immunotherapy. Pediatr Allergy Immunol. 2014;25:611–2.
40. Florack J, Brighetti MA, Perna S, et al. Comparison of six disease severity scores for allergic rhinitis against pollen counts a pro- spective analysis at population and individual level. Pediatr Allergy Immunol. 2016;27(4):382–90. https://doi.org/10.1111/pai.12562.
41. Palmieri L, Dramburg S, Matricardi PM, Tripodi S. Measuring the clinical impact of natural exposure to pollen and molds through e-Diaries. A pilot study in 100 patients with seasonal allergic rhinitis. EAACI. 2022; ePosters
42. Jàcome C, Pereira AM, Sousa Pinto B, Fonseca JA. Digital health and asthma. In: Matricardi PM, Dramburg S, editors. Digital allergology: from theory to practice. Springer; 2024.
43. Caminati M, Vaia R, Furci F, Guarnieri G, Senna G. Uncontrolled asthma: unmet needs in the management of patients. J Asthma Allergy. 2021;14:457–66. https://doi.org/10.2147/jaa.S260604.
44. Eysenbach G. Infodemiology and infoveillance: framework for an emerging set of public health informatics methods to analyze search, communication and publication behavior on the Internet. J Med Internet Res. 2009;11(1):e11. https://doi.org/10.2196/jmir.1157.
45. Lu FS, Hou S, Baltrusaitis K, Shah M, Leskovec J, Sosic R, et al. Accurate influenza monitoring and forecasting using novel internet data streams: a case study in the Boston metropolis. JMIR Public Health Surveill. 2018;4(1):e4. https://doi.org/10.2196/publichealth.8950.
46. Bousquet J, Sousa-Pinto B, Anto JM, Amaral R, Brussino L, Canonica GW, et al. Identification by cluster analysis of patients with asthma and nasal symptoms using the MASK-air® mHealth app. Pulmonology. 2022; https://doi.org/10.1016/j.pulmoe.2022.10.005.
47. Britto MT, Rohan JM, Dodds CM, Byczkowski TL. A randomized trial of user-controlled text messaging to improve asthma outcomes: a pilot study. Clin Pediatr (Phila). 2017;56(14):1336–44. https://doi.org/10.1177/0009922816684857.
48. Van den Wijngaart LS, Roukema J, Boehmer ALM, Brouwer ML, Hugen CAC, Niers LEM, et al. A virtual asthma clinic for children: fewer routine outpatient visits, same asthma control. Eur Respir J. 2017;50(4) https://doi.org/10.1183/13993003.00471-2017.X.
49. Almeida R, Jácome C, Martinho D, Vieira Marques P, Jacinto T, Ferreira A, et al. AIRDOC: smart mobile application for individualized support and monitoring of respiratory function and sounds of patients with chronic obstructive disease. In: 12th IADIS International Conference e-Health 2020, EH 2020, Part of the 14th Multi Conference on Computer Science and Information Systems, MCCSIS 2020: IADIS; 2020. p. 78–88.
50. Jácome C, Almeida R, Pereira AM, Araújo L, Correia MA, Pereira M, et al. Asthma app use and interest among patients with asthma: a multicenter study. J Investig Allergol Clin Immunol. 2020;30(2):137–40. https://doi.org/10.18176/jiaci.0456.
51. Bédard A, Antó JM, Fonseca JA, Arnavielhe S, Bachert C, Bedbrook A, et al. Correlation between work impairment, scores of rhinitis severity and asthma using the MASK-air(®) app. Allergy. 2020;75(7):1672–88. https://doi.org/10.1111/all.14204.
52. WHO Global Observatory for eHealth. mHealth: new horizons for health through mobile technologies: second global survey on eHealth. https://apps.who.int/iris/handle/10665/44607; 2011.

53. Benfante A, Sousa-Pinto B, Pillitteri G, Battaglia S, Fonseca J, Bousquet J, et al. Applicability of the MASK-Air(®) app to severe asthma treated with biologic molecules: a pilot study. Int J Mol Sci. 2022;23(19) https://doi.org/10.3390/ijms231911470.
54. Sousa-Pinto B, Louis R, Anto JM, Amaral R, Sá-Sousa A, Czarlewski W, et al. Adherence to inhaled corticosteroids and long-acting β2-agonists in asthma: a MASK-air study. Pulmonology. 2023; https://doi.org/10.1016/j.pulmoe.2023.07.004.
55. Sousa-Pinto B, Jácome C, Pereira AM, Regateiro FS, Almeida R, Czarlewski W, et al. Development and validation of an electronic daily control score for asthma (e-DASTHMA): a real-world direct patient data study. Lancet Digit Health. 2023;5(4):e227–e38. https://doi.org/10.1016/s2589-7500(23)00020-1.
56. Fathima M, Peiris D, Naik-Panvelkar P, Saini B, Armour CL. Effectiveness of computerized clinical decision support systems for asthma and chronic obstructive pulmonary disease in primary care: a systematic review. BMC Pulm Med. 2014;14:189. https://doi.org/10.1186/1471-2466-14-189.
57. Dramburg S, Marchante Fernández M, Potapova E, Matricardi PM. The potential of clinical decision support systems for prevention, diagnosis, and monitoring of allergic diseases. Front Immunol. 2020;11:2116. https://doi.org/10.3389/fimmu.2020.02116.
58. Bousquet J. Electronic clinical decision support system (eCDSS) in the management of asthma: from theory to practice. Eur Respir J. 2019;53(4) https://doi.org/10.1183/13993003.00339-2019.X.
59. Sá-Sousa A, Fonseca JA, Pereira AM, Ferreira A, Arrobas A, Mendes A, et al. The Portuguese severe asthma registry: development, features, and data sharing policies. Biomed Res Int. 2018;2018:1495039. https://doi.org/10.1155/2018/1495039.
60. Cefaloni F, Passantino L, Di Stasio M, Bonini M. Smart devices and digital therapeutics for asthma care—regulatory challenges. In: Matricardi PM, Dramburg S, editors. Digital allergology: from theory to practice. Springer; 2024.
61. Dierick BJH, Achterbosch M, Eikholt AA, Been-Buck S, Klemmeier T, van de Hei SJ, et al. Electronic monitoring with a digital smart spacer to support personalized inhaler use education in patients with asthma: the randomized controlled OUTERSPACE trial. Respir Med. 2023;218. Available from: https://pubmed.ncbi.nlm.nih.gov/37549796/
62. Do YH, Matricardi PM, Feleszko W, Dramburg S. Digital Health technologies in young children with wheeze or asthma. In: Matricardi PM, Dramburg S, editors. Digital allergology: from theory to practice. Springer; 2024.
63. Brons A, Braam K, Broekema A, et al. Translating promoting factors and behavior change principles into a blended and technology-supported intervention to stimulate physical activity in children with asthma (Foxfit): design study. JMIR Form Res. 2022;6(7):e34121.
64. McDaniel NL, Novicoff W, Gunnell B, Cattell GD. Comparison of a novel handheld telehealth device with stand-alone examination tools in a clinic setting. Telemed J E Health. 2019;25(12):1225–30.
65. Van Houten L, Deegan K, Siemer M, Walsh S. A telehealth initiative to decrease no-show rates in a pediatric asthma mobile clinic. J Pediatr Nurs. 2021;59:143–50.
66. Hsia BC, Singh AK, Njeze O, et al. Developing and evaluating ASTHMAXcel adventures: a novel gamified mobile application for pediatric patients with asthma. Ann Allergy Asthma Immunol. 2020;125(5):581–8.
67. Hosseini A, Buonocore CM, Hashemzadeh S, et al. Feasibility of a secure wireless sensing smartwatch application for the self-management of pediatric asthma. Sensors (Basel). 2017;17(8)
68. Maurer M, Kolkhir P, Ramanauskaite A, Cherrez-Ojeda I. Digital health and chronic urticaria. In: Matricardi PM, Dramburg S, editors. Digital allergology: from theory to practice. Springer; 2024.
69. Poon BY, Shortell SM, Rodriguez HP. Patient activation as a pathway to shared decision-making for adults with diabetes or cardiovascular disease. J Gen Intern Med. 2020;35(3):732–42.

70. Smith SG, Pandit A, Rush SR, Wolf MS, Simon CJ. The role of patient activation in preferences for shared decision making: results from a National Survey of U.S. Adults J Health Commun 2016;21(1):67–75.X.
71. Weller K, Giménez-Arnau A, Grattan C, Asero R, Mathelier-Fusade P, Bizjak M, et al. The Chronic Urticaria Registry: rationale, methods and initial implementation. J Eur Acad Dermatol Venereol. 2021;35(3):721–9.
72. Sitaru S. Digital Health and Atopic Dermatitis. In: Matricardi PM, Dramburg S, editors. Digital allergology: from theory to practice. Springer; 2024.
73. Schuster B, Dugas M, Zink A. Medizinische Apps—Möglichkeiten bei Pruritus. Hautarzt Z Dermatol Venerol Verwandte Geb. 2020;71(7):528–34.
74. Ji J, Venderley J, Zhang H, Lei M, Ruan G, Patel N, et al. Assessing nocturnal scratch with actigraphy in atopic dermatitis patients. NPJ Digit Med. 2023;6(1):72.
75. Sitaru S, Kaczmarczyk R, Erdmann M, Biedermann T, Zink A. 3D whole body scans in dermatology-a new era in clinical practice and research? Dermatol Heidelb Ger. 2022;73(7):575–9.
76. Balato A, Zink A, Babino G, Buononato D, Kiani C, Eyerich K, et al. The impact of psoriasis and atopic dermatitis on quality of life: a literature research on biomarkers. Life Basel Switz. 2022;12(12):2026.
77. Elkhalifa S, Elbashir H, Cerecedo I, Salvo F. Digital health and drug allergies. In: Matricardi PM, Dramburg S, editors. Digital allergology: from theory to practice. Springer; 2024.
78. Elkhalifa S, Bhana R, Blaga A, Joshi S, Svejda M, Kasilingam V, Garcez T, Calisti G. Development and validation of a mobile clinical decision support tool for the diagnosis of drug allergy in adults: the drug allergy app. J Allergy Clin Immunol Pract. 2021;9(12):4410–4418.e4.
79. Greiwe J, Nanda A, Nyenhuis SM. Wearables and sensor technology for allergy care. In: Matricardi PM, Dramburg S, editors. Digital allergology: from theory to practice. Springer; 2024.
80. Castner J, Mammen MJ, Jungquist CR, Licata O, Pender JJ, Wilding GE, et al. Validation of fitness tracker for sleep measures in women with asthma. J Asthma. 2019;56(7):719–30.
81. Koinis-Mitchell D, Kopel SJ, Seifer R, LeBourgeois M, McQuaid EL, Esteban CA, et al. Asthma-related lung function, sleep quality, and sleep duration in urban children. Sleep Health. 2017;3(3):148–56.
82. Anusha AR, Soodi AL, Kumar SP. Design of low-cost hardware for lung sound acquisition and determination of inspiratory-expiratory phase using respiratory waveform. In: 2012 Third International Conference on Computing, Communication and Networking Technologies (ICCCNT'12); 2012. p. 1–5.
83. Liu GZ, Guo YW, Zhu QS, Huang BY, Wang L. Estimation of respiration rate from three-dimensional acceleration data based on body sensor network. Telemed J E Health. 2011;17(9):705–11.
84. Wasserman R, Cunningham-Rundles C, Anderson J, Lugar P, Palumbo M, Patel N, et al. Systemic IgG exposure and safety in patients with primary immunodeficiency: a randomized crossover study comparing a novel investigational wearable infusor versus the Crono pump. Immunotherapy. 2022;14:1315–28.
85. Yang A, Chun KS, Yu L, Walter J, Kim D, Lee JH, et al. Validation of hand-mounted wearable sensor for scratching movements in adults with atopic dermatitis. J Am Acad Dermatol. 2023;88(3):726–9. https://doi.org/10.1016/j.jaad.2022.09.032.
86. Sundhoro M, Agnihotra S, Khan N, Barnes A, BelBruno J, Mendecki L. Rapid and accurate electrochemical sensor for food allergen detection in complex foods. Sci Rep. 2021;11:20831.
87. Popescu F, Dramburg S. Unveiling the potential of social media in allergology: from patient education and support to advocacy and AI integration. In: Matricardi PM, Dramburg S, editors. Digital allergology: from theory to practice. Springer; 2024.
88. Popescu F, Dramburg S. A practical guide to social media in allergic disease management: background, tools, tips and tactics. In: Matricardi PM, Dramburg S, editors. Digital allergology: from theory to practice. Springer; 2024.

89. Chirumamilla S, Gulati M. Patient education and engagement through social media. Curr Cardiol Rev. 2021;17(2):137–43. https://doi.org/10.2174/1573403X15666191120115107.
90. Charles-Smith LE, Reynolds TL, Cameron MA, Conway M, Lau EH, Olsen JM, Pavlin JA, Shigematsu M, Streichert LC, Suda KJ, Corley CD. Using social media for actionable disease surveillance and outbreak management: a systematic literature review. PLoS One. 2015;10(10):e0139701. https://doi.org/10.1371/journal.pone.0139701.
91. Kanchan S, Gaidhane A. Social media role and its impact on public health: a narrative review. Cureus. 2023;15(1):e33737. https://doi.org/10.7759/cureus.33737.
92. Dimov V, Gonzalez-Estrada A, Eidelman F. Social media and allergy. Curr Allergy Asthma Rep. 2018;18(12):76. https://doi.org/10.1007/s11882-018-0822-6.
93. Kaul V, Szakmany T, Peters JI, Stukus D, Sala KA, Dangayach N, Simpson SQ, Carroll CL. Quality of the discussion of asthma on twitter. J Asthma. 2022;59(2):325–32. https://doi.org/10.1080/02770903.2020.1847933.
94. EAACI. EAACI explains food allergy [Video file]; 2018. https://www.youtube.com/watch?v=iaQmGOYW5rg. 2024.
95. Oulee A, Ivanic M, Norden A, Javadi SS, Wu JJ. Atopic dermatitis on TikTok™: a cross-sectional study. Clin Exp Dermatol. 2022;47(11):2036–7. https://doi.org/10.1111/ced.15322.
96. Mueller SM, Hongler VNS, Jungo P, Cajacob L, Schwegler S, Steveling EH, Manjaly Thomas ZR, Fuchs O, Navarini A, Scherer K, Brandt O. Fiction, falsehoods, and few facts: cross-sectional study on the content-related quality of atopic eczema-related videos on YouTube. J Med Internet Res. 2020;22(4):e15599. https://doi.org/10.2196/15599.
97. Dimov V, Gonzalez-Estrada A, Eidelman F. Social media and the allergy practice. Ann Allergy Asthma Immunol. 2016;116(6):484–90. https://doi.org/10.1016/j.anai.2016.01.021.
98. Van Ree R. Databanks and expert systems in allergomics: scientific and clinical implications. In: Matricardi PM, Dramburg S, editors. Digital allergology: from theory to practice. Springer; 2024.
99. Chapman MD, Pomés A, Breiteneder H, Ferreira F. Nomenclature and structural biology of allergens. J Allergy Clin Immunol. 2007;119(2):414–20.
100. Goodman RE, Ebisawa M, Ferreira F, Sampson HA, van Ree R, Vieths S, et al. AllergenOnline: a peer-reviewed, curated allergen database to assess novel food proteins for potential cross-reactivity. Mol Nutr Food Res. 2016;60(5):1183–98.
101. Nakamura R, Teshima R, Takagi K, Sawada J. Development of Allergen Database for Food Safety (ADFS): an integrated database to search allergens and predict allergenicity. Kokuritsu Iyakuhin Shokuhin Eisei Kenkyusho Hokoku. 2005;123:32–6.
102. Nakamura R, Nakamura R, Teshima R. Major revision of the allergen database for food safety (ADFS) and validation of the motif-based allergenicity prediction tool. Kokuritsu Iyakuhin Shokuhin Eisei Kenkyusho Hokoku. 2009;127:44–9.
103. van Ree R, Sapiter Ballerda D, Berin MC, Beuf L, Chang A, Gadermaier G, et al. The COMPARE database: a public resource for allergen identification, adapted for continuous improvement. Front Allergy. 2021;2:700533.
104. Martinez Barrio A, Soeria-Atmadja D, Nistér A, Gustafsson MG, Hammerling U, Bongcam-Rudloff E. EVALLER: a web server for in silico assessment of potential protein allergenicity. Nucleic Acids Res. 2007;35(Web Server issue):W694–700.
105. Goto K, Tamehiro N, Yoshida T, Hanada H, Sakuma T, Adachi R, et al. Novel machine learning method allerStat identifies statistically significant allergen-specific patterns in protein sequences. J Biol Chem. 2023;299(6):104733.
106. Radauer C, Bublin M, Wagner S, Mari A, Breiteneder H. Allergens are distributed into few protein families and possess a restricted number of biochemical functions. J Allergy Clin Immunol. 2008;121(4):847–52.
107. Ivanciuc O, Schein CH, Braun W. SDAP: database and computational tools for allergenic proteins. Nucleic Acids Res. 2003;31(1):359–62.
108. Fleri W, Vaughan K, Salimi N, Vita R, Peters B, Sette A. The immune epitope database: how data are entered and retrieved. J Immunol Res. 2017;2017:5974574.

109. Kadam K, Karbhal R, Jayaraman VK, Sawant S, Kulkarni-Kale U. AllerBase: a comprehensive allergen knowledgebase. Database (Oxford). 2017;2017:bax066.
110. Finn RD, Bateman A, Clements J, Coggill P, Eberhardt RY, Eddy SR, et al. Pfam: the protein families database. Nucleic Acids Res. 2014;42:D222–30.
111. Mari A, Scala E, Palazzo P, Ridolfi S, Zennaro D, Carabella G. Bioinformatics applied to allergy: allergen databases, from collecting sequence information to data integration. The Allergome platform as a model. Cell Immunol. 2006;244(2):97–100.
112. Custovic A, Custovic D, Fontanella S. Machine learning for the management of allergies and asthma in childhood. In: Matricardi PM, Dramburg S, editors. Digital allergology: from theory to practice. Springer; 2024.
113. Custovic D, Fontanella S, Custovic A. Understanding progression from pre-school wheezing to school-age asthma: can modern data approaches help? Pediatr Allergy Immunol. 2023;34(12):e14062.
114. Kothalawala DM, Murray CS, Simpson A, et al. Development of childhood asthma prediction models using machine learning approaches. Clin Transl Allergy. 2021;11(9):e12076.
115. Oksel C, Haider S, Fontanella S, Frainay C, Custovic A. Classification of pediatric asthma: from phenotype discovery to clinical practice. Front Pediatr. 2018;6:258.
116. Haider S, Granell R, Curtin J, et al. Modeling wheezing spells identifies phenotypes with different outcomes and genetic associates. Am J Respir Crit Care Med. 2022;205(8):883–93.
117. Lazic N, Roberts G, Custovic A, et al. Multiple atopy phenotypes and their associations with asthma: similar findings from two birth cohorts. Allergy. 2013;68(6):764–70.
118. Simpson A, Tan VY, Winn J, et al. Beyond atopy: multiple patterns of sensitization in relation to asthma in a birth cohort study. Am J Respir Crit Care Med 2010; 181(11): 1200–6.X.
119. Custovic A, Sonntag H-J, Buchan IE, Belgrave D, Simpson A, Prosperi MCF. Evolution pathways of IgE responses to grass and mite allergens throughout childhood. J Allergy Clin Immunol. 2015;136(6):1645–52.e8.
120. Fontanella S, Frainay C, Murray CS, Simpson A, Custovic A. Machine learning to identify pairwise interactions between specific IgE antibodies and their association with asthma: a cross-sectional analysis within a population-based birth cohort. PLoS Med. 2018;15(11):e1002691.
121. Matricardi PM, Bousquet J. An introduction to clinical decision support systems (CDSS). In: Matricardi PM, Dramburg S, editors. Digital allergology: from theory to practice. Springer; 2024.
122. Courbis AL, Murray RB, Arnavielhe S, Caimmi D, Bedbrook A, Van Eerd M, et al. Electronic clinical decision support system for allergic rhinitis management: MASK e-CDSS. Clin Exp Allergy. 2018;48(12):1640–53.
123. Matricardi PM, Potapova E, Forchert L, Dramburg S, Tripodi S. Digital allergology: towards a clinical decision support system for allergen immunotherapy. Pediatr Allergy Immunol. 2020;31(Suppl. 24):61–4. https://doi.org/10.1111/pai.13165.
124. Chakrabarti B, Kane B, Barrow C, Stonebanks J, Reed L, Pearson MG, Davies L, Osborne M, England P, Litchfield D, McKnight E, Angus RM. The feasibility and impact of implementing a computer-guided consultation to target health inequality in Asthma. NPJ Prim Care Respir Med. 2023;33(1):6. https://doi.org/10.1038/s41533-023-00329-8.
125. Ljungberg H, Carleborg A, Gerber H, Ofverstrom C, Wolodarski J, Menshi F, et al. Clinical effect on uncontrolled asthma using a novel digital automated self-management solution: a physician-blinded randomised controlled crossover trial. Eur Respir J. 2019;54(5)
126. Matui P, Wyatt JC, Pinnock H, Sheikh A, McLean S. Computer decision support systems for asthma: a systematic review. NPJ Prim Care Respir Med. 2014;24:14005. https://doi.org/10.1038/npjpcrm.2014.5.
127. McKibben S, De Simoni A, Bush A, Thomas M, Griffiths C. The use of electronic alerts in primary care computer systems to identify the excessive prescription of short-acting beta2-agonists for people with asthma: a systematic review. NPJ Prim Care Respir Med. 2018;28(1):14. https://doi.org/10.1038/s41533-018-0080-z.
128. Augestad KM, Berntsen G, Lassen K, Bellika JG, Wootton R, Lindsetmo RO, Study Group of Research Quality in Medical Informatics and Decision Support (SQUID). Standards

for reporting randomized controlled trials in medical informatics: a systematic review of CONSORT adherence in RCTs on clinical decision support. J Am Med Inform Assoc. 2012;19(1):13–21. https://doi.org/10.1136/amiajnl-2011-000411. Epub 2011 Jul 29. PMID: 21803926; PMCID: PMC3240766

129. Anto A, Maurer R, Gimenez-Arnau A, Cherrez-Ojeda I, Hawro T, Magerl M, et al. Automatic screening of self-evaluation apps for urticaria and angioedema shows a high unmet need. Allergy. 2021;76(12):3810–3.

130. Nanji KC, Seger DL, Slight SP, et al. Medication-related clinical decision support alert overrides in inpatients. J Am Med Inform Assoc. 2018;25(5):476–81. https://doi.org/10.1093/jamia/ocx115.

131. Antolin-Amerigo D, Alvarez-Perea A, Garriga-Baraut T, Garcia-Gutierrez I. Digital allergology in Spain. In: Matricardi PM, Dramburg S, editors. Digital allergology: from theory to practice. Springer; 2024.

132. Vivo Ocaña A, Bermejo P, Tárraga López PJ. Baja implantación de la teledermatología. J Negativae No Posit Results. 2020;5(3):259–94.

133. González-Pérez R, Sánchez-Machín I, Poza-Guedes P, Matheu V, Álava-Cruz C, Mederos LE. Pertinence of telehealth in a rush conversion to virtual allergy practice during the COVID-19 outbreak. J Investig Allergol Clin Immunol. 2021;31(1):71–80.

134. Bermejo Becerro A, Skrabski F, Pérez Pallisé M, Rodríguez Hermida S, Zubeldia Ortuño J, Alvarez-Perea A. Patient's perceived quality and satisfaction of Teleconsultation Services in an Allergy Department during COVID-19 pandemic era. J Allergy Clin Immunol. 2021;147(Suppl. 2):AB112.

135. Klimek L, Walter U, Becker S, Casper I, Kianfar R, Röseler S, et al. Digital allergology and allergen immunotherapy in Germany. In: Matricardi PM, Dramburg S, editors. Digital allergology: from theory to practice. Springer; 2024.

136. Davies JM. The landscape of digital health approaches to allergy in Australia. In: Matricardi PM, Dramburg S, editors. Digital allergology: from theory to practice. Springer; 2024.

137. Department of Home Affairs. Australian Cyber Security Strategy. In: Department of Home Affairs, editor. Canberra Australia: Commonwealth Department of Home Affairs; 2023. https://www.homeaffairs.gov.au/about-us/our-portfolios/cyber-security/strategy/2023-2030-australian-cyber-security-strategy [2024].

138. Commonwealth Office of the National Data Commissioner. Introducing the DATA Scheme: a scheme for sharing Australian Government data Commonwealth Office of the National Data Commissioner; 2022. https://www.datacommissioner.gov.au/the-data-scheme.

139. Australian Digital Health Agency. My Health Record; Allergies, medicines, adverse reactions. Canberra Australia: Australian Digital Health Agency; 2024. Available from: https://www.digitalhealth.gov.au/initiatives-and-programs/my-health-record/whats-inside/allergies-medicines-adverse-reactions

140. Australian Digital Health Agency. FRED dispense fact sheet: uploading an allergy as an event summary. 2022. https://www.digitalhealth.gov.au/media/1739; [2024].

141. Australian Digital Health Agency. My health record THE BIG picture. Canberra Australia: Australian Digital Health Agency; 2024. https://www.digitalhealth.gov.au/initiatives-and-programs/my-health-record/statistics

142. National Allergy Council National Allergy Strategy. National Allergy Council; 2022. https://nationalallergycouncil.org.au/images/doc/NAS_Document_Final_WEB.pdf.

143. Australian Digital Health Agency, National Allergy Council. Digital Health (My Health Record) project National Allergy Council; 2023 [2024]. Available from: https://nationalallergycouncil.org.au/projects/digital-health.

144. The National Allergy Centre of Excellence. Allergy studies directory 2022 [2024]. Available from: https://www.nace.org.au/allergy-studies-directory/.

145. Australian Bureau of Statistics. National Health Survey: Information on health behaviours, conditions prevalence, and risk factors in Australia 2022. In: The Australian Bureau of Statistics, editor 2024. https://www.abs.gov.au/statistics/health/health-conditions-and-risks/national-health-survey/latest-release.

146. National Health and Medical Research Council. Australian and New Zealand Clinical Trials Registry: National Health and Medical Research Council; 2024. Available from: https://www.anzctr.org.au/Support/AboutUs.aspx.

147. The National Allergy Centre of Excellence. Research to transform the lives of Australians living with allergic disease: Murdoch Childrens' Research Insititute; 2022 [2024]. Available from: https://www.nace.org.au/.

148. James F, Goh MSY, Mouhtouris E, Vogrin S, Chua KYL, Holmes NE, et al. Study protocol: Australasian Registry of Severe Cutaneous Adverse Reactions (AUS-SCAR). BMJ Open. 2022;12:e055906. https://doi.org/10.1136/bmjopen-2021-055906.

149. Centre for Antibiotic Allergy and Research. National Antibiotic Allergy Network 2018; 2024. Available from: https://antibioticallergy.org.au/naan#.

150. The University of Auckland Medical and Health Science. Digital inhaler preferences in health providers and in patients with asthma: a discrete choice experiment 2021 [22/03/2024]. Available from: https://www.auckland.ac.nz/en/fmhs/research/research-study-recruitment/research-study-recruitment-a-l-fmhs/digital-inhaler-preferences.html.

151. Van Haften S, Milic A, Addison-Smith B, Butcher C, Davies JM. Grass Gazers: using citizen science as a tool to facilitate practical and online science learning for secondary school students during the COVID-19 lockdown. Ecol Evol. 2020:1–13. https://doi.org/10.1002/ece3.6948.

152. Douglass JA, Lodge C, Chan S, Doherty A, Tan JA, Jin C, et al. Thunderstorm asthma in seasonal allergic rhinitis: the TAISAR study. J Allergy Clin Immunol. 2021; https://doi.org/10.1016/j.jaci.2021.10.028.

153. Australian Research Data Commons. HeSANDA Development Priorities: Research community consultation report. Canberra, Australia: Australian Research Data Commons; 2021. https://ardc.edu.au/wp-content/uploads/2022/05/HeSANDA-Development-Priorities.pdf

Chapter 2
Digital Health: General Concepts and Terminology

Esther I. Metting and Wieke E. Bouwes

Contents

Abstract Healthcare changed tremendously over the past decades due to the availability and use of technical innovations. The technical support options for diagnosing and managing patients increase by the day and are partly driven by several factors, including the availability of good Internet connection in most Western European regions, storage of all medical data in electronic patient records, and accessibility of most patients to a smartphone, tablet, or computer. Current chal-

E. I. Metting (✉)
Department of Primary and Long-term Care (PLC), University Medical Center Groningen, Groningen, The Netherlands

Data Science Center in Health (DASH), University Medical Center Groningen, Groningen, The Netherlands

Institut für Medizinische Informatik, Charité Universitätsmedizin Berlin, Berlin, Germany
e-mail: e.i.metting@rug.nl; e.i.metting@umcg.nl

W. E. Bouwes
Department of Primary and Long-term Care (PLC), University Medical Center Groningen, Groningen, The Netherlands

Department of Epidemiology, University Medical Center Groningen, Groningen, The Netherlands
e-mail: w.e.bouwes@rug.nl; w.e.bouwes@umcg.nl

© The Author(s), under exclusive license to Springer Nature Switzerland AG 2025
P. M. Matricardi, S. Dramburg, *Digital Allergology*, Health Informatics,
https://doi.org/10.1007/978-3-031-71021-6_2

lenges in healthcare, such as an increase in chronic patients caused by aging of the population, lack of staff, and increasing costs also speed up these technical developments because they are expected to reduce the negative impact of these challenges. Terms such as eHealth, digital health, telehealth, telemedicine, and telemonitoring are often used, and for healthcare professionals it can be difficult to see the forest through the trees. In this paragraph, a pragmatic overview of these concepts will be provided with an explanation. These will be illustrated with examples from scientific literature.

2.1   From Paper Health to Electronic Health

A typical medical practice in the 1980s consisted of large cabinets with health records in paper folders. Computers were not used at that time and therefore all information collected during the assessment was written down by the physician. Assistants used a typewriter to transfer the physician's handwriting into typed documents. Communication between healthcare professionals, e.g., about a clinical case, took place via fax, phone, or regular mail. Documentation activities were time-consuming as electronic health records and e-mail did not exist [1], and medical information or scientific literature could only be found in bookstores or libraries. Dr. Google had not entered the consulting room yet. The role of the physician was more patronizing, and patients were less involved in their own treatment. The way physicians worked is quite different from current clinical practice where patients are expected to take an active role in their disease management process. The role of the clinician is no longer merely patronizing, as shared decision-making has entered the room, placing the patient at the center of care [2].

   The use of technology in healthcare changed medical practice enormously over the past decades. Innovative technologies became available, such as the wide availability of personal computers and the introduction of Internet in the nineties. Nowadays, most of the European citizens have an Internet connection at home and are in possession of a smartphone, tablet, computer, or laptop. This enhanced easy access of citizens to health information, and this impacted the way people cope with their personal health. According to data collected by the European Union, in 2019, 55% of all European citizens use Internet to search for health information [3] and 24% use a wearable or other Internet connected health device to gain insights in their health [4]. Dr. Google now entered the consulting rooms, led to more patient empowerment, and made healthcare less patronizing. Moreover, healthcare patient data are stored in electronic patient records (EPDs) and are in most countries also accessible for patients. Above that, an increasing number of medical devices and applications have been developed to improve patients' self-management, leading to new and exciting possibilities for patient care with more emphasis on patient involvement. Innovations also changed the working processes for healthcare professionals. Information on, for example, guidelines or scientific evidence became easily accessible online, and exchange of data with colleagues was made easier and quicker. The role of healthcare professionals is now slowly changing toward a more coaching position with emphasis on shared decision-making.

These changes are important: rising costs, lack of staff, and an increasing number of complex chronic ill patients force healthcare organizations to implement innovative changes to maintain good quality healthcare that is accessible for all. EHealth offers the potential to make this transition, for example, by improving patients' self-management skills, which can reduce healthcare visits. EHealth contributes to the shift from the traditional model of the physician–patient relationship to the patient becoming a fully integrated member of the health care team by enabling the patient to improve self-management skills [5]. An example of this is the home monitoring of patients' symptoms, which can help to plan medical appointments at the right time. Another example is collecting questionnaire data before consultation, making medical appointments more effective. In short, there is a need to incorporate innovative technology applications in healthcare. During the COVID-19 pandemic, many healthcare organizations implemented technology applications in healthcare which was highly stimulated by the European Union and local governments [6]. We need to make use of this momentum to embrace the available effective technologies to make future healthcare affordable and accessible. The use of technology in healthcare is also called eHealth, digital health, or telehealth. In the next paragraph, an explanation of these concepts will be provided.

2.2 EHealth and Digital Health: How to See the Forest Through the Trees?

The terms eHealth and digital health are used interchangeably in scientific papers and policy reports on technology in healthcare. It is difficult to find clear distinctions between the two concepts because publications on the topic are inconsistent. Moreover, there are many different definitions available, e.g., only for digital health there are ninety-five unique definitions available [7]. In this paragraph, a pragmatic approach is used, starting with a semantic comparison between eHealth and digital health. The "e" in eHealth stands for electronic. Therefore, electronic and digital are compared in Box 2.1.

Box 2.1 Definitions According to the Oxford Languages Dictionary

Electronic:	*accessed by means of a computer or other electronic device especially over a network*
Digital:	*involving or relating to the use of computer technology, using, or storing data/information in the form of digital signals*

According to the information in Box 2.1, digital health can be seen as broad umbrella term for all use of computer technology or storage of data in healthcare, whereas eHealth includes the use of a network, such as Internet. "Digital" comes from the Latin word "digitus," which means "finger" and refers to counting with fingers. It is often used to label tools that use numbers (e.g., an analogous clock with hands versus a digital clock with numbers) or to describe binary coding used by computers (0 and 1). The distinction between digital health and eHealth is vague, but in general one can say that digital health is a broader concept than eHealth [8]. Health applications are always a form of digital health, but if they do not interact with the user, they are not considered to be eHealth. Examples of these are Blockchain, a collection of health data, smart home systems, and artificial intelligence. This difference is also reflected by their definitions in Table 2.1 from the World Health Organization showing that communication is an essential aspect of eHealth but not of digital health [9, 10]

In many publications, the eHealth definition of Eysenbach is used; therefore, it is also mentioned in this paragraph. This definition also shows that communication and sharing of information are essential aspects in eHealth:

> *eHealth is an emerging field in the intersection of medical Informatics, public health, and business, referring to health services and information delivered or enhanced through the Internet and related technologies. In a broader sense, the term characterises not only a technical development, but also a state of mind, a way of thinking, an attitude, and commitments for networked global thinking, to improve healthcare locally, regionally, and worldwide by using information and communication technology* [11].

The definitions of eHealth and digital health show that the concepts are very broad, and both cover many different applications. Figure 2.1 summarizes the relationship and overlap between the different concepts including those on telehealth, social media, artificial intelligence, and big data. It is important to realize that digital health is also applicable outside of healthcare practices, e.g., to improve well-being and lifestyle by using a wearable or app such as Fitbit, Apple Watch, online Weight Watchers app, or food packages scanning apps. In the following paragraphs, more in-depth information will be provided on the other concepts.

Table 2.1 The World Health Organization (WHO) developed separate definitions for eHealth and digital health that reflect the difference between the communication-related aspects of eHealth and the broad focus of digital health, see Table 2.1

Definition of eHealth	Definition of digital health
The cost-effective and secure use of information and communications technologies in support of health and health-related fields, including health-related services, health surveillance, health literature and health education, knowledge and research [9]	*Digital health is a field of knowledge and practice associated with the development and use of digital technologies to improve health.* ***Digital health expands the concept of eHealth to include digital consumers, with a wide range of smart devices and connected equipment.*** It also encompasses other uses of digital technologies for health such as the Internet of Things, advanced computing, big data analytics, artificial intelligence including machine learning, and robotics [10]

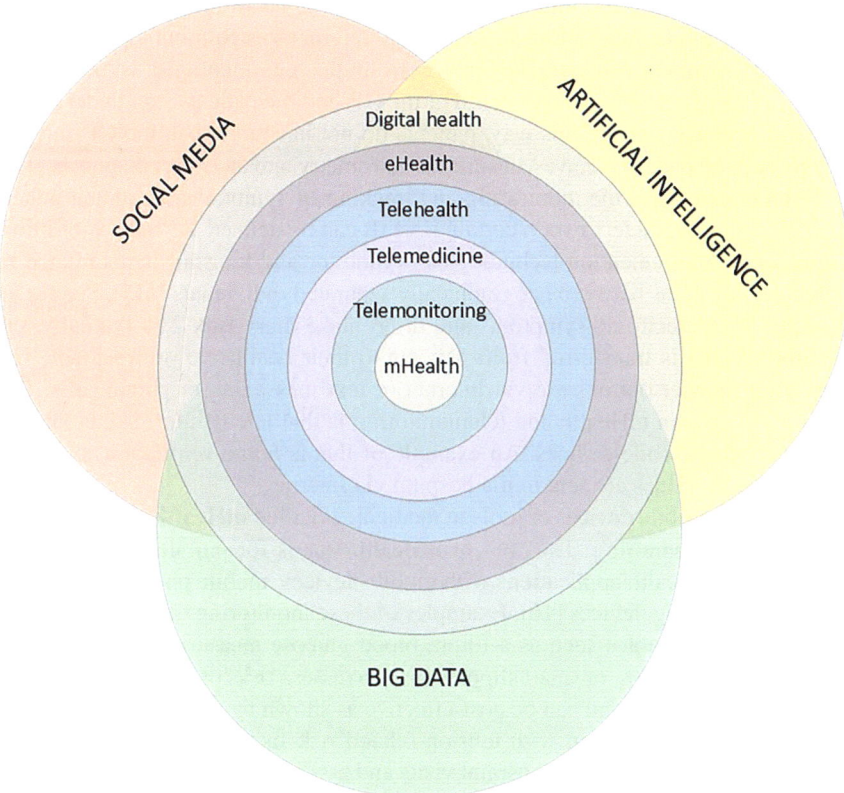

Fig. 2.1 Schematic overview of the concepts discussed in this chapter

2.3 Remote Healthcare: Telemedicine, Telehealth, and mHealth

During the COVID-19 pandemic, many healthcare organizations learned how to provide remote healthcare to avoid infections [12]. This was stimulated by reimbursement programs and governmental subsidies. The umbrella term for remote healthcare is **telehealth** and can be considered as a type of eHealth. **Telemedicine, telemonitoring, and mHealth** are forms of telehealth, and the latter three are all specifically related to healthcare. Telehealth applications address also nonclinical applications (e.g., smartphone reminders for an appointment, or online courses for healthcare professionals).

The term **telemedicine** is often used in healthcare and is a type of telehealth that consists of remote medical diagnostic and/or treatment using telecommunication such as the Internet [13]. An example of telemedicine is the asthma/COPD-service in the Netherlands where GPs can refer patients with respiratory complaints to a diagnostic center close to patients' home. There patients receive a standardized assessment according to current guidelines by a trained laboratory assistant. The data from the assessment is transferred via the Internet to a pulmonologist for diagnosis and treatment advice. The advice from the pulmonologist is transferred directly in the electronic patient record of the GP, and the patients stay under supervision in primary care. In this way, patients do not have to travel, the GP stays in charge, and the patient receives an suitable spirometry and an expert diagnosis [14].

Telemonitoring is the monitoring and tracking of symptoms, treatment adherence, or other parameters over a certain time. It can be defined as "the use of information and communication technologies to monitor and transmit items related to patient health status between geographically separated individuals" [15]. See for an example of an electronic symptom- and drug intake diary Box 2.2. Typically, the monitoring data is transferred from patients to their healthcare professional. The most used transfer options are via Internet or text messaging or phone calls. The difference between mHealth and telemonitoring is that telemonitoring can also be done with non-mobile devices. An example of this is home ventilation of COPD patients where values are sent to the hospital via Internet.

The use of mobile devices or tools in medicine is called **mHealth** and is strongly related to telemonitoring. The "m" of mHealth stands for mobile and is used to describe digital health applications with mobile devices, mobile phones, wearables, or other monitoring devices [16]. Examples of these monitoring devices are regular smartphones, wearables such as a Fitbit, blood glucose measuring patches, home blood-pressure devices, or smart slippers (used to assess risks of falling [14]). Home monitoring is feasible and can be cost-effective as shown by the Safe@Home project where pregnant women with tension-related risk factors measure their blood pressure at home which saves hospital visits and assessments [17]. Sensors become increasingly accurate and smaller which leads to new and exciting mHealth possibilities for the future. It remains however a challenge to determine where the collected data needs to be stored in the Electronic Patient Records (EPRs) and how these data need to be processed. How do you determine whether the data of the patient are reliable? How many measurements need to be stored in the EPR? Above that, clear agreements need to be made with patients and professionals to determine who needs to act on the results of the monitoring and how fast.

Box 2.2 The Impact of Telemonitoring on Adherence to Nasal Corticosteroid Treatment in Children with Seasonal Allergic Rhinoconjunctivitis, Based on Pizulli et al. [18]

To improve adherence in children with allergic rhinoconjunctivitis, a randomized controlled trial was performed to compare an Internet-based telemonitoring program with care as usual. The study was executed during the grass pollen season ($n = 63$, age 5–18 years). Patients were prescribed with a daily dose of nasal corticosteroids and were randomized to intervention or care as usual group. Patients in the intervention group received access to an online electronic diary for daily registration of symptoms and drug intake. The follow-up period was 5 weeks. The diary consisted of daily questions regarding the disease, pollen counts, and a chat option with the physician. Patients received an alert if they did not enter their data. After 5 weeks, patients in the intervention group had a higher daily consumption of nasal corticosteroids compared to patients in the control group.

2.4   Other Forms of eHealth: Online Information, Patient Web Portals, and Social Media

With the use of Internet, **information on health and disease** is easily assessable. There are numerous websites available for patients, but the challenge is to find those who are safe and reliable. The role of patient organizations is essential to provide this information. These organizations can also help patients to get in touch in online peer sessions or via social media (e.g., Facebook). One example of this is the website patientslikeme.com with more than 850,000 members worldwide who can find online information about their disease and share experiences with peers. On this website, patients can see opinions of peers regarding effectiveness and side-effects of specific medication which can help them to make decisions regarding their treatment. Providing reliable online patient information can also help to reduce work pressure of healthcare professionals. The launch of the freely available patient information website developed by the Dutch College of Primary Care led to a 12% decrease in primary care usage nationwide. This website contains information regarding symptoms, diseases and provides advice when to contact your general practitioner or call the emergency department [19]. Nowadays, patients are more involved in their treatment and sufficient knowledge regarding their disease is the keystone for good self-management.

Compared to the 1980s and 1990s, both patients' demand and actual access to their medical records have increased, driven by two primary factors. First, the shift from paper-based records to electronic health records has made it easier for patients to access their health information. Second, the growing need for patient autonomy and empowerment has initiated a more patient-centered healthcare model, in which access to medical data is no longer seen as unnecessary. Technology developments along with increased patient empowerment and more focus on self-management changed the general opinion regarding accessibility of patients' medical records. Technically, it is now feasible to provide patients' direct **access to their own medical records**, although this is not available in every country or healthcare organization. Typically, electronic data of patients is accessible via patient web portals linked to healthcare organizations. These are websites or applications that provide secured access to patients' medical data and often also to other applications. Examples of these applications are monitoring of symptoms via questionnaires or wearables, sending messages to healthcare professionals, having insights in the communication between physicians, and more. The effect of accessibility to electronic health records health outcomes is limited. And although it might lead to feelings of empowerment, it also can lead to confusion or anxiety. Unfortunately, studies on this topic are difficult to compare, due to large heterogeneity of study design [20], therefore it is difficult to draw hard conclusions. There are indications that patient training might lead to more positive results [21].

Communication between healthcare professionals and patients changed tremendously due to the implementation of eHealth. An important reinforcer for digital communication was the COVID-19 pandemic which led to a worldwide increase of video consultations and digital meetings [22]. Online meetings reduce travel time and environmental impact transportation, but it can also make communication with different healthcare professionals from distinct locations at the same time easier. Communication can also take place via messaging platforms, which are offered by electronic patient records or are stand-alone secured messaging programs. Patients can use this to ask short and simple questions that are non-urgent. This saves patients waiting time at the phone, and healthcare professionals can answer questions at a convenient time [23]. Sending messages such as an SMS to patients can also be very practical. This can be used to send reminders regarding upcoming medical visits to avoid no-shows. EHealth communication also provides the opportunity to treat patients remotely [24].

2.5   Social Media, Good for Your Health?

Social media, including Twitter, Facebook, YouTube, LinkedIn, and Instagram, are used by healthcare professionals and patients to share opinions, updates, or to contact peers. Scientists sometimes use social media to recruit patients for their studies [25, 26]. Social media can also be helpful for organizations or healthcare organizations to share information regarding information of the clinical practice such as opening times, staff, announcements, and other relevant news. For example, the European Academy of allergy and clinical immunology (EAACI) is active on Facebook and shares information on allergy on different topics telemedicine, air pollution, or allergy education. An example of the content EEACI shares is presented in Box 2.3. During international conferences, many delegates and presenters share their experiences at professional platforms such as LinkedIn or on Twitter. This can lead to interesting discussions with colleagues that are visible for all users of that platform. Unfortunately, there is also a downside to social media, it can be complicated to make sure that your messages and posts remain up-to-date, privacy and confidentiality of patients and colleagues should be maintained and the boundaries between professionalism and personal life can become blurry [26].

Box 2.3 Social Media and EAACI
EAACI is active at social media on Twitter, LinkedIn, and on Facebook. The organization has several Facebook pages: information page, EAACI patients, EAACI junior members, and EAACI Zurich. All these pages provide relevant up-to-date information for professionals and patients regarding allergy and

asthma. LinkedIn is used to communicate with professionals and regularly provides more in-depth information regarding, for example, publications, conference presentations, or topics for discussion. Short messages can be shared with Tweed on Twitter, and this is extremely popular during conferences to share pictures, announcements, or news items. During the EAACI conference in 2022, the hashtag #EAACI2022 was used to post Tweets regarding the conference. Below a Facebook and Twitter post are shown [27, 28].

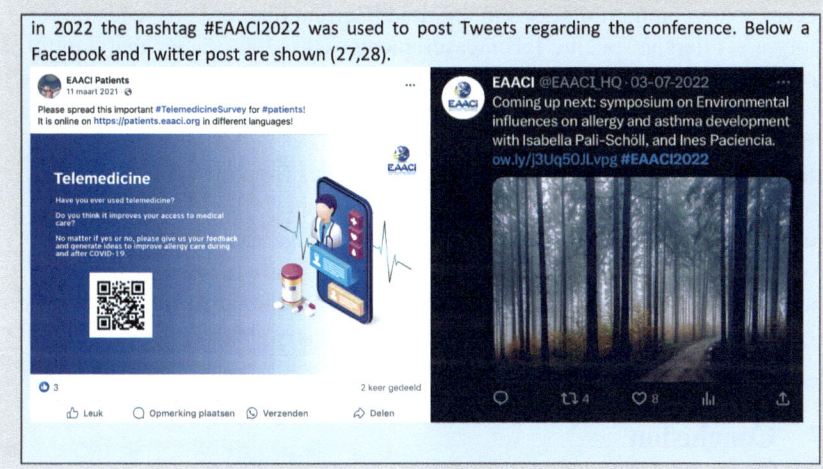

2.6   Big Data and Artificial Intelligence

The use of Electronic Patient Records (EPRs) has consequences for patients and healthcare organizations. On the one hand, patient records lead to the availability of large databases, which can be used for research and evaluation purposes. Data from ERPs of large healthcare organizations can be seen as big data. According to the IBM, big data can be defined as "data sets whose size or type is beyond the ability of traditional relational databases to capture, manage and process the data with low latency" [29]. Big data can be used to develop prediction models based on patient characteristics, risk factors, chosen treatments, and disease outcomes. These models can be implemented in clinical decision support systems (CDSS) that help to make clinical choices. An example of a prediction model based on data is presented in Box 2.4. **Artificial Intelligence (AI)** is already widely used in imaging, where it can help radiologists to interpret visual data. Types of AI can help to distinguish benign tumors from malignant and thereby improving diagnostics [30]. EPRs can provide extensive data, for which AI can be used to perform a cluster analysis to discover different patient phenotypes. This can be relevant to predict the efficacy of certain treatment-specific types of patients. In this way, unnecessary and ineffective treatments can be prevented, and it improves personalized medicine [31]. Big data and AI are related to digital health because they make use of digital databases and the models that are built upon big data can be used by eHealth applications to create personalized advice based on specific demographic and medical risk factors.

> **Box 2.4 Nasal DNA Methylation at Three CpG Sites Predicts Childhood Allergic Disease, Based on van Breugel et al. [32]**
> This is an excellent example of how databases generated by ERPs can be used to derive at relevant insights for daily clinical practise. Asthma, rhinitis, and eczema are common diseases in children. Current diagnosis depends on history and allergen specific IgE measurements. This study shows that a multiomics model can accurately predict whether a child has allergic disease. The researchers developed a machine learning prediction model by using data from genome, DNA methylome of blood and nasal cells, and environmental factors. This prediction model was built upon data from the Dutch prevention and incidence of asthma and mite allergy birth cohort [PIAMA] and was validated in three other cohorts. This study showed that nasal DNA methylation on itself is already a strong predictor of allergic disease in the presence of IgE sensitization. This is relevant because there is a huge need for non-invasive biomarkers to improve diagnosis, especially in early childhood.

2.7 Conclusion

The introduction of the personal computer and later the use of Internet changed the organization of healthcare importantly. Computers and other technology are inevitable in current clinical practice. Technology keeps evolving and leads to new innovations that will impact the way patients are treated in the coming decades. Patients are more actively involved in their own disease management, and the availability of huge databases with anonymous patient records can be used to improve personalized care. The self-management of patients becomes easier with the help of smart applications, e.g., to scan food packages or to provide pollen warnings. These innovations are expected to reduce the negative impact of the aging population, workload, lack of staff, and increasing costs. Different health technology concepts are used inconsistently in literature and guidelines, and there is a need for a clear and pragmatic explanation. This chapter provided a brief overview of the most used concepts in digital health research along with some practical examples from allergy management.

References

1. Campanella P, Lovato E, Marone C, Fallacara L, Mancuso A, Ricciardi W, et al. The impact of electronic health records on healthcare quality: a systematic review and meta-analysis. Eur J Public Health. 2016;26(1):60–4.

2. Timmermans S. The engaged patient: the relevance of patient–physician communication for twenty-first-century health. J Health Soc Behav. 2020;61(3):259–73.
3. Eurostat—Internet Activities. 2019 [cited 2020 Nov 19]. Available from: https://ec.europa.eu/eurostat/cache/infographs/ict/vis/internet_activities/index.html.
4. Eurostat—Data Explorer. [cited 2021 May 8]. Available from: https://appsso.eurostat.ec.europa.eu/nui/submitViewTableAction.do.
5. Ahern DK, Kreslake JM, Phalen JM. What is eHealth (6): perspectives on the evolution of eHealth research. J Med Internet Res. 2006;8(1)
6. Akay M, Subramaniam S, Brennan C, Bonato P, Waits CMK, Wheeler BC, et al. Healthcare innovations to address the challenges of the COVID-19 pandemic. IEEE J Biomed Health Inform. 2022;26(7):3294–302.
7. Fatehi F, Samadbeik, M, Kazemi, A. What is Digital Health? Review of Definitions. Studies in health technology and informatics. 2020;275, 67–71. Available from: https://pubmed.ncbi.nlm.nih.gov/33227742/
8. Scott R, Mars M. Here we go again—"Digital Health". J Int Soc Telemed eHealth. 2019;7(1)
9. World Health Organization. www.emro.who.int/health-topics/ehealth/. eHealth.
10. World Health Organization. Digital health. https://www.who.int/health-topics/digital-health.
11. Eysenbach G. What is e-health? J Med Internet Res. 2001;3:1–5. JMIR Publications Inc.
12. Doraiswamy S, Abraham A, Mamtani R, Cheema S. Use of telehealth during the COVID-19 pandemic: scoping review. J Med Internet Res. 2020;22. JMIR Publications Inc.
13. Roy J, Levy DR, Senathirajah Y. Defining telehealth for research, implementation, and equity. J Med Internet Res. 2022;24. JMIR Publications Inc.
14. Metting EI, Riemersma RA, Kocks JH, Piersma-Wichers MG, Sanderman R, Van Der Molen T. Feasibility and effectiveness of an Asthma/COPD service for primary care: a cross-sectional baseline description and longitudinal results. NPJ Prim Care Respir Med. 2015;25
15. Maric B, Kaan A, Ignaszewski A, Lear SA. A systematic review of telemonitoring technologies in heart failure. Eur J Heart Fail. 2009;11(5):506–17.
16. Chan J. Exploring digital health care: eHealth, mHealth, and librarian opportunities. J Med Libr Assoc. 109(3):374–81.
17. van den Heuvel JFM, van Lieshout C, Franx A, Frederix G, Bekker MN. SAFE@HOME: cost analysis of a new care pathway including a digital health platform for women at increased risk of preeclampsia. Pregn Hypertens. 2021;24:118–23.
18. Pizzulli A, Perna S, Florack J, Pizzulli A, Giordani P, Tripodi S, et al. The impact of telemonitoring on adherence to nasal corticosteroid treatment in children with seasonal allergic rhinoconjunctivitis. Clin Exp Allergy. 2014;44(10):1246–54.
19. Spoelman WA, Bonten TN, De Waal MWM, Drenthen T, Smeele IJM, Nielen MMJ, et al. Effect of an evidence-based website on healthcare usage: an interrupted time-series study. BMJ Open. 2016;6(11):e013166. Available from: http://bmjopen.bmj.com/
20. Zhou J, Arriaga RI, Liu H, Huang M. A tale of two perspectives: harvesting system views and user views to understand patient portal engagement. In: Proceedings—2022 IEEE 10th International Conference on Healthcare Informatics, ICHI 2022. Institute of Electrical and Electronics Engineers Inc.; 2022. p. 373–83.
21. Leb I, Magnin S, Prokosch HU, Boeker M. Patient portals: objectives, acceptance, and effects on health outcome—a scoping review of reviews. In: Studies in health technology and informatics. IOS Press BV; 2021. p. 194–201.
22. Shanbehzadeh M, Kazemi-Arpanahi H, Kalkhajeh SG, Basati G. Systematic review on telemedicine platforms in lockdown periods: lessons learned from the COVID-19 pandemic. J Educ Health Promotion. 2021;10. Wolters Kluwer Medknow Publications
23. Yoo W, Kim SY, Hong Y, Chih MY, Shah DV. Gustafson DH. Patient-clinician mobile communication: aanalyzing text messaging between adolescents with asthma and nurse case managers. Telemed e-Health 2015;21(1):62–69.
24. Dantas LF, Fleck JL, Cyrino Oliveira FL, Hamacher S. No-shows in appointment scheduling—a systematic literature review. Health Policy. 2018;122(4):412–21.

25. van der Worp H, Loohuis AMM, Flohil IL, Kollen BJ, Wessels NJ, Blanker MH. Recruitment through media and general practitioners resulted in comparable samples in an RCT on incontinence. J Clin Epidemiol. 2020;119:85–91.
26. Dimov V, Gonzalez-Estrada A, Eidelman F. Social media and the allergy practice. Ann Allergy Asthma Immunol. 2016;116:484–90. American College of Allergy, Asthma and Immunology
27. EAACI (Twitter). Coming up next. 2022, July 3. Available from: https://twitter.com/search?q=symposium%20on%20environmental%20influences%20on%20allergy8tsrc=typed_query.
28. EAACI Patients (Facebook). Please spread this. 2021. https://www.facebook.eom/EAACIPatients/photos/a.16291681473142Sl/291802800842825.
29. IBM. Big data analytics [Internet]. 2023 [cited 2023 Sep 6]. Available from: https://www.ibm.com/analytics/big-data-analytics#:~:text=It%20can%20be%20defined%20as,high%20velocity%20and%20high%20variety.
30. Hosny A, Parmar C, Quackenbush J, Schwartz LH, Aerts HJWL. Artificial intelligence in radiology. Nat Rev Cancer. 2018;18:500–10. Nature Publishing Group
31. Tang HHF, Sly PD, Holt PG, Holt KE, Inouye M. Systems biology and big data in asthma and allergy: recent discoveries and emerging challenges. Eur Respir J. 2020;55(1)
32. van Breugel M, Qi C, Xu Z, Pedersen CET, Petoukhov I, Vonk JM, et al. Nasal DNA methylation at three CpG sites predicts childhood allergic disease. Nat Commun. 2022;13(1)

Chapter 3
Legal and Regulatory Challenges for Digital Health Technologies with a Focus on the European Legal Situation

Sebastian Dramburg

Contents

In the current healthcare context, medical applications, including apps, software solutions, smart devices, wearables, artificial intelligence (AI), digital decision support systems, telemedicine, remote monitoring, and patient training have revolutionized the provision and administration of healthcare services.

Medical applications now function as potent tools for managing and monitoring health and harnessing smart devices and wearables to obtain real-time data on vital signs, activity levels, and other health indicators. These applications play a crucial part in preventative healthcare by enabling individuals to take charge of their health maintenance. Through fostering a proactive approach, they encourage active engagement in well-being.

The integration of artificial intelligence has significantly enhanced the diagnostic and decision-making capacities of medical applications. AI algorithms can analyze vast datasets, aiding in the interpretation of medical images, identifying patterns, and providing valuable insights to healthcare professionals. This not only expedites the diagnostic process but also contributes to more personalized and efficient treatment strategies.

S. Dramburg (✉)
Law Office DSK Dramburg PartGmbB, Berlin, Germany
e-mail: post@dskdramburg.de

© The Author(s), under exclusive license to Springer Nature
Switzerland AG 2025
P. M. Matricardi, S. Dramburg, *Digital Allergology*, Health Informatics,
https://doi.org/10.1007/978-3-031-71021-6_3

Digital decision support systems have become integral to clinical workflows, offering evidence-based guidance to healthcare practitioners in areas such as diagnosis, treatment planning, and medication management. These tools augment clinical expertise, fostering more informed and standardized decision-making across healthcare settings.

Telemedicine has emerged as a transformative force, enabling remote consultations between patients and healthcare providers. This not only facilitates timely access to healthcare services but also extends medical expertise to underserved or remote areas. The advent of telemedicine has been particularly impactful in improving healthcare accessibility and reducing barriers to timely medical interventions.

Remote monitoring, facilitated by medical apps and connected devices, allows healthcare providers to track patients' health parameters outside traditional clinical settings. This is particularly beneficial for individuals managing chronic conditions, as it enables continuous monitoring and early detection of potential health issues, leading to more proactive and personalized interventions.

Patient training applications have evolved to provide accessible and personalized educational resources to individuals seeking to better understand and manage their health conditions. These tools empower patients to actively participate in their care, fostering health literacy and promoting self-management.

In essence, the contemporary array of medical applications represents a paradigm shift in healthcare delivery, leveraging technology to enhance preventive care, diagnostics, treatment personalization, and patient engagement. As these technologies continue to advance, they hold the promise of further optimizing healthcare outcomes and fostering a more patient-centric and data-driven approach to medicine.

3.1 What Makes an App a Health App?

In the dynamic landscape of mobile health applications, it has become increasingly vital to discern the nuanced differences between applications that confer genuine medical benefits and those that predominantly cater to lifestyle preferences. The prolific emergence of health-related apps spans a broad spectrum, encompassing tools dedicated to the management of chronic conditions, diagnostic support, treatment adherence, and those focusing on general fitness tracking and well-being.

A quintessential characteristic that distinguishes a medical application is its capacity to deliver evidence-based and clinically validated benefits, directly contributing to the diagnosis, treatment, or ongoing monitoring of health conditions. Such applications typically undergo rigorous testing and validation processes and adhere to established regulatory standards to ensure not only their efficacy but also their safety in diverse clinical scenarios. This level of scrutiny is fundamental to instil confidence among healthcare practitioners, regulators, and users regarding the reliability and utility of the application in the realm of medical decision-making.

Conversely, lifestyle-oriented applications primarily target personal preferences and lifestyle choices. While they may incorporate features that contribute to general wellness, fitness tracking, or nutrition management, they often lack the comprehensive validation necessary for integration into clinical practices. These applications are designed to enhance aspects of daily life rather than providing the substantiated, medically validated benefits required for making critical healthcare decisions.

Therefore, the critical differentiator lies in the depth of medical validation and the application's adherence to stringent regulatory standards. A truly medical application goes beyond merely enhancing lifestyle aspects and ensures that its features are underpinned by robust scientific evidence, meeting the high standards necessary for genuine medical utility and contributing meaningfully to the broader healthcare ecosystem.

3.2   Which Certification Process Must a Health App Undergo?

Certifications and legal restrictions for medical applications are essential safeguards. They ensure patient safety by validating adherence to rigorous standards, confirming clinical validity, and promoting interoperability and data security. Additionally, these measures standardize quality, establish legal compliance, and mitigate liability. By providing market access and facilitating global trade, certifications contribute to a trustworthy and accountable integration of technology into healthcare, aligning innovation with patient well-being and system integrity.

The Medical Device Regulation (MDR) is an all-encompassing and revised regulatory system of the European Union pertaining to medical devices, which became effective on 26 May 2021.[1] It is a modernized version of the Medical Devices Directive (MDD). The rationale for the MDR lies in the imperative to adjust regulatory protocols in response to the constant advancements in technology and the growing intricacy of medical devices. The foremost goal is to guarantee the safety and functionality of medical devices, while concurrently augmenting public trust in these items.

The MDR sets out stricter protocols for assessing conformity, clinically evaluating, and monitoring medical devices. It also prioritizes transparency concerning the efficiency and safety of these products, providing superior information for patients

---

[1] Regulation (EU) 2017/745 of the European Parliament and of the Council of 5 April 2017 on medical devices, amending Directive 2001/83/EC, Regulation (EC) No 178/2002 and Regulation (EC) No 1223/2009 and repealing Council Directives 90/385/EEC and 93/42/EEC.

and healthcare providers alike. It also prioritizes transparency concerning the efficiency and safety of these products, providing superior information for patients and healthcare providers alike. The regulation emphasizes the importance of manufacturers implementing quality management systems and enforces rigorous standards for documentation and traceability of medical devices. The MDR aims to establish a regulatory framework that is both comprehensive and current, guaranteeing that medical devices meet the highest standards while conforming to safety and effectiveness requirements.

The MDR mandates the CE marking for digital healthcare equipment as a primary outcome.[2] This marking is a crucial regulatory requirement for mobile health devices in the European Union. It indicates compliance with EU safety and performance standards, allowing legal marketing and sales within the EU. Mobile health developers must ensure that their devices comply with the relevant directives and regulations, such as the Medical Devices Regulation (MDR) or In Vitro Diagnostic Regulation (IVDR),[3] depending on the nature of the device. For digital medical applications, obtaining the CE marking involves a comprehensive conformity assessment process that evaluates aspects such as the application's safety, performance, and intended purpose. The responsibility of compiling technical documentation, including risk assessments, clinical evaluations, and details regarding the application's design and functionality, lies with the manufacturer.

Notably, the CE marking for medical applications is not only about the product itself but also extends to the quality management system of the manufacturer. Compliance with ISO 13485, an international standard for medical device quality management systems, is often a prerequisite for obtaining and maintaining the CE marking.[4] The standard specifies requirements for a quality management system (QMS) for organizations involved in the design, development, production, installation, and servicing of medical devices and related services.[5]

In addition, certain digital health applications may fall under the category of medical devices without an intended medical purpose. These products still need to adhere to applicable regulations and may require CE marking.

In summary, obtaining the CE marking for digital medical applications involves a thorough evaluation of their safety, performance, and adherence to regulatory requirements. It not only ensures compliance with EU directives but also

---

[2] The "CE marking" is a symbol affixed to products to indicate compliance with EU directives and approval for sale within the European Economic Area.

[3] European Commission. "Regulation (EU) 2017/746 of the European Parliament and of the Council of 5 April 2017 on in vitro diagnostic medical devices and repealing Directive 98/79/EC and Commission Decision 2010/227/EU." Available online: https://eur-lex.europa.eu/eli/reg/2017/746/oj.

[4] The "ISO" (International Organization for Standardization) is a globally recognized body that develops and publishes international standards for various industries and sectors to ensure quality, safety, and efficiency in products, services, and systems worldwide.

[5] International Organization for Standardization provides detailed information about the content and application of ISO 13485, as well as access to the full text of the standard and related resources: www.iso.org/standard/59752.html.

underscores the commitment to delivering safe and effective healthcare solutions in the European market.

3.3 Who Is Liable for Damages Caused by Health Apps and Other Digital Medical Devices?

The legal obligations of a publisher of mobile software applications and electronic devices include ensuring compliance with a range of regulations and protecting the interests of users. A crucial aspect involves following data protection laws by implementing strong privacy policies and obtaining explicit user consent for the collection, processing, and storage of personal information. Failure to comply with these regulations can result in significant fines[6] and harm to reputation.

Digital medical products may be subject to medical product regulations, such as the EU's Medical Device Regulation (MDR). Under MDR, manufacturers of medical devices have clear responsibilities regarding liability. They are liable for damages caused by their products, including those related to design, production, or instructions for use. It is therefore essential to comply with these regulations, as non-compliance may result in legal repercussions.

Moreover, the publisher is responsible for the content that the platform hosts. It is crucial to be diligent in monitoring user-generated content to avoid violations of intellectual property rights, defamation, or unlawful activities. The incorporation of appropriate content moderation procedures and the formulation of unambiguous guidelines for user behavior are crucial in fulfilling legal obligations. Regular updates to the terms of service, together with transparent communication of any alterations to users, assist in maintaining legal compliance and reducing potential risks linked to the mobile application.

With the implementation of sales law reforms that extend consumer rights when purchasing digital products, application providers are obligated to provide updates that maintain product functionality, data processing procedures, and data security. The product provider is responsible for offering regular updates throughout the contractual relationship or for a period of time that is reasonably expected by the consumer upon purchasing the app. This ensures that the consumer receives the necessary updates.

The participation of "Notified Bodies" is also a key facet of the MDR. Manufacturers are obligated to collaborate with these bodies to evaluate and confirm the conformity of their products with regulatory requirements.

Manufacturers are required to report any serious incidents associated with their medical devices that could cause harm. This mandatory reporting is vital for upholding transparency and facilitating swift action in response to potential issues.

---

[6] The website www.enforcementtracker.com provides a Europe-wide overview of fines imposed by data protection authorities for corresponding violations.

The precise requirements regarding liability regulations may depend on the specific context and the nature of the medical device. Manufacturers must be thoroughly informed about the specific requirements of the MDR and guarantee that their products comply with these rules to mitigate liability risks.

When using digital health technology, the conventional doctor–patient relationship may be disrupted. It is essential to establish clear agreements and employ transparent communication to clarify potential liability issues and prevent liability risks. The involvement of multiple organizations can escalate the likelihood of liability, even triggering liability for third parties under your responsibility.

3.4 Data Protection and Data Security: Basics for Health Care Professionals Using Digital Technologies

In modern medicine, the intersection of privacy and healthcare presents unique challenges. The ever-increasing digitization of patient records, diagnostic tools, and treatment modalities has led to an unprecedented accumulation of sensitive medical information. Ensuring the privacy and security of this data is paramount given the potential consequences of unauthorized access or misuse.

Patients entrust healthcare providers with intimate details about their health, so it is imperative that robust safeguards are in place to protect against breaches. Striking a balance between the seamless exchange of medical data for research and treatment purposes and the protection of individual privacy rights is a complex task. The intricacies of navigating this delicate balance make privacy a central and complicated challenge in the landscape of modern medicine.

In the rapidly changing world of digital medical devices, it is crucial to prioritize user privacy and comply with data protection regulations, especially the General Data Protection Regulation (GDPR). One of the main challenges in data protection law for digital medical products is the categorization of health-related data as special personal data.[7] The classification as special data reflects the need for stringent regulation and heightened protection mechanisms, given the potential implications of unauthorized access or misuse on individuals' privacy, autonomy, and well-being. Consequently, companies that process health data must comply with additional legal and ethical obligations. They must adhere to strict data protection requirements, obtain explicit consent, ensure robust data security measures, and promptly report any breaches. Regular risk assessments and privacy impact assessments are essential. Non-compliance can result in substantial fines and damage to the company's reputation. Proper handling of health data is crucial to maintain integrity and legality.

---

[7] Art. 9 Nr. 1 GDPR.

Ethical data handling is guided by two fundamental principles: purpose limitation[8] and data minimization.[9] These principles promote the careful gathering of relevant information that is directly related to a device's intended purpose. This approach aims to strike a balance between technological advancement and the need to safeguard individuals' privacy rights. A thorough comprehension and application of data minimization and purpose limitation not only ensures compliance with regulations but also enhances transparency and trust in the creation and use of digital health technologies.

Another important aspect of privacy law is the informed consent from affected users. Developers must prioritize obtaining explicit and informed consent from users before collecting and processing their health data. This involves transparently communicating the purpose, scope, and duration of data processing, ensuring that users fully comprehend how their information will be utilized.[10] The consent process should be clear, easily accessible, and provide users with the option to grant or deny consent freely. Upholding the principles of informed consent is not only a legal obligation but also establishes a foundation of trust between users and developers. This promotes ethical data practices in the dynamic landscape of digital health.

Cross-border processing presents a unique challenge in terms of data protection law. When navigating the global landscape of digital medical devices, it is important to carefully consider international data transfers, particularly in the context of the GDPR. If health data is transmitted across borders, developers must ensure compliance with the GDPR's strict requirements for such transfers. To safeguard the privacy and security of the data during its journey, it is recommended to implement mechanisms such as Standard Contractual Clauses[11] or Binding Corporate Rules.[12] It is essential to communicate transparently about the international nature of data

---

[8] Art. 5 No. 1 (c) GDPR: "Personal data shall be [...] collected for specified, explicit and legitimate purposes and not further processed in a manner that is incompatible with those purposes; further processing for archiving purposes in the public interest, scientific or historical research purposes or statistical purposes shall, in accordance with Article 89(1), not be considered to be incompatible with the initial purposes ('purpose limitation'); [...].

[9] Art. 5 No. 1 (c) GDPR: "Personal data shall be [...] adequate, relevant and limited to what is necessary in relation to the purposes for which they are processed ('data minimisation'); [...]".

[10] Art. 13 GDPR provides an overview of the scope of the minimum content of the privacy policy.

[11] "Standard Contractual Clauses" (SCCs) are standardized contractual terms provided by the European Commission. They serve as a mechanism for ensuring the lawful transfer of personal data from the European Union to countries outside the EU that may not have an adequate level of data protection. Organizations use SCCs as a legal framework to establish safeguards and protect the privacy rights of individuals when engaging in international data transfers. These clauses set out obligations for both the data exporter and the data importer, providing a standardized and recognized approach to meeting the requirements of data protection laws.

[12] "Binding Corporate Rules" (BCRs) are internal privacy policies adopted by multinational companies to facilitate secure cross-border data transfers. They serve as a framework for consistent data protection practices within the organization, ensuring compliance with privacy regulations, especially in the absence of adequate safeguards in certain countries. BCRs are legally binding and approved by relevant data protection authorities under the GDPR.

processing and the safeguards in place to obtain informed consent from users. By addressing the complexities of international data transfers, developers not only fulfil their legal obligations but also demonstrate a commitment to protecting user data on a global scale. This fosters trust and compliance with the evolving standards of data protection.

These points are the foundation of a data protection-compliant application, but they are only a part of the many requirements that publishers of digital medical devices must adhere to. By considering these aspects, developers of digital medical devices can enhance compliance with data protection regulations and contribute to the responsible and ethical use of health data.

3.5   The Use of Artificial Intelligence in Healthcare: Legal and Ethical Considerations

In the case of AI-based medical applications, data protection must meet even more stringent legal requirements, even if the applicable data protection law does not contain specific provisions for the processing of personal data by AI.[13,14]

Due to this specificity of AI-based software, the data subject must be informed in advance of the proposed processing in a transparent and comprehensible manner. Providers face the problem that AI-based processing, in particular, requires extensive explanation of the algorithm used; after all, the health data is usually used to train the AI model.

The federated learning method is therefore used to fulfil the principle of data minimisation.[15] Instead of centralizing all available data for training a unified algorithm, a version of the algorithm is deployed on individual devices, undergoing training exclusively with locally available data. At predefined intervals, the locally trained data is transmitted to the service provider, where it is amalgamated into an aggregated model. This design ensures that the trained algorithm inherently lacks any personal data, thereby exempting its transfer and subsequent processing from the purview of GDPR regulations. However, it is essential to acknowledge a drawback associated with this methodology—it results in a more intricate algorithm and incurs substantially higher development costs.

In the context of potential liability for an AI medical device, the primary question that arises pertains to the responsible parties for a defective AI within the medical sector. Generally, numerous parties are involved in the life cycle of an AI. For instance, if an AI medical device were to malfunction, the programmer, the

---

[13] van den Hoven van Genderen, European Data Protection Law Review, 2017;338(346).

[14] Only the prohibition of automated decision making in Art. 22 GDPR addresses the functional basis of AI to a certain extent.

[15] See Footnote 5.

manufacturer, the supplier/distributor, the operator/user (i.e., the doctor or hospital), and the notified body may all face liability.

Liability issues are a significant concern for AI app providers, in addition to their general obligations. All providers must address the challenge of organizing liability and warranty frameworks.

Malfunctioning AI results may result in severe harm to consumers, with medical AI apps being of particular concern. If a user were to rely on a diagnosis issued by the app and fail to seek timely further treatment, causal attribution of health damage to the app may arise. It is important to note that the AI itself cannot be held liable, and therefore the manufacturer remains liable in such cases.

The issue's relevance is highlighted by the EU Commission's initiative to "adapt liability laws to the digital age, circular economy and global value chains." The initiative offers various evidentiary rule options, including a complete reversal of the burden of proof, which could pose a challenge for manufacturers seeking to evade liability. To minimize any potential risks, manufacturers must provide comprehensive and precise definitions of their product's capabilities and usage guidelines. It is imperative that apps serve solely as sources of information, and the user or their doctor should make all decisions regarding the product's use.

Chapter 4
Digital Health for Patients with Pollen Allergy: The Pollen App Experience and Beyond

Markus Berger, Katharina Bastl, Maximilian Bastl, Lukas Dirr, and Uwe E. Berger

Contents

Abstract Experiences with the services of the Austrian Pollen Information Service formerly located at the Medical University of Vienna show the multiple benefits of digital health. The pollen diary supports patients/users and/or practitioners in pollen

M. Berger (✉)
Department of Oto-Rhino-Laryngology, Klinik Landstraße, Wiener Gesundheitsverbund, Vienna, Austria
e-mail: markus.berger@pollenresearch.com

K. Bastl · M. Bastl
Department of Oto-Rhino-Laryngology, Medical University of Vienna, Vienna, Austria
e-mail: katharina.bastl@meduniwien.ac.at; maximilian.bastl@meduniwien.ac.at

L. Dirr
Department of Botany, University of Innsbruck, Innsbruck, Austria

Department of Botany and Biodiversity Research, University of Vienna, Vienna, Austria
e-mail: lukas.dirr@univie.ac.at

U. E. Berger
Department of Botany, University of Innsbruck, Innsbruck, Austria
e-mail: uwe.berger@pollenresearch.com

© The Author(s), under exclusive license to Springer Nature
Switzerland AG 2025
P. M. Matricardi, S. Dramburg, *Digital Allergology*, Health Informatics,
https://doi.org/10.1007/978-3-031-71021-6_4

49

allergy diagnosis. The symptom report generated by the pollen diary shows all the significant positive correlations between personal symptoms and certain pollen types resulting in further indications for pollen allergy diagnosis. The Pollen+ app unites information, forecasts, the pollen diary, and different maps under one roof to empower patients/users to make informed decisions and to support them in allergen avoidance. In addition, pollen forecasts are personalized for those who use the pollen diary. The Ragweed Finder collects reports all over Austria and distributes the ones verified by experts to local and regional authorities to curb the spread of ragweed and thus limit the burden of concerned pollen allergy sufferers and to raise the awareness for ragweed. All services are free of charge, grant easy access (Internet and mobile device/computer required) and comply with the latest General Data Protection Regulation (GDPR). The digital health benefits addressed encompass personalization, (self-) management, cost-effectiveness, affordability, confidentiality, and equity. While the benefits from digital health as illustrated by the experiences described herein are evident, the transformation of digital health continues, and ethical issues should be kept in view.

Abbreviations

API   Application programming interface
EU   European Union
PHD   Patients Hayfever Diary
REST   Representational state transfer
SQL   Structured Query Language

This chapter summarizes hands-on experiences with the digital health services of the Austrian Pollen Information Service formerly located at the Medical University of Vienna (www.pollenwarndienst.at). As typical digital health services, they improve access to information, reduce costs, increase quality, and personalize forecasts. We present herein the pollen diary (www.pollendiary.com or in the Pollen+ App), the symptom report, the Pollen+ App, and the Ragweed Finder (App; www.ragweed-finder.at) and show how they can empower patients and/or practitioners to make better-informed decisions, to manage their pollen allergies, to facilitate allergy diagnosis and to help curb the spread of ragweed (*Ambrosia artemisiifolia*) in Austria.

4.1   Short History of the Austrian Pollen Information Service on Its Road to Digital Health

The development and innovations of the Austrian pollen information service can be taken as an object lesson for the road to digital health. One of the first pollen traps in Austria was installed in Vienna, the capital of Austria, in 1977. In the 1980s, first pollen forecasts were recorded on tape which were accessible by phone followed by pollen information distribution to practitioners in the 1990s. Finally, pollen information was presented online in the late 1990s. The pollen diary was developed in 2009 as an online platform for symptom documentation, followed by the first version of the Pollen App (now Pollen+ App) in 2012. This was the first step toward digital health. An app distributing pollen information and including the pollen diary as well was an innovation. The first personalized pollen information was made available in 2013 [1]. The Ragweed Finder was developed in 2017, and the symptom report was developed in 2022 [2]. A key aim of the digital health services should be "easy access." Therefore, only Internet access via a PC or a smartphone is a prerequisite to use the services provided by the Austrian Pollen Information Service. The services are free of charge for the same reason and to ensure affordability. This approach grants that health inequalities within the population play a minor role. Free and continuous access to high-quality pollen information is a major pillar for allergen avoidance and nowadays can only be achieved with digital solutions.

4.2 The Pollen Diary Experience

The Pollen Diary referred to herein is the one available via www.pollendiary.com and is also called "Patient's Hayfever Diary" (PHD). It is online since 2009 and grew in terms of countries and languages until it was well spread over Europe [3]. Later it was included in the Pollen App (now Pollen+ App) available to an even wider public [1]. It is a pool for crowdsourced symptom data—managing nearly 230.000 users (status in March 2023) in 13 different European countries—as well as a tool for patients/users with a suspected pollen allergy and for practitioners if patients/users make their data available. The generated symptom data was and is a treasure to in-depth studies on the calculation of symptom scores [3], the pattern of allergies [4], the formulation of pollen season definitions [5, 6] and as comparison to pollen data [7], allergen data [8], phenological data [9], or air pollution parameters [10]. Those studies would not have been possible without the symptom data of the pollen diary. It should be noted that the symptom data generated is gained from users and not from initially diagnosed patients (although users can be patients), because of privacy and data protection issues. Anonymity is granted to every user including complete deletion of all data if requested. The pollen diary fulfills the European Union (EU) regulation on data privacy (regulation EU 2016/679). This includes that it collects only a minimum of personal data (e.g., email address) and adheres to the General Data Protection Regulation, Directive 95/46/EC, and Council of the EU for data protection. The symptom data can be filtered with certain measures to allow a high quality of the data [3].

The pollen diary is composed of symptom documentation and symptom visualization: it starts with a simple questionnaire of eleven questions and the possibility to document additional notes of personal interest (other symptoms like headache or skin itching, or activities on that day like cycling). The questions address the general well-being on that day, the location time was spent most on that day, organ specific burden (from none to severe), organ specific symptoms, the medication intake, the time frame of experienced symptoms on that day (e.g., in the morning, during the night, the whole day), and how the performance was impaired on that day (from no impaired performance to strong impaired performance). The organs asked for are eyes, nose, and lungs, which are typically involved in a pollen allergy. It should be noted that other organ specific symptoms might also occur, and that allergy should be also seen as a systemic disease [11]. There is a calendar function to help users to have an overview on which days they already entered their data. It is important to use the pollen diary continuously in order to receive significant results. The pollen diary therefore offers a reminder service that can be activated in the personal settings.

Every user has the possibility to view his/her data via the visualization option (Fig. 4.1). There, the personal symptom data is viewed together with the regional pollen data of the locations chosen for the selected time period. Those graphs are comparison graphs and inform the patient/user about a possible uniform or heterogenous occurrence of symptoms with a specific selected pollen type. A uniform occurrence might be a first step toward the suspicion of a specific pollen allergy. This feature is helpful for bringing persons concerned by health problems to practitioners, but also when the patient is already in professional care to promote pollen allergy diagnosis. Therefore, also practitioners benefit from the pollen diary. The data (if made available from the patient) gives indications and helps to isolate the possible cause of the pollen allergy. This option should not be underestimated since a wide range of pollen types are included for selection: alder, ash, birch, cultivated rye, the cypress family, elm, grasses, hazel, mugwort, the nettle family, oak, olive tree, plane tree, ragweed, and willow. The symptom report goes one step further in supporting the diagnosis (see below).

In addition, practitioners and patients may use the documentation and visualization of symptoms to track the success of a therapy. Is the new medication adequate? Is the immunotherapy already showing relief? Such questions can be answered with personal symptom data because it is more objective than the memory of the patient especially when comparing different years and pollen seasons. Pollen seasons can

Fig. 4.1 Visualization of personal symptoms together with regional pollination from alder and birch in 2019 (anonymized user from the region Vienna)

Country	Downloads
Austria	282,830
Germany	204,691
France	122,263
Sweden	103,796
Switzerland	31,786
Spain	23,765
United Kingdom	23,326
Italy	15,219
Belgium	14,775
The Netherlands	10,037
Total	**832,488**

be very different from each other with "mast years" (= a year in which an unusually high amount of flowers, thus pollen and seeds, is produced) of certain plants or less intense blooms depending on various factors like allergen production, climate, geography, and air pollution [12]. Therefore, to our experience, the pollen diary empowers patients/users to make more informed decisions together with their practitioner on allergy diagnosis, medication intake, and therapy success.

4.3 The Symptom Report Experience

The symptom report is an automatic and user-friendly summary and visualization of the most important symptom data from the pollen diary. It compares the entered symptom data with the pollen data of the chosen year and shows only significant positive correlations that might be an indication for an allergic reaction. It does not contain any personal data. It is an additional tool for patient/user and practitioner, but not a pollen allergy diagnosis itself. It can be requested either via the website of the pollen diary (www.pollendiary.com) or via the Pollen App. The symptom report describes the start date, end date, and the duration of entered symptoms and shows the pattern of symptom severity together with the regional pollination of one or more significant positive correlated pollen type(s). This report therefore does not show all comparisons with all pollen types, only the significant positive ones. A significant positive correlation can be a hint for the source of the pollen allergy. The results are therefore established mathematically using a correlation factor and visually using a comparison graph that is easy to interpret. All other (irrelevant) data are not shown to minimize confusion. However, there might occur other pollen type(s) simultaneously, that falsify the situation or cross-reactions may interfere. Therefore, the symptom report should be discussed with the practitioner in order to attain an appropriate pollen allergy diagnosis (including the indispensable skin and blood tests).

4.4 The Pollen App Experience

The Pollen App was developed and first distributed in 2012. It was designed for Apple iOS and Android operating systems. Since 2023 it is named "Pollen+," but referred to herein as "Pollen App." This new version includes weather-related asthma and a weather alert to help avoid thunderstorm asthma besides the previous functions as listed below:

- The allergy risk (calculated based on the intensity of pollination, weather parameters, and atmospheric chemical forecast data).
- The pollen forecast information.
- The pollen diary.
- The load map (anonymized symptom data from the pollen diary displayed on a map).

- Forecast maps (derived from different pollen forecast models).
- A search for practitioners.
- An encyclopedia for various allergenic plants.
- The settings.

Not all options or services may be available for the selectable countries (depending on the access to data of certain countries). Total download numbers and download numbers by individual country are shown in Fig. 4.2. The allergy risk and the pollen forecast information are automatically personalized if the user/patient is logged in and uses the pollen diary. The pollen forecast information can be selected via cities, postal code, regions, or the current location (if GPS is enabled). The calculation of the personalized pollen information compares the most recent personal symptom data with the regional anonymized symptom data and then adjusts the pollen forecast information accordingly (e.g., load is decreased or raised). More precise and put in statistical terms, this regional anonymized symptom data is defined as the median symptom level and its interquartile range of all users who entered symptom data on a corresponding day [1]. A screen window of 5 days is used so that the changes of the symptom levels can be tracked accurately and renewed for each day [1].

The quality of the pollen forecasts is important since the forecasts are the core of the app and as such directly influence the measures taken by persons concerned and consequently their success in allergen avoidance. Not many scientific evaluations were undertaken to study the accurateness and reliability of pollen forecasts. The hitherto information points to the need for improvement and quality control for pollen forecasts [13]. Most pollen forecasts failed to reach a hit rate (=the rate of correct forecasts) of 60%, even when a higher tolerance was calculated [13]. The forecasts of the Pollen App performed significantly better and achieved 80% accuracy. Thus, it is possible to distribute high quality pollen forecasts, although they are based on many sources and must be tailored by well-trained personnel [14]. Pollen allergy sufferers strongly rely on the forecasts and deserve the most accurate information possible. The Pollen App cooperates with the country pollen information services and provides their forecasts for their country to grant the most accurate information, since models alone do not perform well enough. Patients/users personal symptom data is integrated in certain forecast models (the personalized pollen information). The diversity of information made available via the Pollen App empowers patients to make informed decisions concerning their allergen avoidance.

The Pollen App is one of the few apps that was reviewed in scientific literature [15]. It was the blueprint for a similar app in Germany, the "Husteblume," also one of the few apps reviewed for validation [15]. Furthermore, the Pollen App was the template for the app of the EU project PASYFO. So, the pioneering role, the transferability and impact of the Pollen App on the scientific field are significant.

The Pollen App provides a date for the readiness to flower for the most important allergenic plants [13]. Such "countdowns" are important when planning the medication intake timely before the start of the season. The Pollen App may also support patients in adherence of an immunotherapy by providing information, symptom documentation, and medical assistance under one roof. However, the patient must

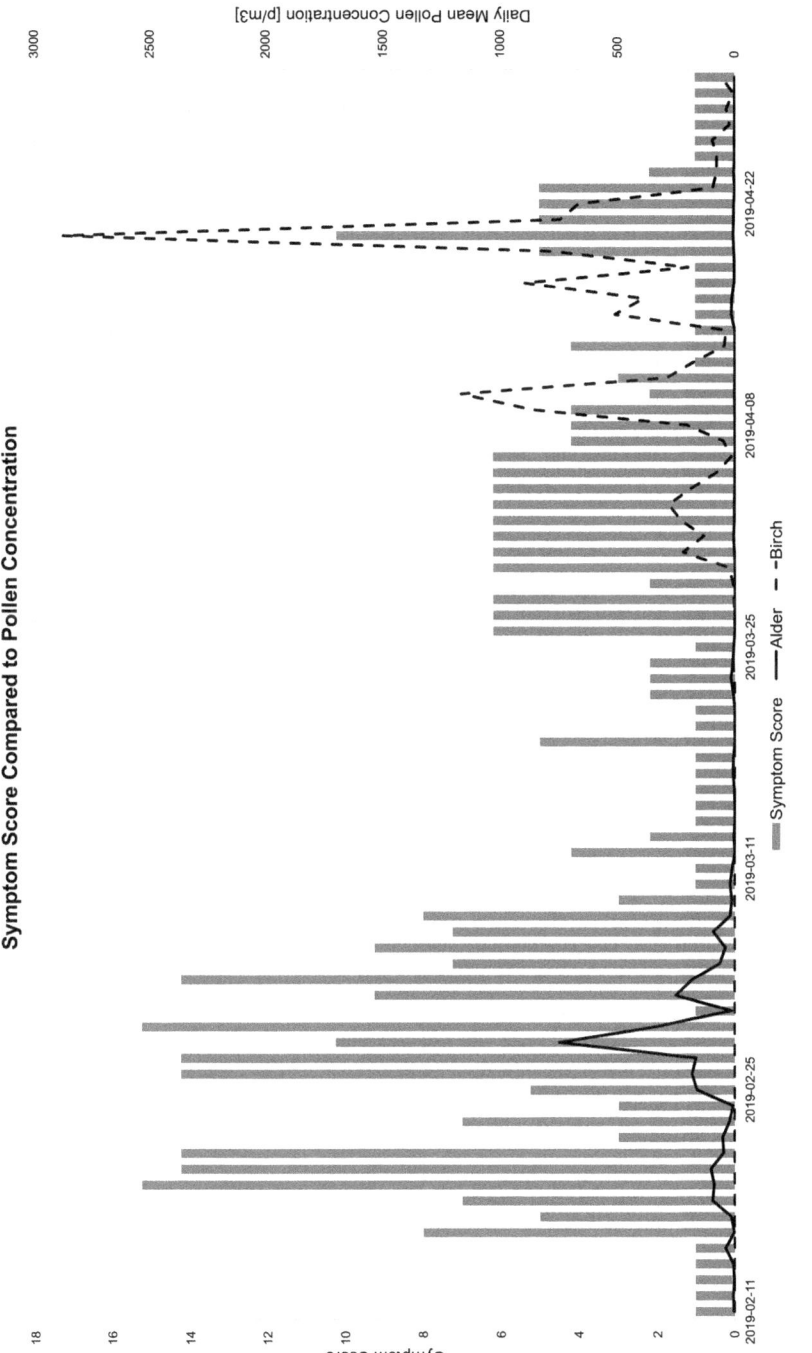

Fig. 4.2 Map with total download numbers of the Pollen App in all available European countries

share his/her data of the pollen diary with the practitioner for this purpose to allow better interpretation and monitoring of the therapy. The first noticeable relief should motivate the patient to continue and complete the therapy with the practitioner. In conclusion, there is still unused potential of the App and the pollen diary. Strategies need to be developed to encourage patients to make use of these possibilities. The Pollen App was attested to be one of the few apps that are of interest in diagnosis, management, and cost-effectiveness in allergic rhinitis [15].

4.5   The Ragweed Finder Experience

The Ragweed Finder was made available in 2017 via www.ragweedfinder.at. It is a Citizen Science project with the aim to curb the distribution of the neophyte rag-weed (*Ambrosia artemisiifolia*) in Austria. Later it was distributed as an App ("Ragweed Finder") for Apples operating system iOS and Android in 2019. It uses GPS data (if granted by the user) once for the report of the location of the ragweed plant(s). The Ragweed Finder provides the following components: a map displaying all verified reports of a given season (Fig. 4.3), historical reports, information about ragweed, a tutorial how to identify ragweed correctly and best practice tips.

Attention was paid especially to the education of users and to support them in correct identification with a detailed and easy to follow description and photos for comparison combined with a checklist prior to submission of a report. In addition, every submitted report is reviewed by an expert. A photo is required for every report for this purpose. The user is contacted in either case if the report was falsified or verified. If the report was verified, it is forwarded to the regional authorities who may use this data to take suitable measures to eradicate ragweed or to improve the situation. It is evident that not every report can lead to an eradication. However, the reports help to find hot spots and to prioritize certain spots and/or measures (eradi-cation, mowing, etc.).

The Ragweed Finder was immediately accepted by the Austrian population and soon the numbers of submitted reports changed from hundreds to thousands (Table 4.1). It is noteworthy, that the rate of correct identification was high through the whole time period (Table 4.1). However, the positivity rate improved most after the implementation of the previously mentioned checklist that is displayed before a report can be submitted. The Ragweed Finder is therefore one of the few Citizen Science projects on nature observations that works with reports verified by experts.

A scientific evaluation of the data from the Ragweed Finder is on its way [16]. First results show that reported ragweed is mostly located in fields, followed by roadside. Most verified reports concern the federal state Burgenland, followed by Lower Austria and Styria [16]. This is not surprising when considering that ragweed is a major problem in the East of Austria, while the West of Austria is much less affected (although ragweed has arrived there as well). Results to which degree the Ragweed Finder leads to a decrease of the ragweed population need to be awaited.

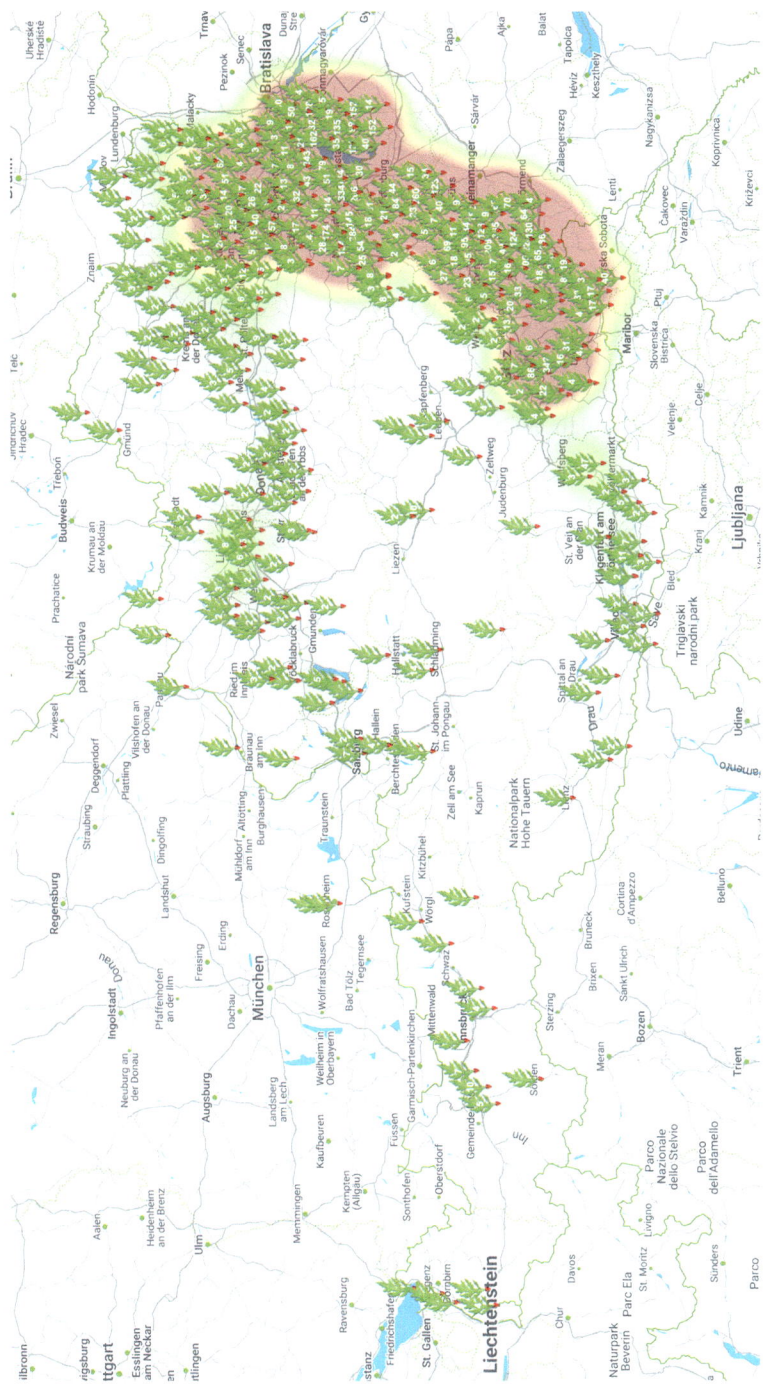

Fig. 4.3 Ragweed Finder reports from 2017 to 2023. Each dot marks one report. Borders of Austria Data source: Statistik Austria—data.statistik.gv.at

Table 4.1 Total submitted reports, verified reports, and rate of correct identification of ragweed via the Ragweed Finder from the years 2017 until 2023

Year	Total reports	Verified reports	Correct identification rate
2022	2432	2343	96%
2021	1552	1458	93%
2020	931	853	92%
2019	1643	1468	89%
2018	635	579	91%
2017	410	324	79%

The Ragweed Finder is a tool that helps to reduce or curb the ragweed population in Austria and therefore helps ragweed pollen allergy sufferers to recognize the plant and causally contribute to limit its distribution. In addition, it raises the awareness in the general population for this invasive neophyte.

4.6 Technical Background of the Services

The technical background for the pollen diary includes state-of-the-art security routines [3] which are described in the following:

1. Pollen Diary

   The system runs a Java-based app on a server located in an ISO-certified data center of Hetzner Finland Oy. Data are stored in a Structured Query Language (SQL) database, and a daily encrypted backup is stored off-site. Interaction with the pollen diary follows via a multilingual web user interface that can be used with any modern web browser. A representational state transfer (REST)-based application programming interface (API) is used by the Pollen App to provide the same functionality as the web user interface. In addition, the pollen diary gathers information via APIs from the European Aeroallergen Network (EAN) database for regional pollen data and an internal data exchange platform for providing personalized forecasts in the Pollen App. Communication is secured via HTTP secure/transport layer security (Web user interface and REST API) and where possible, access to the REST API is restricted by an Internet protocol address.

2. Pollen App

   The smartphone app is built using the JavaScript Framework vue.js and Apache Cordova for using native Smartphone functions. The app is available for the operating systems Apple iOS and Android. As the app is based on web technologies, there is only one code base for both platforms. The smartphone app communicates with the pollen diary using a dedicated REST-API.

3. Ragweed Finder

   The Ragweed Finder is a website and companion smartphone app and provides a backend system for administrative users to view and manage ragweed findings. It is built using the latest .NET technologies on the server side. The smartphone app is built using the JavaScript Framework vue.js and Apache Cordova for using native Smartphone functions. The Ragweed Finder app is based on web technologies, there is only one code base for both platforms. It communicates with the server using a dedicated REST-API. The Ragweed Finder is hosted in professional cloud datacenters in the European Union.

4.7   Pollen Allergy and Digital Health services: State-of-the-Art and Future Milestones

Ethics in digital health is a separate topic but must be debated for services like the ones presented herein and included in all developments for services alike. The principles of equity, privacy, confidentiality, ownership, personal respect, responsibility, accountability, and informed consent are essential. However, there are several concerns that need to be addressed for every service, among them affordability, education, safety, and security in data exchange and use or access to data. The scientific and medical responsibility of a pollen information service and its handling of data has been discussed and proposed to at best fulfill the following requirements [14]:

– Inclusion of high-quality pollen data (from regional/country pollen information services).
– Inclusion of phenological data inclusion of forecast models especially those that can estimate long range transport of pollen.
– Medical and allergological expertise.
– Access to symptom data such as the pollen diary.
– Co-operations with acknowledged meteorological institutions.
– Expertise in forecasting the pollen load.

Therefore, only independent, nonprofit institutions with the required expertise should disseminate pollen information in order to provide accurate and reliable forecasts.

The focus of the Austrian Pollen Information Service, namely the herein discussed pollen diary, the Pollen App, and the Ragweed Finder, lie on responsibility, privacy, equity, affordability, personalization, and reducing costs in the health care sector caused by pollen allergies such as prolonged times of suffering (until diagnosis or treatment), reduced work force/performance in school, sick leaves, or medication costs. All services ensure an easy access and provide benefits typical for digital health (Table 4.2).

The future will hold transformations in digital health for pollen allergy sufferers for certain. The impact of mobile technologies and big data is already visible [17]. The next milestones will probably address a higher degree of personalization. Institutions involved in the care for persons concerned by pollen allergies should be ready to accompany them on the road to digitalization and take all measures possible to ensure to keep the ethical principles in digital health.

Table 4.2 The described services of the Austrian Pollen Information Services are checked regarding the most important digital health benefits

Digital health benefits	Pollen diary	Pollen+app	Ragweed Finder
Access/equity	Mobile device/computer internet	Mobile device, internet	Mobile device/ computer internet
Affordability	Free	Free	Free
Easy documentation	Yes	Yes	Yes
Personalization	Only personal symptom data	Yes, forecasts are personalized if the pollen diary is used	No
Confidentiality/ privacy	Yes	Yes	Yes
Facilitation of diagnosis	Yes, if shared with practitioner and/or if the symptom report is used	Yes, via the pollen diary	No
Reduction of costs	Yes, if discussed and planned with the practitioner (adaptation of medication or therapy)	Yes, if (personalized) pollen forecasts are used for allergen avoidance	Yes, by action of local authorities curbing reported ragweed findings

References

1. Kmenta M, Bastl K, Jäger S, Berger U. Development of personal pollen information—the next generation of pollen information and a step forward for hay fever sufferers. Int J Biometeorol. 2014;58(8):1721–6.
2. Bastl K, Berger M. Pollen und allergie. Wien: MANZ Verlag; 2021. p. 204.
3. Bastl K, Bastl M, Bergmann KC, Berger M, Berger U. Translating the burden of pollen allergy into numbers using electronically generated symptom data from the patient's hayfever diary in Austria and Germany: 10-year observational study. J Med Internet Res. 2020;22(2)
4. Bastl M, Bastl K, Dirr L, Berger M, Berger U. Variability of grass pollen allergy symptoms throughout the season: Comparing symptom data profiles from the Patient's Hayfever Diary from 2014 to 2016 in Vienna (Austria). World Allergy Org J. 2021;14(3):100518. https://doi.org/10.1016/j.waojou.2021.100518.
5. Bastl K, Kmenta M, Berger UE. Defining pollen seasons: background and recommendations. Curr Allergy Asthma Rep. 2018;18(12)
6. Pfaar O, Karatzas K, Bastl K, Berger U, Buters J, Darsow U, et al. Pollen season is reflected on symptom load for grass and birch pollen-induced allergic rhinitis in different geographic areas—an EAACI Task Force Report. Allergy: Eur J Allergy Clin Immunol. 2020;75(5):1099–106.
7. Bastl K, Kmenta M, Berger M, Berger U. The connection of pollen concentrations and crowd-sourced symptom data: New insights from daily and seasonal symptom load index data from 2013 to 2017 in Vienna. World Allergy Org J. 2018;11(1):24. https://doi.org/10.1186/s40413-018-0203-6.
8. Bastl K, Kmenta M, Pessi AMAM, Prank M, Saarto A, Sofiev M, et al. First comparison of symptom data with allergen content (Bet v 1 and Phl p 5 measurements) and pollen data from four European regions during 2009–2011. Sci Total Environ. 2016;548–549:229–35.
9. Kmenta M, Bastl K, Kramer MF, Hewings SJ, Mwange J, Zetter R, et al. The grass pollen season 2014 in Vienna: a pilot study combining phenology, aerobiology and symptom data. Sci Total Environ. 2016;566–567:1614–20. https://doi.org/10.1016/j.scitotenv.2016.06.059.

10. Berger M, Bastl K, Bastl M, Dirr L, Hutter HPP, Moshammer H, et al. Impact of air pollution on symptom severity during the birch, grass and ragweed pollen period in Vienna, Austria: importance of O3 in 2010–2018. Environ Pollut. 2020;263:1–9. Available from: https://linkinghub.elsevier.com/retrieve/pii/S0269749119373038
11. Pucci S, Incorvaia C. Allergy as an organ and a systemic disease. Clin Exp Immunol. 2008;153(Suppl. 1):1–2.
12. D'Amato G, Cecchi L, Bonini S, Nunes C, Annesi-Maesano I, Behrendt H, et al. Allergenic pollen and pollen allergy in Europe. Allergy: Eur J Allergy Clin Immunol. 2007;62(9):976–90.
13. Bastl K, Berger U, Kmenta M. Evaluation of Pollen apps forecasts: the need for quality control in an eHealth service. J Med Internet Res. 2017;19(5):1–8.
14. Bastl K, Berger M, Bergmann KC, Kmenta M, Berger U. The medical and scientific responsibility of pollen information services. Wien Klin Wochenschr. 2017;129(1–2):70–4.
15. Sousa-Pinto B, Anto A, Berger M, Dramburg S, Pfaar O, Klimek L, et al. Real-world data using mHealth apps in rhinitis, rhinosinusitis and their multimorbidities. Clin Transl Allergy. 2022;12(11)
16. Dirr L, Bouchal JM, Bastl K, Bastl M, Berger M, Berger UE, et al. Ragweed finder app—a tool to document the spreading of a Neophyte. CitSciHelvetia'23; 2023.
17. Matricardi PM, Dramburg S, Alvarez-Perea A, Antolín-Amérigo D, Apfelbacher C, Atanaskovic-Markovic M, et al. The role of mobile health technologies in allergy care: an EAACI position paper. Allergy: Eur J Allergy Clin Immunol. 2020;75(2):259–72.

Chapter 5
Automated Pollen Monitoring and Exposure Prediction for Pollen Allergic Patients Care

Mariel Suarez-Suarez, Monica Gonzalez-Alonso, Paolo Maria Matricardi, Stephanie Dramburg, and Jeroen Buters

Contents

M. Suarez-Suarez · M. Gonzalez-Alonso · J. Buters (✉)
Center of Allergy & Environment (ZAUM), Member of the German Center for Lung Research (DZL), Technical University and Helmholtz Center Munich, Munich, Germany
e-mail: buters@tum.de

P. M. Matricardi
Department of Pediatric Respiratory Medicine, Immunology and Critical Care Medicine, Charité–Universitätsmedizin Berlin, a corporate member of Freie Universität Berlin and Humboldt–Universität zu Berlin, Berlin, Germany

Institute of Allergology, Charité—Universitätsmedizin Berlin, Corporate Member of Freie Universität Berlin and Humboldt-Universität zu Berlin, Berlin, Germany

Fraunhofer Institute for Translational Medicine and Pharmacology ITMP, Allergology and Immunology, Berlin, Germany

S. Dramburg
Department of Pediatric Respiratory Medicine, Immunology and Critical Care Medicine, Charité–Universitätsmedizin Berlin, a corporate member of Freie Universität Berlin and Humboldt–Universität zu Berlin, Berlin, Germany

© The Author(s), under exclusive license to Springer Nature Switzerland AG 2025
P. M. Matricardi, S. Dramburg, *Digital Allergology*, Health Informatics,
https://doi.org/10.1007/978-3-031-71021-6_5

5.1 Is Pollen Important?

Millions of people are familiar with runny noses, red and watery eyes, sneezing during spring and summer, and allergic symptoms caused by seasonal pollen allergens, thus allergies are a major global public health concern [1, 2]. Airborne allergens are the major cause of allergies and can lead to rhinoconjunctivitis, eosinophilic bronchitis, or allergic asthma [3]. The situation for patients is worsening because climate change is increasing pollen concentrations of the most allergic taxa in Europe, with a longer pollen season, and earlier start of the season [4–7].

Allergens from pollen are proteins that induce immunoglobulin E (IgE) responses in humans. Pollen is released from male flowers like catkins and easily transported by wind. Upon contact to wet surfaces, pollen rapidly releases several compounds (proteins, lipids, etc.), including allergens [8]. As a result, allergic symptoms can arise in sensitized individuals and there is a need to find tools to support allergic individuals in coping with their disease. To do so, these individuals need to know their exposure, as this information enables them to optimally plan daily activities and medication intake. Also dose-finding studies with provocation tests as primary endpoints are conducted to establish a dose–response relationship for clinical effects of airborne allergens [9].

5.2 How to Measure Pollen Exposure?

Airborne pollen concentration data are being regularly obtained using manual methodologies since the 1950s. Figure 5.1 shows the most common manual pollen traps, including the Hirst-type pollen trap, which is the worldwide most widely used manual device. The advantage of this method is that it allows identification of different pollen taxa and spores [10] with an established and certified methodology [11]. Although well-established and commonly used, manual methods have several drawbacks, limiting their efficacy to help patients avoid allergen exposure or take preventive measures regarding their symptoms. Some of these disadvantages are: a time delay of up to 10 days after sample collection due to the manual counting, a time resolution of mostly one value per 24 h [12], and sampling flow errors [13–15]. A variability in manual accuracy within pollen monitoring networks of about 30% is common and thus accepted [16].

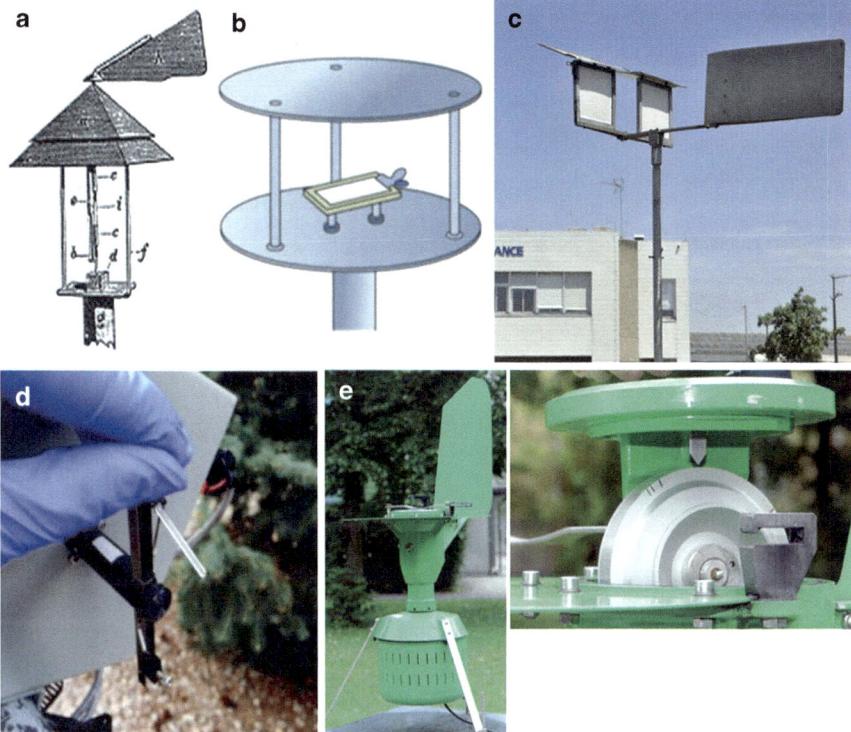

Fig. 5.1 Depictions of the most common manual pollen traps according to (**a**) Blackley, (**b**) Durham, (**c**) Cour, (**d**) a Rotorod (especially used in the USA), (**e**) Hirst-type pollen and spore trap with a detailed image of the inside: a sticky tape on a rotation drum. The Hirst-type trap is the worldwide most used trap

The available pollen data is mostly organized in national networks or single stations, with little contact between the stations. Thus, whether somebody was measuring pollen in a location was often known only to a few people. To improve contact between stations, the interactive pollen monitoring "map of the world" app was created after conducting a review on pollen and spores monitoring stations worldwide in 2018 (Fig. 5.2). As a result, more than 879 active pollen monitoring stations in the world were identified, with more than 500 being located in Europe [17]. This map is currently able to discriminate between manual and automatic devices, it can be modified by the user according to his needs and was recently updated (URL https://www.zaum-online.de/pollen/pollen-monitoring-map-of-the-world.html). The map does not contain pollen data but contains links to the individual stations supplying the data. It enables stakeholders to access worldwide pollen data.

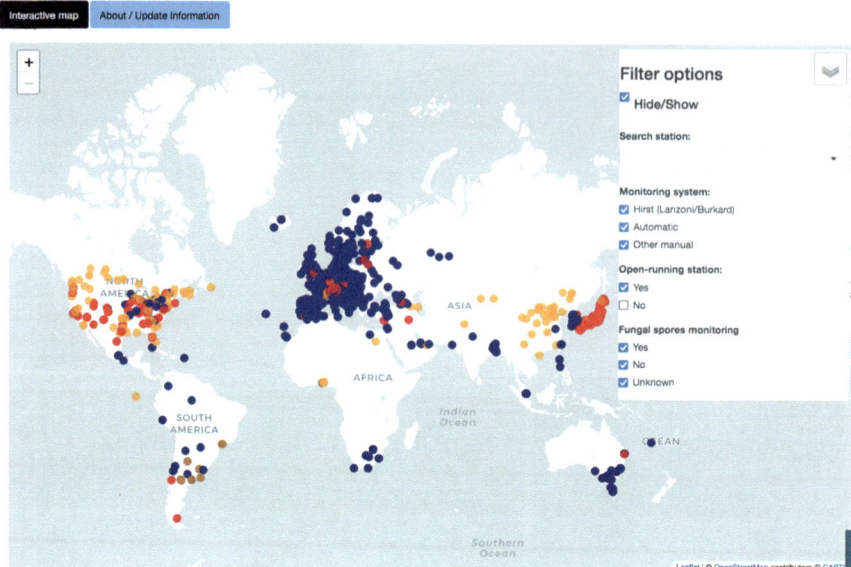

Fig. 5.2 Map of pollen monitoring station in the world (accessible at https://www.zaum-online. de/pollen/pollen-monitoring-map-of-the-world.html, access in March 2025)

5.3 Automatic Pollen Monitoring

Automatic pollen monitors have the potential to provide (near)-real-time data to support the management of seasonal allergic diseases [12]. Different types of automatic devices emerged in the last decade, with the latest technologies exploiting two main techniques: (1) image recognition and (2) airflow cytometry [18]. Both provide real-time data within 1–3 h of the measurement and a resolution of 3 h or less [12].

5.3.1 Pros and Cons of Different Automatic Instruments

A summary of the evolution and breakthroughs of automated pollen monitoring technologies was published [19]. Further, a comparison between nine automatic pollen monitors and four manual Hirst-type traps under the same conditions yielded heterogeneous results [20]. In short, some devices were able to reliably identify birch pollen concentrations in different time periods (1 hour, 3 hours, or 24 hours) while the recognition of grass pollen seemed to be more challenging. Currently, the most common pollen monitors are the manual Hirst-type traps, followed by the automatic monitor Hund BAA500 (Hund GmbH, Germany) and the automatic monitor Poleno (Swisens, Emmen, Switzerland). Automatic monitors of these types together make up about 10% of all monitors in Europe. As depicted in the pollen monitoring map of the world, most manual and automatic pollen monitors can be found in Central and Northern Europe. In the USA, the most common automatic monitor is the Pollensense, which in Europe, when compared to the other monitors, did not perform well yet. The most used automatic pollen monitor in Asia is the Yamatronics KH3000 (Yamatronics, Kanagawa, Japan) (see below). Below, we present short summaries on instruments which are frequently used.

5.3.2 KH-3000 (Yamatronics, Kanagawa, Japan)

Yamatronics KH-3000 is an automatic pollen monitor based on an optical system that uses a semiconductor laser with a wavelength of 780 nm and an output power of 3 mW. The scattered light from the particle in the ribbon beam is detected by forward and sideways scattering signal at a flow of 4.1 L/min. This instrument has been used in Japan since 2002 across the "Hanakosan" network to monitor especially the dominant allergic pollen of the Japanese cedar, *Cryptomeria japonica* and *Cupressaceae* [21, 22]. The system is not able to (sufficiently) discriminate between other pollen types [20]. This is of little concern in Japan as the major allergenic pollen is from Japanese cedar [23].

5.3.3 BAA500 (Hund GmbH, Wetzlar, Germany)

The Helmut Hund BAA500 (Bio Aerosol Analyzer) is an automated device based on image recognition, which essentially automates the current standard manual Hirst-type process [12]. Figure 5.3a shows the design of the Hund BAA500. The instrument samples ambient air intermittently with a virtual 3-stage impactor. The sampling flow is 1120 L/min (high volume sampling), sampled for 1 min every 10 min (adjustable). This cycle of 1 out of 10 min is run for 3 h but can also be adjusted between 1 (minimum) and 24 h. Common is the 3 h interval. The pollen is deposited on gel-covered sample carriers, moved to a heating station where the gel is liquefied, thus hydrating the pollen grains. Then, the sample is transferred to a digital microscope equipped with a camera that photographs about 144 different areas of the carrier, which is about 33% of the surface area, and a stack of images is generated from each area. Every image stack consists of approximately 210 images at different positions along the *z*-axis and is used to produce one synthetic 2D image. The constructed 2D image is then compared with a library of validated images from known pollen. The algorithms of this device are constantly being improved, but a sufficiently high accuracy was already obtained [24]. The instrument can identify 35 pollen classes [20, 25] and *Alternaria* spores [26], although not all with the same accuracy.

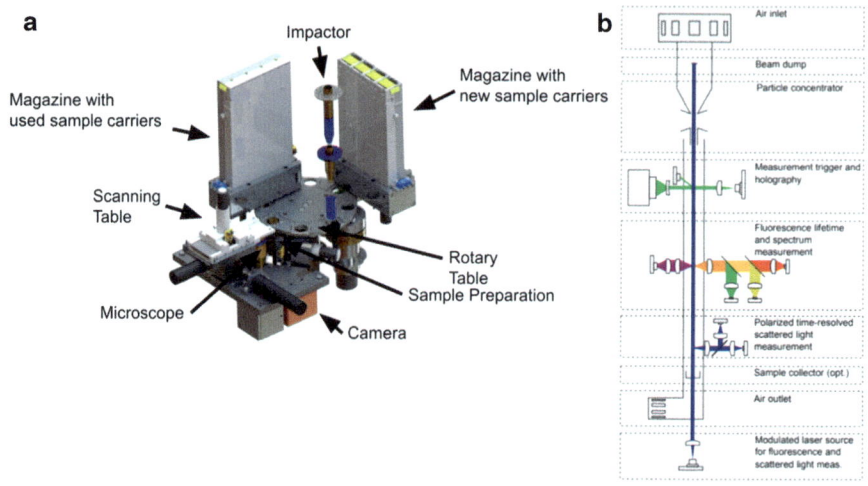

Fig. 5.3 Image of the most common comprehensive automatic pollen monitors: (**a**) The Hund BAA502 (with permission). (**b**) The Swisens Poleno (copyright Swisens AG, with permission)

5.3.4 Poleno (Swisens, Emmen, Switzerland)

Swisens Poleno is an automated pollen monitoring system based on airflow cytometry. It identifies pollen particles by using digital holography and may also use fluorescence (and hypothetically also light polarization). Figure 5.3b shows the schematic structure of the instrument: it samples ambient air at a rate of 40 L/min and uses a virtual impactor to concentrate particles larger than 10 μm, thereby including most clinically relevant pollen types. A laser light scattering triggers the measurement providing a first estimation of particle size, velocity, and alignment. Then two holography cameras focused at 90° to each other are triggered to obtain the hologram of the particle. Additionally, UV-induced fluorescence of the same particle provides information on particle composition, which is measured at three different excitation wavelengths (405, 365, and 280 nm) and five measurement emission windows from 320 to 750 nm [22, 27]. The hologram and optionally also the fluorescence results (currently not used) are then analyzed by AI algorithms, and pollen concentrations are delivered. A challenge of this system is that it needs to be calibrated to a manual Hirst-type pollen trap, which has accuracy problems itself (see above). These uncertainties are then partly transferred to the automatic device.

5.4   Crowd-Sourcing or the "Allergic Nose as Pollen Biosensor" Concept

The usual scientific and clinical approach to pollen allergy is to monitor pollen concentrations for short-term prediction of allergy symptoms in individual patients or an examined population. A somewhat contra-intuitive possibility to assess and predict pollen exposure based on the collection of daily symptom information from pollen allergic patients was recently proposed [28]. This "allergic nose as pollen biosensor" concept (Fig. 5.4) is based on short daily symptom questionnaires collected via e-Diary apps to produce daily symptom-medication scores, time trajectories, and descriptive reports of the severity of allergic rhinitis in pollen allergic patients [32]. In line with the crowd-sensing concept, proposed by Bernd Resch in 2013 [33], the allergic nose is proposed as a "pollen detector" whose outcome can be integrated into data obtained by pollen monitoring stations, thus contributing individual measurements and symptoms perception [28]. If this hypothesis is validated by prospective studies, monitoring of seasonal allergic rhinoconjunctivitis could be easily and cost-effectively expanded to geographic areas lacking pollen monitoring stations.

A scientific basis to this approach has been already given by studies showing that pollen forecasts improve when pollen data are integrated with information on patients' symptoms, based on a citizen science approach [30, 31, 34]. Moreover, the respiratory symptoms of pollen allergic patients have been used to validate criteria for pollen season definitions [35] and to cluster patients by disease severity [36]. Last, by activating GPS geolocation on e-Diaries apps, it is possible to produce a map of the territory based on real-time patients' symptoms reporting in an approach defined Volunteered Geographic Information (VGI) [37], thus adding spatial distribution to the time trends of pollen dispersion [28].

As the collection of intentionally patient-generated data may be challenging, particularly among heterogeneous populations and over longer time periods, information from Google Trends, a web-based surveillance tool, has been proposed, to monitor individuals searching for specific topics on Google when suffering from pollen allergy symptoms [38]. However, the obtained results had limited granularity, and more research is needed before prediction models based on search term analyses will yield reliable results. By contrast, a high correlation between social media posts on allergy symptoms and the spatial and temporal distribution of pollen has been observed in several cohorts [39, 40]. After removing confounders, such as bot-generated accounts, re-postings, and irrelevant content, AI may allow the prediction of pollen exposure based on social sensing data in the future [41]. This does not eliminate the need for measurements, as human noses could react to concomitant exposures (many exposures, one nose), and it might not always be possible to discriminate which exposure does what. Having measured single exposures (pollen, molds, pollution, etc.) might then resolve the mayor allergic symptoms provoking factor. Having both symptoms and measurements is the optimal situation.

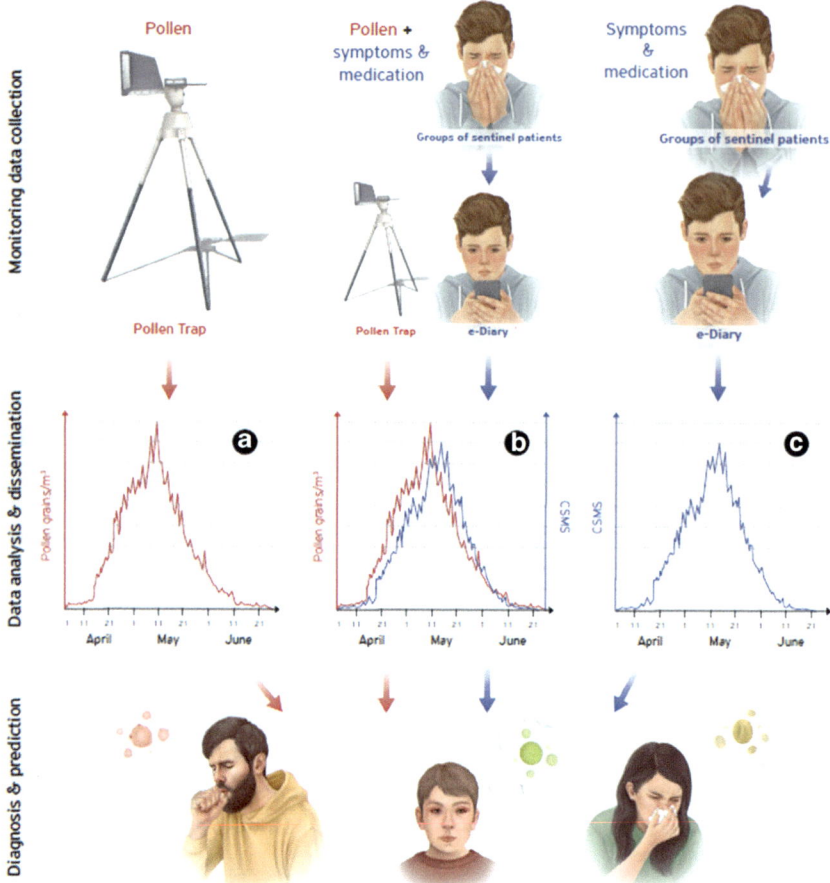

Fig. 5.4 The "allergic nose as pollen-biosensor" concept. Monitoring environment and/or sentinel patients for diagnosis and short-term prediction of seasonal allergic rhinitis. (**a**) Diagnosis and short-term prediction of seasonal allergic rhinitis are supported for decades by networks of pollen stations monitoring the concentration of allergenic pollen grains dispersed in the local outdoor air. Pollen data, collected through manual or automated pollen traps, are analyzed to produce not only retrospective pollen calendars but also prospective time trajectories whose shape changes by geographic area and year of registration. These data are useful for etiological diagnosis and short-term prediction of seasonal allergic rhinoconjunctivitis and asthma. (**b**) The allergenicity and clinical impact of pollen grains are greatly influenced by several co-factors, including meteorologic, pollution, allergen content, and patient's sensitivity. Therefore, for about 10 years, mathematical models have been used to integrate both pollen (and meteo−/pollution) data and patients' symptoms data, to provide more accurate prospective information on the trends of clinically relevant exposure [29–31]. (**c**) The "allergic nose as pollen detector" concept proposes that only data collected with e-Diaries from groups of well-characterized, mono-sensitized, sentinel patients may be efficient enough to support etiological diagnosis and prediction of seasonal allergic rhinoconjunctivitis. If this hypothesis will be validated by prospective studies, monitoring of seasonal allergic rhinoconjunctivitis could be easily and cost-effectively expanded to geographic areas deprived of pollen monitoring stations (reproduced from [28], permission to be asked)

5.5 Pollen Data and Their Dissemination

5.5.1 Dissemination of Pollen Data

How to obtain the correct and timely pollen data is a major concern, as discussed above. However, the task of getting these data to the individuals who need them is equally important. Around the world, there are several pollen monitoring networks.

(a) Pollen networks based on Hirst-type pollen traps. The European data obtained with manual procedures (mainly Hirst-type pollen traps) are, with exceptions, centrally stored at the EAN Database in Vienna, Austria. However, as manual traps are mostly privately owned, the data are not publicly available, but often at a cost. The data are not used to generate pollen exposure predictions, but only used to calibrate numerical prediction models retrospectively. These numerical models for future exposure predictions then run independently of the current Hirst-trap measurements.

(b) Pollen networks based on automatic pollen monitors New developments are the networks of automatic pollen monitors. These include MeteoSwiss using Poleno as main automatic pollen monitor in Switzerland, or www.pollen-science.eu and www.ePIN.bayern.de using the Hund BAA500 in Bavaria (Germany). In Japan, a network is composed by KH-3000, in Serbia two automatic instruments are installed [42].

(c) A new way to disseminate pollen information is in development. The EU-funded environmental data base EBAS is currently being adjusted to accommodate pollen values. This platform allows free access to all public data on pollen (and other parameters) in Europe.

5.5.2 Networks

MeteoSwiss (Switzerland). Meteo Swiss operates the national pollen monitoring network, collecting data of different monitoring stations covering Switzerland's most important climatic and vegetation regions. This network is composed by mostly manual pollen traps and 14 additional automatic devices, in this case Swisens Poleno instruments. More information about the network can be found at www.meteoswiss.admin.ch.

Pollen Science (Bavaria, Germany). Pollen science displays near real-time pollen concentrations (Fig. 5.5) via a graphical interface showing the data collected at different pollen measurement stations. It contains data of the Hund BAA500

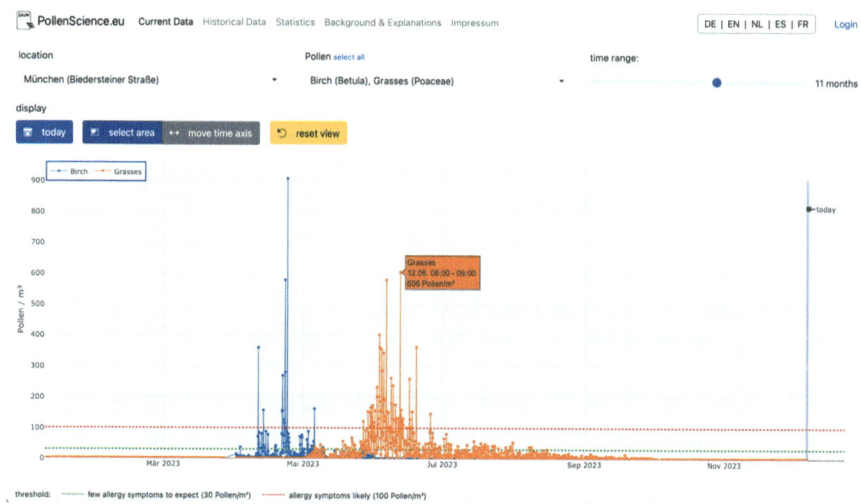

Fig. 5.5 Graphical interface webpage www.PollenScience.eu. The website (in 5 different languages) is interactive, i.e., the location, date and pollen type can be picked up by the user

automatic devices as well as from manual Hirst-type pollen traps. The aim is to gradually add data from many more pollen measuring stations in Europe. More information can be found at https://pollenscience.eu/.

ePIN (Bavaria, Germany). ePIN was the first automatic pollen monitoring network worldwide that offered a real-time species specific pollen information to the public [43]. More information can be found at https://epin.lgl.bayern.de/.

Hanakosan network (Japan). The Hanakosan network includes more than 120 sites using the laser optic KH-3000 [44], and it is monitored by the Ministry of the Environment, Government of Japan (http://kafun.taiki.go.jp/ (currently offline). In Japan, the major allergenic pollen is from Japanese Cedar, which produces rather large pollen (32–35 μm, in comparison birch pollen are 21 μm) [45]. The network mainly can detect large particles, which by default are then pollen. The system is not good at discriminating between different pollen taxa (see above).

EBAS (Norway) is a database with atmospheric measurement data. The infrastructure is operated by NILU-Norwegian Institute for Air Research. The aim of this platform is to handle, store, and disseminate atmospheric composition data generated by international and national frameworks. The database has been adapted to accommodate pollen concentrations, especially from automatic pollen monitors, but is currently showing only 5 of automatic stations. This number is expected to grow in the near future.

5.6 Pollen Prediction

Some research groups in charge of pollen monitoring provide a forecast for the following days (between 1 and 7 days), based on regression models developed with the time series of pollen records in their cities [46–48]. Also, some groups have used artificial intelligence (AI) algorithms to make predictions [47, 49–51]. Nevertheless, these forecasts are provided with data from several days before due to the delay on sampling analysis [34].

The appearance of automatic monitors opens the possibility to produce more accurate forecasts based on almost real-time data [12]. In the future, the automatic pollen data will be incorporated online into the pollen forecasts which may greatly improve pollen flight prediction [52].

5.6.1 Many Forecasting Apps, No Data

The digitization of everyday life has given access to an enormous amount of data, and instantaneously, especially to anyone with a smartphone at hand. This accessibility is beneficial for a wide variety of uses in many different fields, also for people suffering from allergies [53]. For example, many phone apps that have been developed provide information about pollen counts and/or exposure risk levels.

However, the vast amount of information available on the Internet has also some drawbacks, especially the lack of validation of the data sources [34]. Some Pollen Apps have been developed by official surveillance institutions, i.e., "Pollen+ App" from the European Aeroallergen Network (EAN) (https://www.polleninfo.org/FR/fr/gratis-pollen-app.html). But for many other apps, it is difficult to identify the source of pollen data and information.

Hence, despite offering very practical information for patients, the lack of source information for the forecasted data should alarm users. While some services use historical data to predict future pollen flights, the sources of others remain unclear. However, in times of changing climate conditions and biodiversity, even historical data might not represent the most accurate basis to predict the future situation. It is expected that (near) real-time measurements will improve the accuracy of prediction models and forecasts with these measurements are currently being developed.

Although manual and automatic pollen monitors are important data sources, having a tightly knit automatic monitoring network is not affordable. In addition, the manual system also faces the lack of experienced personnel to analyze so many air samples, thus a tightly knit network of cheaper manual systems is not likely either. For an allergic individual living in an area with pollen monitors the question arises, which pollen monitoring station is the right station representing his situation. One solution is to calculate pollen levels with interpolation methodologies, enabling allergic individuals to know their exposure in their hometowns, therefore avoiding the problem of not knowing which monitoring station is representative for their area. Different statistical interpolation methods exist, such as kriging [54], inverse distance weighting [55], or splines [56]. These techniques will soon be available in areas with automatic pollen monitors.

Whatever the model, the availability of (near) real-time data of real-world measurements is a great advantage to allergic individuals. Patients can check online what the actual pollen flight is right now (see websites above).

5.6.2   Including Automatic Pollen Monitors in Predictions

It is a great advantage to have real-time data to inform allergy sufferers, but it is even better to have a prediction to advise patients to minimize their future exposure. Numerical models that can forecast pollen flight in Europe are COSMO-ART [57], SILAM (System for Integrated modeLling of Atmospheric coMposition) [58], and Google   https://storage.googleapis.com/gmp-maps-demos/pollen/index. html#heatmap among others. These prediction models are based on the use of weather variables relevant for pollen and fungal spore seasons [12]. However, these current models rely on historical climatology to produce the pollen flight predictions, they do not use actual pollen or spore concentration data, so the quality of the forecast could be affected [19, 59]. It is to be expected that (near) real-time data will improve this situation by including a correction to the model with current pollen information.

Tests were performed with assimilating (near) real-time pollen concentration data into the models, but assimilation showed little effect on the forecast due to relaxation time of the systems, meaning that the assimilation is forgotten within a few hours of prediction [52]. Based on this experience, another approach was made to calibrate the pollen forecast model [59]. In both cases, the pollen concentration data were from manual equipment (Hirst-type trap). It will be an advance to introduce data generated by automatic pollen monitors as input to the model.

5.7   Future Fields in Aeroallergen Exposure

5.7.1   Allergenicity

Humans do not react to the whole pollen but to the allergens released by pollen [60]. This means that the concentration of airborne pollen is an indirect indicator, a proxy of exposure [61]. Monitoring the airborne allergens (mostly pollen) and determining their concentrations have been done worldwide for decades. The amount of allergen released by one pollen is not constant, but varies according to the year of observation, day of release, temperature, location, and humidity [61–64].

Indeed, depending on the day of sampling or origin of pollen, birch pollen differ ten-fold in allergen (Bet v 1)-release [61], 12-fold for Ole e 1 release from olive pollen [63], and 10 to 20-fold in Phl p 5 release from grass pollen, the major grass pollen allergen [62]. Similar effects were reported for Art v 1 from *Artemisia* pollen [64]. Like any natural product, pollens vary in ripening. Pollen grains ripen in male flowers like catkins, and, for instance, birch pollen dramatically increases their Bet v 1 content one week before being released from the catkin. The catkin can release the pollen whenever the weather is good for pollination. Depending on the day of release, (birch) pollen contains more allergen than the same pollen that would have been released earlier [65].

Over the last two decades, the correlation of allergen exposure with symptoms has been studied; the reaction of human immune cells (mast cells and basophils) correlated better with allergen Phl p 5 release from grass [62] or Bet v 1-release from birch pollen [61] than with pollen count. The same was true for symptoms in allergic individuals [60]: patients react more tightly regulated to the allergen in ambient air than to the pollen carrying these allergens. The pollen potency (the amount of allergen released by one pollen) may be different depending on geographical location [61]. The pollen potency also can vary from year to year, during the mean pollen season, and from location to location [61–63, 66]. Drivers affecting pollen potency were detected and modeled [67]. Levels of the major grass pollen allergen, Phl p 5, were positively associated with reported allergy symptoms and medication intake and much better correlated than with daily pollen counts [60]. Thus, it would be wise to monitor airborne allergen instead of airborne pollen. Still, monitoring released allergen by pollen is tedious and expensive. Because the airborne allergens stem exclusively from pollen, airborne pollen counts are currently the best proxy for allergen exposure.

5.7.2 New Algorithms

Most automatic pollen monitors rely on AI algorithms to detect and analyze pollen types. New algorithms are constantly being developed for existing instruments. To measure the accuracy of the algorithm, each new algorithm is being tested against Hirst-type traps, showing a good correlation so far [67]. As there are several different new instruments and many new algorithms, an app was developed in order to compare and test the accuracy of new algorithms. This app is an update of the EUMETNET-Autopollen campaign [20]. With this app, it is possible to compare between algorithms from different devices. The app can be found here: https://autopollen.shinyapps.io/APP_AUTOPOLLEN_COMPARE/.

Until now the current algorithms of the different instrument are showing at least equal results identifying different pollen types as Hirst-type traps. With time AI and computational resources will improve, thus in the near future the automatic pollen monitors will give better results than Hirst-type traps. It is highly recommended to enable re-analysis of the pollen already counted with the old algorithm, in order to avoid blaming climate change for a changed pollen exposure, when a change in algorithm was the underlying culprit (climate change by algorithm change).

5.7.3   Co-exposure

Generally, people are exposed to different components of the atmosphere on a daily basis, so it is unlikely that a person is exposed to a pure allergen alone. As a result, the patients' symptoms may be different depending on co-exposure to non-pollen components of ambient air, like air pollution, bacteria, and ozone, among others.

For example, the combination of pollen with certain bacteria can influence the allergic sensitization, as was the case for endotoxin released from gram-negative bacteria in combination with artemisia pollen. Artemisia pollen has the highest capacity among pollen to carry certain bacteria. Without these bacteria, the Artemisia pollen was less allergenic, i.e., it did not sensitize experimental animals to the Art v 1 allergen. However, the same pollen was quite effective in inducing a Th2 sensitization when associated with certain bacteria [68]. Also, organic pollutants, like diesel emission (polycyclic aromatic hydrocarbons), can interact with pollen and/or the human immune system, aggravating allergic diseases. For example, diesel particle extracts induced proallergic effects on basophils from birch pollen allergic individuals [69] and were shown to enhance allergic sensitizations [70].

Another study found that pollen-associated lipid mediators shift the human immune system toward a Th2-dominated response [71]. Evidence also shows that chemical pollutants may facilitate pollen allergen release, thereby modify pollen potency, or act as adjuvants to stimulate IgE-mediated responses: for example, urban residents who are more exposed to environmental pollution tend to experience more respiratory allergies than rural individuals [72].

5.8   Conclusions

The public focus on airborne allergen exposure is still rudimentary as until now the focus in ambient air quality is toward man-made pollution (i.e., diesel particles, ozone, nitrogen oxides). The understanding that also the biological components of ambient air are important for the health of a population, and that a large part of the population needs this information on biological components like pollen, is slowly increasing. At the same time, a revolution on ambient biological particle monitoring is taking place: instead of good but time-consuming pollen data depending on human labor, data of reliable automatic instruments are now available. The combination of the awareness that air quality is not only affected by chemical man-made components but also contains important biological particles, and new reliable ways to measure and disseminate this information will make air quality monitoring much better in the near future.

References

1. Pawankar R. Allergic diseases and asthma: a global public health concern and a call to action. World Allergy Org J. 2014;7 https://doi.org/10.1186/1939-4551-7-12.
2. Schmidt CW. Pollen overload: seasonal allergies in a changing climate. Environ Health Perspect. 2016;124:A70–5. https://doi.org/10.1289/ehp.124-A70.
3. Candeias J, Schmidt-Weber C, Buters J. Dosing intact birch pollen grains at the air-liquid interface (ALI) to the immortalized human bronchial epithelial cell line BEAS-2B. PLoS One. 2021;16 https://doi.org/10.1371/journal.pone.0259914.
4. Anderegg WRL, Abatzoglou JT, Anderegg LDL, Bielory L, Kinney PL, Ziska L. Anthropogenic climate change is worsening North American pollen seasons. Proc Natl Acad Sci U S A. 2021;118:e2013284118. https://doi.org/10.1073/pnas.2013284118.
5. Glick S, Gehrig R, Eeftens M. Multi-decade changes in pollen season onset, duration, and intensity: a concern for public health? Sci Total Environ. 2021;781:146382. https://doi.org/10.1016/j.scitotenv.2021.146382.
6. Rojo J, Picornell A, Oteros J, Werchan M, Werchan B, Bergmann K-C, Smith M, Weichenmeier I, Schmidt-Weber CB, Buters J. Consequences of climate change on airborne pollen in Bavaria. Central Europe Reg Environ Change. 2021;21:9. https://doi.org/10.1007/s10113-020-01729-z.
7. Zhang Y, Steiner AL. Projected climate-driven changes in pollen emission season length and magnitude over the continental United States. Nat Commun. 2022;13:1234. https://doi.org/10.1038/s41467-022-28764-0.
8. Platts-Mills TAE, Woodfolk JA. Allergens and their role in the allergic immune response. Immunol Rev. 2011;242:51–68. https://doi.org/10.1111/j.1600-065X.2011.01021.x.
9. Pfaar O, Hohlfeld JM, Al-Kadah B, Hauswald B, Homey B, Hunzelmann N, Schliemann S, Velling P, Worm M, Klimek L. Dose-response relationship of a new Timothy grass pollen allergoid in comparison with a 6-grass pollen allergoid. Clin Exp Allergy. 2017;47:1445–55. https://doi.org/10.1111/cea.12977.
10. Hirst JM. An automatic volumetric spore trap. Ann Appl Biol. 1952;39:257–65. https://doi.org/10.1111/j.1744-7348.1952.tb00904.x.
11. EN 16868 2019. EN 16868—Ambient air—sampling and analysis of airborne pollen grains and fungal spores for networks related to allergy—Volumetric Hirst method.
12. Tummon F, Arboledas LA, Bonini M, Guinot B, Hicke M, Jacob C, Kendrovski V, McCairns W, Petermann E, Peuch V-H, Pfaar O, Sicard M, Sikoparija B, Clot B. The need for Pan-European automatic pollen and fungal spore monitoring: a stakeholder workshop position paper. Clin Transl Allergy. 2021b;11:e12015. https://doi.org/10.1002/clt2.12015.
13. Oteros J, Buters J, Laven G, Röseler S, Wachter R, Schmidt-Weber C, Hofmann F. Errors in determining the flow rate of Hirst-type pollen traps. Aerobiologia. 2017;33:201–10. https://doi.org/10.1007/s10453-016-9467-x.
14. Suarez-Suarez M, Maya-Manzano JM, Clot B, Graber M-J, Sallin C, Tummon F, Buters J. Accuracy of a hand-held resistance-free flowmeters for flow adjustments of Hirst-type pollen traps. Aerobiologia. 2023;39:143–8. https://doi.org/10.1007/s10453-023-09782-x.
15. Triviño, M.M., Maya-Manzano, J.M., Tummon, F. et al. Variability between Hirst-type pollen traps is reduced by resistance-free flow adjustment. Aerobiologia 2023;39:257–273. https://doi.org/10.1007/s10453-023-09790-x
16. Smith M, Oteros J, Schmidt-Weber C, Buters JTM. An abbreviated method for the quality control of pollen counters. Grana. 2019;58(3):185–90.
17. Buters JTM, Antunes C, Galveias A, Bergmann KC, Thibaudon M, Galán C, Schmidt-Weber C, Oteros J. Pollen and spore monitoring in the world. Clin Transl Allergy. 2018;8:9. https://doi.org/10.1186/s13601-018-0197-8.
18. Huffman JA, Perring AE, Savage NJ, Clot B, Crouzy B, Tummon F, Shoshanim O, Damit B, Schneider J, Sivaprakasam V, Zawadowicz MA, Crawford I, Gallagher M, Topping D, Doughty DC, Hill SC, Pan Y. Real-time sensing of bioaerosols: review and current perspectives. Aerosol Sci Technol. 2020;54:465–95. https://doi.org/10.1080/02786826.2019.1664724.

19. Clot B, Gilge S, Hajkova L, Magyar D, Scheifinger H, Sofiev M, Bütler F, Tummon F. The EUMETNET AutoPollen programme: establishing a prototype automatic pollen monitoring network in Europe. Aerobiologia. 2020; https://doi.org/10.1007/s10453-020-09666-4.

20. Maya-Manzano JM, Tummon F, Abt R, Allan N, Bunderson L, Clot B, Crouzy B, Daunys G, Erb S, Gonzalez-Alonso M, Graf E, Grewling Ł, Haus J, Kadantsev E, Kawashima S, Martinez-Bracero M, Matavulj P, Mills S, Niederberger E, Lieberherr G, Lucas RW, O'Connor DJ, Oteros J, Palamarchuk J, Pope FD, Rojo J, Šaulienė I, Schäfer S, Schmidt-Weber CB, Schnitzler M, Šikoparija B, Skjøth CA, Sofiev M, Stemmler T, Triviño M, Zeder Y, Buters J. Towards European automatic bioaerosol monitoring: comparison of 9 automatic pollen observational instruments with classic Hirst-type traps. Sci Total Environ. 2023;866:161220. https://doi.org/10.1016/j.scitotenv.2022.161220.

21. Kawashima S, Clot B, Fujita T, Takahashi Y, Nakamura K. An algorithm and a device for counting airborne pollen automatically using laser optics. Atmos Environ. 2007;41:7987–93. https://doi.org/10.1016/j.atmosenv.2007.09.019.

22. Tummon F, Adamov S, Clot B, Crouzy B, Gysel-Beer M, Kawashima S, Lieberherr G, Manzano J, Markey E, Moallemi A, O'Connor D. A first evaluation of multiple automatic pollen monitors run in parallel. Aerobiologia. 2021a; https://doi.org/10.1007/s10453-021-09729-0.

23. Yamada T, Saito H, Fujieda S. Present state of Japanese cedar pollinosis: the national affliction. J Allergy Clin Immunol. 2014;133:632–639.e5. https://doi.org/10.1016/j.jaci.2013.11.002.

24. Oteros J, Weber A, Kutzora S, Rojo J, Heinze S, Herr C, Gebauer R, Schmidt-Weber CB, Buters JTM. An operational robotic pollen monitoring network based on automatic image recognition. Environ Res. 2020;191:110031. https://doi.org/10.1016/j.envres.2020.110031.

25. Oteros J, Pusch G, Weichenmeier I, Heimann U, Möller R, Röseler S, Traidl-Hoffmann C, Schmidt-Weber C, Buters JTM. Automatic and online pollen monitoring. Int Arch Allergy Immunol. 2015;167:158–66. https://doi.org/10.1159/000436968.

26. González-Alonso M, Boldeanu M, Koritnik T, Gonçalves J, Belzner L, Stemmler T, Gebauer R, Grewling Ł, Tummon F, Maya-Manzano JM, Ariño AH, Schmidt-Weber C, Buters J. Alternaria spore exposure in Bavaria, Germany, measured using artificial intelligence algorithms in a network of BAA500 automatic pollen monitors. Sci Total Environ. 2023;861:160180. https://doi.org/10.1016/j.scitotenv.2022.160180.

27. Sauvageat E, Zeder Y, Auderset K, Calpini B, Clot B, Crouzy B, Konzelmann T, Lieberherr G, Tummon F, Vasilatou K. Real-time pollen monitoring using digital holography. Atmos Measure Techn. 2020;13:1539–50. https://doi.org/10.5194/amt-13-1539-2020.

28. Matricardi PM, Hoffmann T, Dramburg S. The "allergic nose as a pollen detector" concept: e-Diaries to predict pollen trends. Pediatr Allergy Immunol. 2023;34:e13966. https://doi.org/10.1111/pai.13966.

29. Bastl K, Kmenta M, Berger M, Berger U. The connection of pollen concentrations and crowd-sourced symptom data: new insights from daily and seasonal symptom load index data from 2013 to 2017 in Vienna. World Allergy Org J. 2018;11:24. https://doi.org/10.1186/s40413-018-0203-6.

30. Bastl K, Kmenta M, Geller-Bernstein C, Berger U, Jäger S. Can we improve pollen season definitions by using the symptom load index in addition to pollen counts? Environ Pollut. 2015;204:109–16. https://doi.org/10.1016/j.envpol.2015.04.016.

31. Damialis A, Häring F, Gökkaya M, Rauer D, Reiger M, Bezold S, Bounas-Pyrros N, Eyerich K, Todorova A, Hammel G, Gilles S, Traidl-Hoffmann C. Human exposure to airborne pollen and relationships with symptoms and immune responses: Indoors versus outdoors, circadian patterns and meteorological effects in alpine and urban environments. Sci Total Environ. 2019;653:190–9. https://doi.org/10.1016/j.scitotenv.2018.10.366.

32. Tripodi S, Giannone A, Sfika I, Pelosi S, Dramburg S, Bianchi A, Pizzulli A, Florack J, Villella V, Potapova E, Matricardi PM. Digital technologies for an improved management of respiratory allergic diseases: 10 years of clinical studies using an online platform for patients and physicians. Ital J Pediatr. 2020;46:105. https://doi.org/10.1186/s13052-020-00870-z.

33. Resch B. People as sensors and collective sensing-contextual observations complementing geosensor network measurements. In: Krisp JM, editor. Progress in location-based services. Berlin, Heidelberg: Springer; 2013. p. 391–406. https://doi.org/10.1007/978-3-642-34203-5_22.

34. Bastl K, Berger U, Kmenta M. Evaluation of Pollen Apps forecasts: the need for quality control in an eHealth service. J Med Internet Res. 2017;19:e7426. https://doi.org/10.2196/jmir.7426.

35. Karatzas K, Katsifarakis N, Riga M, Werchan B, Werchan M, Berger U, Pfaar O, Bergmann K-C. New European Academy of Allergy and Clinical Immunology definition on pollen season mirrors symptom load for grass and birch pollen-induced allergic rhinitis. Allergy. 2018;73:1851–9. https://doi.org/10.1111/all.13487.

36. Voukantsis D, Karatzas K, Jaeger S, Berger U, Smith M. Analysis and forecasting of airborne pollen–induced symptoms with the aid of computational intelligence methods. Aerobiologia. 2013;29:175–85. https://doi.org/10.1007/s10453-012-9271-1.

37. Goodchild MF. Citizens as sensors: the world of volunteered geography. GeoJournal. 2007;69:211–21. https://doi.org/10.1007/s10708-007-9111-y.

38. Iinuma T, Yonekura S, Sakurai D, Inaba Y, Kawasaki Y, Okamoto Y. Investigating Japanese cedar pollen-induced allergic rhinitis and related terms using Google trends. Allergol Int. 2020;69:616–8. https://doi.org/10.1016/j.alit.2020.03.006.

39. Sitaru S, Wecker H, Buters J, Biedermann T, Zink A. Social media to monitor prevalent diseases: Hay fever and Twitter activity in Germany. Allergy. 2023;78:2777–80. https://doi.org/10.1111/all.15787.

40. Wakamiya S, Matsune S, Okubo K, Aramaki E. Causal relationships among pollen counts, tweet numbers, and patient numbers for seasonal allergic rhinitis surveillance: retrospective analysis. J Med Internet Res. 2019;21:e10450. https://doi.org/10.2196/10450.

41. Cowie S, Arthur R, Williams HTP. @choo: Tracking Pollen and Hayfever in the UK Using Social Media. Sensors (Basel). 2018;18:4434. https://doi.org/10.3390/s18124434.

42. Tešendić D, Boberić Krstićev D, Matavulj P, Brdar S, Panić M, Minić V, Šikoparija B. RealForAll: real-time system for automatic detection of airborne pollen. Enterprise Inform Syst. 2022;16:1793391. https://doi.org/10.1080/17517575.2020.1793391.

43. Kutzora S, Strasser A, Grenzebach K, Ramona G, Gebauer R, Weinberger A, Szperalski J, Herr C, Quartucci C, Heinze S. Establishment, operation and development of the electronic Pollen Information Network (ePIN) in Bavaria, Germany; 2023. https://doi.org/10.21203/rs.3.rs-3760963/v1.

44. Miki K, Fujita T, Sahashi N. Development and application of a method to classify airborne pollen taxa concentration using light scattering data. Sci Rep. 2021;11:1–12. https://doi.org/10.1038/s41598-021-01919-7.

45. Kakui H, Tsurisaki E, Sassa H, Moriguchi Y. An improved pollen number counting method using a cell counter and mesh columns. Plant Methods. 2020;16:124. https://doi.org/10.1186/s13007-020-00668-4.

46. Lara B, Rojo J, Fernández-González F, Pérez-Badia R. Prediction of airborne pollen concentrations for the plane tree as a tool for evaluating allergy risk in urban green areas. Landsc Urban Plan. 2019;189:285–95. https://doi.org/10.1016/j.landurbplan.2019.05.002.

47. Lops Y, Choi Y, Eslami E, Sayeed A. Real-time 7-day forecast of pollen counts using a deep convolutional neural network. Neural Comput Appl. 2020;32:11827–36. https://doi.org/10.1007/s00521-019-04665-0.

48. Scheifinger H, Belmonte J, Buters J, Celenk S, Damialis A, Dechamp C, García-Mozo H, Gehrig R, Grewling L, Halley JM, Hogda K-A, Jäger S, Karatzas K, Karlsen S-R, Koch E, Pauling A, Peel R, Sikoparija B, Smith M, Galán-Soldevilla C, Thibaudon M, Vokou D, de Weger LA. Monitoring, modelling and forecasting of the Pollen season. In: Sofiev M, Bergmann K-C, editors. Allergenic pollen: a review of the production, release, distribution and health impacts. Netherlands, Dordrecht: Springer; 2013. p. 71–126. https://doi.org/10.1007/978-94-007-4881-1_4.

49. Goudarzi G, Birgani YT, Assarehzadegan M-A, Neisi A, Dastoorpoor M, Sorooshian A, Yazdani M. Prediction of airborne pollen concentrations by artificial neural network and their

relationship with meteorological parameters and air pollutants. J Environ Health Sci Eng. 2022;20:251–64. https://doi.org/10.1007/s40201-021-00773-z.

50. Grinn-Gofroń A, Nowosad J, Bosiacka B, Camacho I, Pashley C, Belmonte J, De Linares C, Ianovici N, Manzano JMM, Sadyś M, Skjøth C, Rodinkova V, Tormo-Molina R, Vokou D, Fernández-Rodríguez S, Damialis A. Airborne *Alternaria* and *Cladosporium* fungal spores in Europe: forecasting possibilities and relationships with meteorological parameters. Sci Total Environ. 2019;653:938–46. https://doi.org/10.1016/j.scitotenv.2018.10.419.

51. Picornell A, Hurtado S, Antequera-Gómez ML, Barba-González C, Ruiz-Mata R, de Gálvez-Montañez E, Recio M, del Mar Trigo M, Aldana-Montes JF, Navas-Delgado I. A deep learning LSTM-based approach for forecasting annual pollen curves: *Olea* and Urticaceae pollen types as a case study. Comput Biol Med. 2024;168:107706. https://doi.org/10.1016/j.compbiomed.2023.107706.

52. Sofiev M. On possibilities of assimilation of near-real-time pollen data by atmospheric composition models. Aerobiologia. 2019;35:523–31. https://doi.org/10.1007/s10453-019-09583-1.

53. Kmenta M, Zetter R, Berger U, Bastl K. Pollen information consumption as an indicator of pollen allergy burden. Wien Klin Wochenschr. 2016;128:59–67. https://doi.org/10.1007/s00508-015-0855-y.

54. Krige DG. A statistical approach to some basic mine valuation problems on the Witwatersrand. J Southern Afr Inst Mining Metall. 1951;52:119–39. https://doi.org/10.10520/AJA0038223X_4792.

55. Shepard D. A two-dimensional interpolation function for irregularly-spaced data. In: Proceedings of the 1968 23rd ACM National Conference, ACM '68. New York, NY: Association for Computing Machinery; 1968. p. 517–24. https://doi.org/10.1145/800186.810616.

56. Hämmerlin G, Hoffman K-H. Splines. In: Hämmerlin G, Hoffman K-H, editors. Numerical mathematics. New York, NY: Springer; 1991. p. 229–71. https://doi.org/10.1007/978-1-4612-4442-4_6.

57. Vogel B, Vogel H, Bäumer D, Bangert M, Lundgren K, Rinke R, Stanelle T. The comprehensive model system COSMO-ART—radiative impact of aerosol on the state of the atmosphere on the regional scale. Atmos Chem Phys. 2009;9:8661–80. https://doi.org/10.5194/acp-9-8661-2009.

58. Sofiev M, Vira J, Kouznetsov R, Prank M, Soares J, Genikhovich E. Construction of the SILAM Eulerian atmospheric dispersion model based on the advection algorithm of Michael Galperin. Geosci Model Dev. 2015;8:3497–522. https://doi.org/10.5194/gmd-8-3497-2015.

59. Adamov S, Pauling A. A real-time calibration method for the numerical pollen forecast model COSMO-ART. Aerobiologia. 2023;39:327–44. https://doi.org/10.1007/s10453-023-09796-5.

60. Fuertes E, Jarvis D, Lam H, Davies B, Fecht D, Candeias J, Schmidt-Weber CB, Douiri A, Slovick A, Scala E, Smith TEL, Shamji M, Buters JTM, Cecchi L, Till SJ. Phl p 5 levels more strongly associated than grass pollen counts with allergic respiratory health. J Allergy Clin Immunol. 2024;153:844–51. https://doi.org/10.1016/j.jaci.2023.11.011.

61. Buters JTM, Thibaudon M, Smith M, Kennedy R, Rantio-Lehtimäki A, Albertini R, Reese G, Weber B, Galan C, Brandao R, Antunes CM, Jäger S, Berger U, Celenk S, Grewling Ł, Jackowiak B, Sauliene I, Weichenmeier I, Pusch G, Sarioglu H, Ueffing M, Behrendt H, Prank M, Sofiev M, Cecchi L. Release of Bet v 1 from birch pollen from 5 European countries. Results from the HIALINE study. Atmos Environ. 2012;55:496–505. https://doi.org/10.1016/j.atmosenv.2012.01.054.

62. Buters J, Prank M, Sofiev M, Pusch G, Albertini R, Annesi-Maesano I, Antunes C, Behrendt H, Berger U, Brandao R, Celenk S, Galan C, Grewling Ł, Jackowiak B, Kennedy R, Rantio-Lehtimäki A, Reese G, Sauliene I, Smith M, Thibaudon M, Weber B, Cecchi L. Variation of the group 5 grass pollen allergen content of airborne pollen in relation to geographic location and time in season. J Allergy Clin Immunol. 2015;136:87–95. https://doi.org/10.1016/j.jaci.2015.01.049.

63. Galan C, Antunes C, Brandao R, Torres C, Garcia-Mozo H, Caeiro E, Ferro R, Prank M, Sofiev M, Albertini R, Berger U, Cecchi L, Celenk S, Grewling Ł, Jackowiak B, Jäger S, Kennedy R,

Rantio-Lehtimäki A, Reese G, Sauliene I, Smith M, Thibaudon M, Weber B, Weichenmeier I, Pusch G, Buters JTM. HIALINE Working Group. Airborne olive pollen counts are not representative of exposure to the major olive allergen Ole e 1. Allergy. 2013;68:809–12. https://doi.org/10.1111/all.12144.

64. Grewling Ł, Bogawski P, Kostecki Ł, Nowak M, Szymańska A, Frątczak A. Atmospheric exposure to the major *Artemisia* pollen allergen (Art v 1): seasonality, impact of weather, and clinical implications. Sci Total Environ. 2020;713:136611. https://doi.org/10.1016/j.scitotenv.2020.136611.

65. Buters JTM, Weichenmeier I, Ochs S, Pusch G, Kreyling W, Boere AJF, Schober W, Behrendt H. The allergen Bet v 1 in fractions of ambient air deviates from birch pollen counts. Allergy. 2010;65:850–8. https://doi.org/10.1111/j.1398-9995.2009.02286.x.

66. Buters JTM, Kasche A, Weichenmeier I, Schober W, Klaus S, Traidl-Hoffmann C, Menzel A, Huss-Marp J, Kramer U, Behrendt H. Year-to-year variation in release of Bet v 1 allergen from birch pollen: evidence for geographical differences between West and South Germany. Int Arch Allergy Immunol. 2008;145:122–30. https://doi.org/10.1159/000108137.

67. Maya-Manzano JM, Oteros J, Rojo J, Traidl-Hoffmann C, Schmidt-Weber C, Buters J. Drivers of the release of the allergens Bet v 1 and Phl p 5 from birch and grass pollen. Environ Res. 2022;214:113987. https://doi.org/10.1016/j.envres.2022.113987.

68. Oteros J, Bartusel E, Alessandrini F, Núñez A, Moreno DA, Behrendt H, Schmidt-Weber C, Traidl-Hoffmann C, Buters J. Artemisia pollen is the main vector for airborne endotoxin. J Allergy Clin Immunol. 2019;143:369–77. https://doi.org/10.1016/j.jaci.2018.05.040.

69. Lubitz S, Schober W, Pusch G, Effner R, Klopp N, Behrendt H, Buters JTM. Polycyclic aromatic hydrocarbons from diesel emissions exert proallergic effects in birch pollen allergic individuals through enhanced mediator release from basophils. Environ Toxicol. 2010;25:188–97. https://doi.org/10.1002/tox.20490.

70. Diaz-Sanchez D, Garcia MP, Wang M, Jyrala M, Saxon A. Nasal challenge with diesel exhaust particles can induce sensitization to a neoallergen in the human mucosa. J Allergy Clin Immunol. 1999;104:1183–8. https://doi.org/10.1016/s0091-6749(99)70011-4.

71. Gilles S, Mariani V, Bryce M, Mueller MJ, Ring J, Behrendt H, Jakob T, Traidl-Hoffmann C. Pollen allergens do not come alone: pollen associated lipid mediators (PALMS) shift the human immune systems towards a T(H)2-dominated response. Allergy Asthma Clin Immunol. 2009;5:3. https://doi.org/10.1186/1710-1492-5-3.

Chapter 6
Digital Solutions for Pollen Allergy and Allergen Immunotherapy: The AllergyMonitor Experience

Salvatore Tripodi, Simone Pelosi, and Paolo Maria Matricardi

Contents

Abstract Digital healthcare technologies, particularly given the fast developments in artificial intelligence, can assist doctors in making well-informed diagnostic and therapeutic choices. In the treatment of allergies, electronic clinical diaries have recently been used to prospectively collect patient data and improve diagnostic accuracy.

S. Tripodi (✉)
Allergology Service, Policlinico Casilino Hospital, Rome, Italy

S. Pelosi
TPS Production, Rome, Italy

P. M. Matricardi
Department of Pediatric Respiratory Medicine, Immunology and Critical Care Medicine, Charité–Universitätsmedizin Berlin, a corporate member of Freie Universität Berlin and Humboldt–Universität zu Berlin, Berlin, Germany

Institute of Allergology, Charité—Universitätsmedizin Berlin, Corporate Member of Freie Universität Berlin and Humboldt-Universität zu Berlin, Berlin, Germany

Fraunhofer Institute for Translational Medicine and Pharmacology ITMP, Allergology and Immunology, Berlin, Germany

P. M. Matricardi, S. Dramburg, *Digital Allergology*, Health Informatics,
https://doi.org/10.1007/978-3-031-71021-6_6

83

This review summarizes the clinical and scientific experience gathered with a digital platform for patients with pollen allergies. The AllergyMonitor® (AM) mobile application and back-office enable patients to record their daily allergy symptoms, as well as the intake of symptomatic medication and immunotherapy and possible side effects. Results can be viewed by both the patient and the treating physician in concise reports via smartphone or computer.

Many clinical studies and routine experience have shown that (A) the etiological diagnosis of seasonal allergic rhinitis (SAR) is often challenging in polysensitized patients living in areas with high levels and diversity of pollen exposure; (B) the diagnostic work-up of these patients can be aided by matching prospectively recorded symptom and pollen data in a Clinical Decision Support System (CDSS), (C) adherence to daily symptom monitoring can remain high (>80%) for several weeks if prescribed and carefully explained by the treating physician, in a blended care approach; (D) the use of mobile technology can improve adherence to symptomatic drugs and allergen-specific immunotherapy.

Trials and clinical practice based on the use of AM have demonstrated the reliability and positive impact of a digital platform that includes an electronic diary (e-Diary) on allergic rhinitis patient care.

6.1 Introduction

6.1.1 Allergy to Pollen

Allergic rhinitis (AR) is, along with asthma, one of the most common manifestations of pollen allergy, a highly prevalent condition affecting approximately 20% of the global population, including children and adolescents, with an increasing incidence over the last few decades [1–3].

Pollen allergy can manifest as seasonal allergy rhinitis (SAR), in which the allergic reaction occurs during the plant flowering season, or as perennial allergy, in which the allergic reaction occurs throughout the year due to constant exposure to inhalant allergens.

Patients are affected by nasal and ocular symptoms (e.g., sneezing, rhinorrhea, nasal congestion, itching, tearing), systemic symptoms (e.g., fatigue, irritability, headache), and treatment side effects (e.g., sedation from antihistamines). Pollen allergy can have a significant economic and social burden, as it can affect the quality of life of individuals and their daily activities. People with pollen allergy may miss work or school due to symptoms and may be forced to limit outdoor activities during the plant flowering season, and often, AR coexists with asthma and other comorbidities. In addition, the management of pollen allergy can entail significant costs for patients and the healthcare system, for example, for diagnosis, medication, and immunotherapy interventions [3, 4].

6.2   Allergen-Specific Immunotherapy

The only causal treatment option for AR and allergic asthma is allergen-specific immunotherapy (AIT), which is mostly administered as repeated subcutaneous injections or daily intake of sublingual tablets/drops.

AIT should be considered in the presence of:

- Evidence of IgE sensitization (positive skin prick tests and/or specific IgE) to one or more clinically relevant allergens.
- Moderate to severe symptoms that interfere with regular daily activities or sleep despite regular and appropriate pharmacotherapy and/or avoidance strategies.

To be effective with a medium- to long-term perspective, AIT must be performed on a regular basis for at least 3 years [4].

6.2.1   Digital Solutions for Allergic Rhinitis

Many apps are widely used for AR and chronic rhinosinusitis (CRS). They can help better understand these diseases and their management, but among the over 1,500 apps available on Google Play and Apple App stores, only six apps for AR (AirRater, AllergyMonitor, AllerSearch, Husteblume, MASK-air, and Pollen App) are validated by rigorous scientific publications [5, 6].

6.2.2   AllergyMonitor® Description: App for the Patient and Back-Office for the Physician

AM (TPS software production, Rome, Italy) is an online service developed in 2009 with the aim of allowing the registration of clinical symptoms, medication intake, and adherence to allergen-specific sublingual immunotherapy (SLIT), as well as monitoring the effectiveness and side effects of SLIT or subcutaneous immunotherapy (SCIT) in patients with allergic rhinoconjunctivitis and/or asthma. The system, which is available to everyone and easy to use, consists of two parts: a patient app (front-end) and a website for the treating physician (back-office), which is a unique feature compared to other validated apps. The app, which patients can freely download from Google Play and Apple App Store, is available in several languages. Every day, users are asked to complete a short and graphically supported questionnaire (using emoticons in a categorical visual analogue scale) on their symptoms of eyes, nose and lungs, as well as a visual analog scale on their general allergic conditions. Once activated by the physician through the back-office, the app user can also record daily medication intake, adherence to sublingual immunotherapy, and potentially detectable side effects. To provide a summary and feedback to the user, all entered data can be easily viewed within the app in summary graphs that show the evolution of symptoms over time.

Through their back-office, physicians can access all registered data of individual patients, which can be viewed as different internationally validated graphs of symptoms and medications (Rhinoconjunctivitis Total Symptom Score (RTSS), Adjusted Mean Symptom Score (AdSS), Rescue Medication Score (RMS), and Adjusted Combined Score (ACS)) [7, 8]. These graphs can be combined with local pollen monitoring data, which are automatically imported into the back-office by retrieving them from the databases of the Italian Aerobiological Monitoring Network "POLLnet," ISPRA (Istituto per la Protezione e la Ricerca Ambientale). From a telemedicine perspective, the back-office allows physicians to individually configure the front-end of each patient, for example, by adding symptomatic drugs or adding sublingual immunotherapy and monitoring side effects.

A messaging system between physician and patient based on e-mail, chat, or short message service (SMS) facilitates direct communication, and an automatic alert system reports missed registration days to both front-end and back-office users. This blended approach has allowed for better adherence to patient recordings, significantly higher than that of other apps downloaded independently by patients [9, 10].

6.2.3   Etiological Diagnosis for AIT in SAR

The efficacy of AIT depends not only on the standardization and quality of the products used for this therapy but also on the selection of clinically relevant allergens for the patient [11].

Selecting appropriate treatment becomes challenging for individuals with multiple sensitivities, a growing occurrence, especially in regions like the Mediterranean. The complexity arises due to the simultaneous presence of various pollens in the air. This was highlighted in the @IT.2020 multicenter observational study, involving 348 pediatric patients and 467 adults with Seasonal Allergic Rhinitis (SAR). The study encompassed nine urban centers across seven Southern European/Mediterranean countries: Porto, Portugal; Valencia, Spain; Marseille, France; Rome and Messina, Italy; Tirana, Albania; Athens, Greece; Istanbul and Izmir, Turkey. Polysensitization, even for the allergens' major molecules, was present in 71.3% of all cases. The pediatric cohort from Rome was found to be the most polysensitized, with an average number of 3.8 sIgE to major allergenic molecules per patient [12].

In such cases, the etiological diagnosis based on retrospective clinical history, which is inevitably affected by recall bias, and on sensitization to whole extracts, both through skin prick tests and specific serum IgE assays, often leads to equivocal results. Component resolved diagnosis (CRD) has certainly simplified the selection by allowing the detection of IgE sensitization to the specific molecules, and therefore allowing modification of the etiological diagnosis, based only on clinical history and skin prick test (SPT), in about 47% of cases [13]. However, sometimes even CRD fails to identify the clinically relevant allergens for a given patient and therefore which ones to choose for AIT.

Monitoring the patient's symptoms recorded during exposure to airborne allergens (pollens and alternaria) with AM and correlating them with pollen curves has been shown to be fundamental, both confirming the severity of symptoms not adequately controlled by pharmacological therapy, and allowing the selection of which allergens to choose for the most appropriate AIT [14].

Figure 6.1 shows a paradigmatic case of a 17-year-old boy at the time of study inclusion, who lives in Rome, with a history of persistent moderate-severe SAR since the age of 5 years (ARIA criteria [15]) which has worsened in recent years mainly in the months from January to June. The patient is part of the multicenter study @IT2020 [12] an observational clinical study on the impact of CRD and digital symptoms recording for the diagnosis of pollen allergy. The figure shows that RTSS and SPT demonstrate polysensitization, particularly to Alternaria, Cypress, Timothy and Bermuda Grass, and Pellitory. All allergens, based on the local pollen calendar, were compatible with the patient's rhinitis symptoms. The assay of specific IgE toward extracts and molecules was performed with the multiplex ESEP (Euroline Southern European Profile) test (EUROIMMUN AG, Lübeck, Germany, [16, 17]), which confirmed the patient's polysensitization to the same allergens even at the molecular level. The patient performed symptom monitoring with AM, demonstrating high adherence from February to September, which clearly showed that the ~~only~~ clinically relevant allergen was only grass pollen.

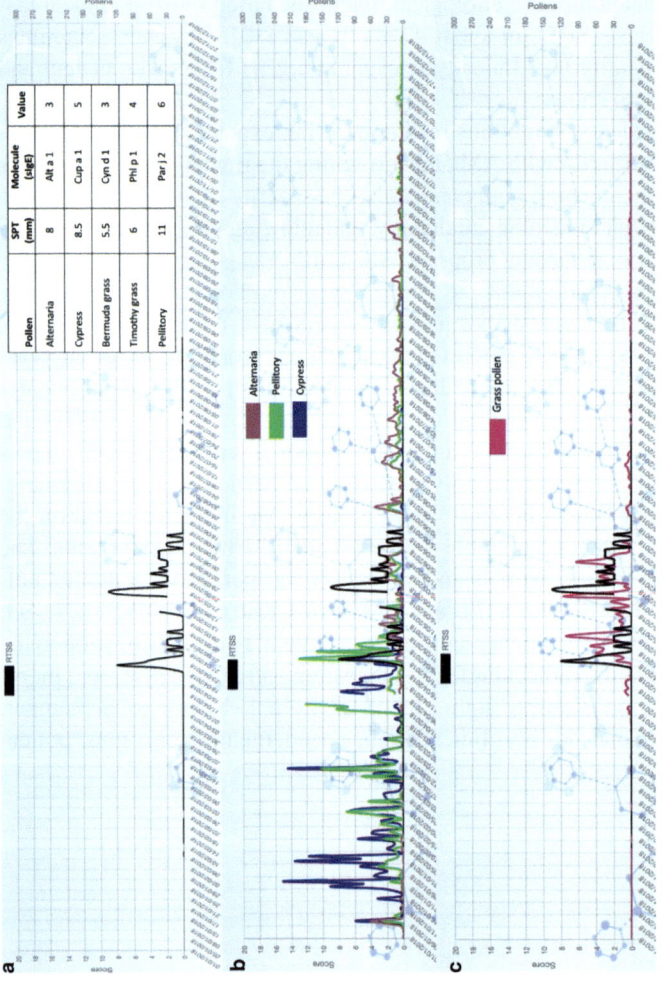

Fig. 6.1 Representative summary of a patient, living in Rome and suffering from SAR in the @IT.2020 multicenter study. (**a**) Summary of clinical and diagnostic information combined with longitudinal symptom monitoring between 1/02/2018 and 30/08/2018 via the AM app. RTSS = rhinoconjunctivitis total symptoms score (range 0–18), SPT = wheal medium diameter of the skin prick test results, sIgE = serum specific IgE antibodies directed against the major allergenic molecule of each allergen source. IgE results are expressed as classes from 0 to 6 corresponding to the following concentrations (all expressed in kU/L): class $0 < 0.35$; class $1 < 0.7$; $0.7 \leq$ class $2 < 3.5$; $3.5 \leq$ class $3 < 17.5$; $17.5 \leq$ class $4 < 50.0$; $50.0 \leq$ class $5 < 100.0$; class $6 \geq 100.0$. (**b**) RTSS matched with normalized airborne concentrations of *Alternaria*, Cypress pollen, and pollen of Wall pellitory. (**c**) RTSS matched with normalized airborne concentration of grass pollen

6.3 Clinical Decision Support System (CDSS)

This mismatch between patients' symptoms and their specific pollen sensitivities prompted the development of a computerized tool (CDSS) that helps doctors better diagnose allergies. This is crucial for effective treatment, as allergen immunotherapy's success depends on identifying the exact allergen triggering the allergic reaction [13, 18]. An algorithm for a CDSS (@IT2020-CDSS) [16, 19] was developed for seasonal allergic rhinitis and its diagnostic phases (anamnesis, skin prick test or serum sIgE, CRD diagnosis, and real-time and prospective symptom recording via AM), and this approach was evaluated in a study assessing the accuracy of physicians´ decisions on AIT prescription [16]. The @IT2020-CDSS algorithm (Fig. 6.2) is based on clinical data progressively considered in three phases: phase 1—clinical history and sensitization to whole extracts (SWE) [i.e., SPT and/or serum sIgE to a panel of allergens that includes timothy grass, cypress, birch, olive, ragweed, mugwort, pellitory, alternaria]; phase 2—addition of specific IgE dosages to molecular allergen components (CRD); phase 3—addition of data on symptoms recorded through AM with comparison to pollen trajectories [16].

After training on the @IT2020-CDSS algorithm, 46 physicians (18 allergists (AS) and 28 general practitioners (GP)) proposed a hypothetical AIT prescription for 10 index clinical cases. The decisions were repeatedly recorded at different

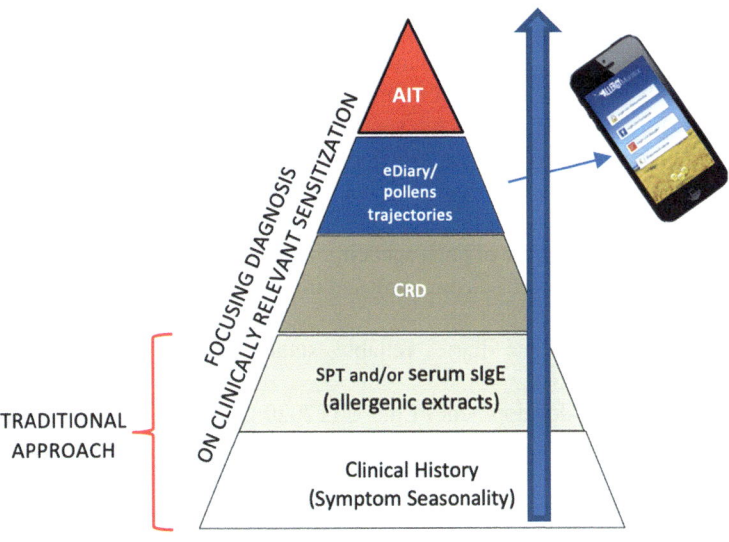

Fig. 6.2 @IT2020: Algorithm for a potential Clinical Decision Support System (CDSS) for seasonal allergy, "Pyramid model". The successive steps of the diagnostic algorithm of @IT2020-CDSS develop vertically as a "pyramid". In most clinical cases, excluding step by step more and more seasonal allergens, the 'pyramid' algorithm proceeds from a large basis toward a narrow top, allowing the recognition of only one or a few relevant allergen(s) among the many putative considered by the traditional diagnostic approach. Modified from Matricardi PM et al. [19]

phases of the algorithm. The prescription of AIT for pollen and alternaria allergy based on anamnesis and SWE was heterogeneous but converging toward a consensus after the integration of CRD and e-Diary information. The combined use of CRD and AM increased the number and the accuracy of hypothetical AIT prescriptions in both groups ($p < .01$). The participating physicians in the study rated the algorithm as useful to optimize the classical diagnostic work-up. In conclusion, the implementation of CRD and e-Diary in the @IT2020-CDSS algorithm improved consensus on AIT prescription for SAR between AS and GP [16].

The same analysis was repeated in the multicenter @IT-2020 study [20, 21], and data are being processed and published, but preliminary results are in line with those of the pilot study [S. Dramburg, personal communication].

Trajectories of daily symptom scores (dSS) collected from 100 polysensitized patients with seasonal allergic rhinitis during 2018 in Rome (Italy) and matched with the concentration of pollen grains (Cypress, Timothy and Bermuda Grass, Pellitory), and Alternaria spores in the air were analyzed (Fig. 6.3). Observing the graphs of each patient and following internally developed and shared guidelines, three independent experts evaluated, with a score class ranging from 0 (null) to 4 (maximum): (1) data completeness, (2) average symptom severity, (3) overall symptom impact, (4) allergen priority, and (5) overall clinical relevance, referred to each patient for each allergen. Consensus was considered achieved when scores attributed by different experts to the same item fell into two contiguous classes [22].

Full consensus on data completeness by the three experts was achieved in 531/600 (88.5%) evaluations, of which 495 met the criteria for subsequent analysis. Among these, full consensus was found in 439 (90.1%) for average symptom severity, 467 (94.3%) for overall symptom impact, 381 (77.0%) for allergen priority, and 381 (77.0%) for allergen clinical relevance.

In conclusion, visual analysis and interpretation of graphs generated by electronic diaries of patients with SAR and pollen curves, supported by specific guidelines, allow for correct data interpretation in most cases; however, it is not possible to eliminate a certain degree of heterogeneity in subjective interpretation by experts. This visual analysis, which is demanding and time-consuming, could be replaced by mathematical algorithms and machine-learning techniques, making reading and interpretation of electronic diaries reliable, standardized, fast, and user-friendly even in everyday practice.

Further phases of development of the @IT2020-CDSS are ongoing and include subsequent implementation of various steps of the algorithm (SWE>CRD>AM and pollen curves), first with a visual mode similar to the previously described one but applied to the entire case series of the multicenter study @IT2020 [20, 21], and then through statistical algorithms and AI techniques, in order to make the system user-friendly for both patients and physicians.

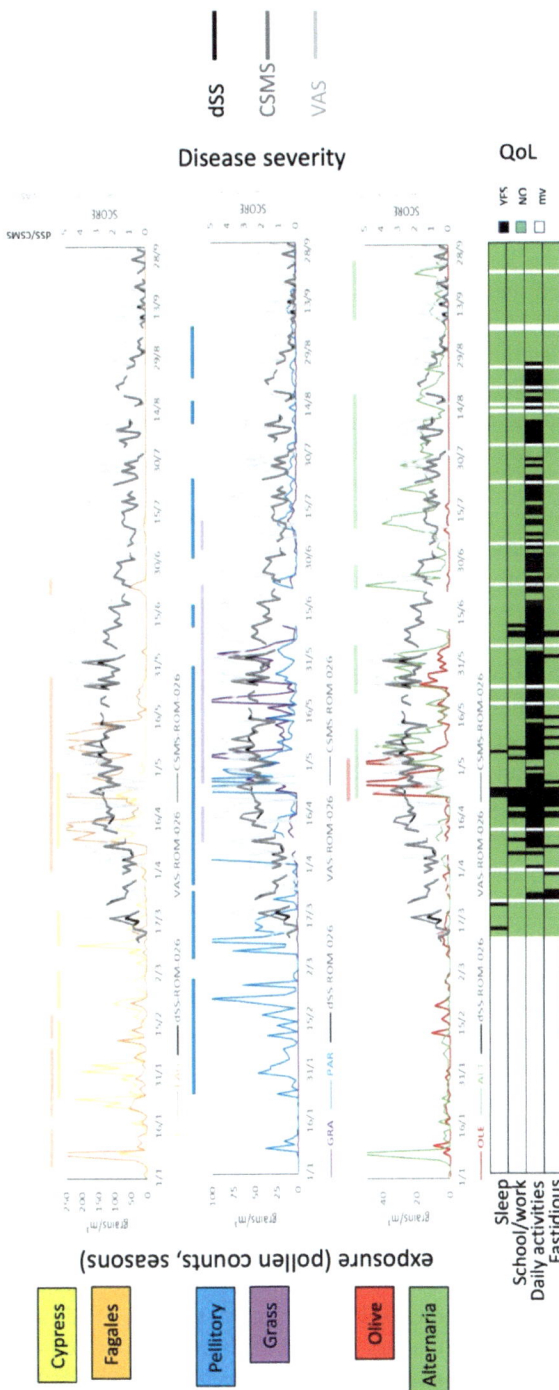

Fig. 6.3 Data recorded by a patient living in Rome, in the @IT2020 multicenter study from March to September 2018 *dSS* daily symptoms score, *CSMS* combined symptoms medication score, *VAS* visual analogue scale; and the pollen trajectories, also shown as bars with the method of pollen fragmented season [21]. Pollen seasons were defined according to EAACI criteria, but resulting in multiple segments (fragments), after the application of start and stop signals based on daily and cumulative pollen counts within a short sequence of days, also within the season and not only at its start and end QoL = symptoms impacting the quality of life according to ARIA criteria [12]; Sleep = sleep disturbed the night before; School/work = limitation in school or work activities; Daily activities = limitation in usual activities; Fastidious = intensity of the disturbance; mv = missing value

None of the mentioned technologies aim to replace healthcare providers. Their goal is to support collaborative decision-making and ensure timely access to specialist healthcare.

6.3.1   Adherence to Pharmacological Therapy and Sublingual Immunotherapy (SLIT)

It is widely demonstrated that adherence to therapy in chronic conditions such as AR and asthma is poor [23, 24], and digital technologies, particularly mHealth, while facilitating the collection of large amounts of data independent of geographical location and social differences, have not always been able to improve adherence, not only to therapies, but also to electronic diaries, which sometimes have fallen below 10% after only 2 weeks [10]. A positive influence on such aspects is certainly a blended care approach [25], as demonstrated in a study with the AM app, in which 67 patients were adequately instructed on the use of AM and received personalized reminders via phone, in addition to automatic warning messages in case of non-registration, adherence to daily symptom monitoring remained high (>80%) for several weeks [9].

In another study, the impact of telemonitoring via AM on adherence to daily topical corticosteroid treatment in children with severe hay fever was analyzed. The study showed an improvement in both adherence to daily pharmacological treatment and knowledge of the disease [26].

One of the most significant problems related to long-term daily administration of sublingual immunotherapy (SLIT) is poor compliance and a high dropout rate. Only 50% and 20% of patients who start treatment with SLIT continue daily administration in the second and third year of treatment, respectively [27]. In a pilot study, the long-term adherence of a small group of patients undergoing SLIT with usual care support was compared with a group of patients receiving SLIT plus digital adherence monitoring via AM, and a marked reduction in the dropout rate was observed in the second year of therapy among the 28 patients using the app [28].

6.4   Conclusions and Perspectives

Studies and clinical practice based on the use of AM have demonstrated the reliability of prospective collection of digital data via an e-Diary and its impact on patient adherence to both pharmacological treatment and allergen immunotherapy. The role of the attending physician is fundamental, not only for optimal adherence to digital technologies, but also in a collaborative context of blended care. Over time, the interaction between doctors and patients will progressively change with the increasing use of digital opportunities. Exploring the potential of using e-Diaries and mobile health platforms, along with CDSS, can enhance diagnostic accuracy, particularly for patients with multiple sensitivities. This approach can also predict and prevent exposure to adverse conditions like high pollen levels, increased air pollution, and the use of symptomatic drugs for individual patients. Surely, the new AI technologies will play a fundamental role, promising to revolutionize many sectors of human life, including healthcare. To implement these technologies in clinical practice to improve patient participation and care, clinical studies are needed to demonstrate positive impact, especially on clinical outcomes, but also regulatory infrastructures, as recognized by international organizations such as the World Health Organization (WHO), and adequate training for physicians.

References

1. Passali D, Cingi C, Staffa P, et al. The International Study of the Allergic Rhinitis Survey: outcomes from 4 geographical regions. Asia Pac Allergy. 2018;8:e7. https://doi.org/10.5415/apallergy.2018.8.e77.
2. Greiner AN, Hellings PW, Rotiroti G, Scadding GK. Allergic rhinitis. Lancet. 2011;378:2112-22. https://doi.org/10.1016/S0140-6736(11)60130-X. Epub 2011 Jul 23. PMID: 21783242.
3. Wise SK, Lin SY, Toskala E, Orlandi RR, et al. International Consensus statement on allergy and rhinology: allergic rhinitis. Int Forum Allergy Rhinol. 2018;8:108–352. https://doi.org/10.1002/alr.22073.
4. Roberts G, Pfaar O, Akdis CA, et al. EAACI Guidelines on Allergen Immunotherapy: allergic rhinoconjunctivitis. Allergy. 2018;73(4):765–98. https://doi.org/10.1111/all.13317.
5. Tripodi S, Giannone A, Sfika I, et al. Digital technologies for an improved management of respiratory allergic diseases: 10 years of clinical studies using an online platform for patients and physicians. Ital J Pediatr. 2020;46(1):105. https://doi.org/10.1186/s13052-020-00870-z.
6. Sousa-Pinto AA, Berger M, et al. Real-world data using mHealth apps in rhinitis, rhinosinusitis and their multimorbidities. Clin Transl Allergy. 2022;12(11):e12208. https://doi.org/10.1002/clt2.12208.
7. Canonica GW, Baena-Cagnani CE, Bousquet J, et al. Recommendations for standardization of clinical trials with Allergen Specific Immunotherapy for respiratory allergy. A statement of a World Allergy Organization (WAO) taskforce. Allergy. 2007;62(3):317–24. https://doi.org/10.1111/j.1398-9995.2006.01312.x.
8. Florack J, Brighetti MA, Perna S, et al. Comparison of six disease severity scores for allergic rhinitis against pollen counts a prospective analysis at population and individual level. Pediatr Allergy Immunol. 2016;27(4):382–90. https://doi.org/10.1111/pai.12562.
9. Di Fraia M, Tripodi S, Arasi S, et al. Adherence to prescribed E-diary recording by patients with seasonal allergic rhinitis in the @IT-2020 project: observational study. J Med Internet Res. 2019;22(3):e16642.
10. Bédard A, Basagaña X, Anto JM, et al. Mobile technology offers novel insights into the control and treatment of allergic rhinitis: the MASK study. J Allergy Clin Immunol. 2019;144:135–43.
11. Muraro A, Roberts G, Halken S, et al. EAACI guidelines on allergen immunotherapy: Executive statement. Allergy. 2018;73(4):739–43.
12. Dramburg S, Grittner U, Potapova E, et al. Heterogeneity of sensitization profiles and clinical phenotypes among patients with seasonal allergic rhinitis in Southern European Countries – the @IT.2020 multicenter study. Allergy. 2024 Apr;79(4):908–923. https://doi.org/10.1111/all.16029. Epub 2024 Feb 5. PMID: 38311961.

13. Stringari G, Tripodi S, Caffarelli C, et al. The effect of component-resolved diagnosis on specific immunotherapy prescription in children with hay fever. J Allergy Clin Immunol. 2014;134(1):75–81. https://doi.org/10.1016/j.jaci.2014.01.042.
14. Bianchi A, Tsilochristou O, Gabrielli F, Tripodi S, Matricardi PM. The smartphone: a novel diagnostic tool in pollen allergy? J Investig Allergol C47lin Immunol. 2016;26:204–7.
15. Bousquet J, Bedbrook A, Czarlewski W, et al. Guidance to 2018 good practice: ARIA digitally-enabled, integrated, person-centred care for rhinitis and asthma. Clin Transl Allergy. 2019;9:16.
16. Arasi S, Castelli S, Di Fraia M, et al. @IT2020: An innovative algorithm for allergen immunotherapy prescription in seasonal allergic rhinitis. Clin Exp Allergy. 2021;51:821–8. https://doi.org/10.1111/cea.13867.
17. Di Fraia M, Arasi S, Castelli S, et al. A new molecular multiplex IgE assay for the diagnosis of pollen allergy in Mediterranean countries: a validation study. Clin Exp Allergy. 2019;49(3):341–9.
18. Canonica GW, Bachert C, Hellings P, et al. Allergen immunotherapy (AIT): a prototype of precision medicine. World Allergy Organ J. 2015;10(8):31.
19. Matricardi PM, Potapova E, Forchert L, et al. Digital allergology: towards a clinical decision support system for allergen immunotherapy. Pediatr Allergy Immunol. 2020;31(Suppl. 24):61–4.
20. Lipp T, Acar Şahin A, Aggelidis X, et al. Heterogeneity of pollen food allergy syndrome in seven Southern European countries: the @IT.2020 multicenter study. Allergy. 2021;76(10):3041–52. https://doi.org/10.1111/all.14742.
21. Hoffmann TM, Travaglini A, Brighetti MA, et al. @IT.2020 study team. Cumulative pollen concentration curves for pollen allergy diagnosis. J Investig Allergol Clin Immunol. 2021;31(4):340–3. https://doi.org/10.18176/jiaci.0646.
22. Palmieri L, Dramburg S, Matricardi PM, Tripodi S. Measuring the clinical impact of natural exposure to pollen and molds through e-Diaries. A pilot study in 100 patients with seasonal allergic rhinitis. EAACI 2022, ePosters
23. Braido F, Brusselle G, Guastalla D, et al. Determinants and impact of suboptimal asthma control in Europe: The International Cross-sectional and Longitudinal Assessment on Asthma Control (Liaison) study. Respir Res. 2016;17:51.
24. Bousquet J, Murray R, Price D, et al. The allergic allergist behaves like a patient. Ann Allergy Asthma Immunol. 2018;121(6):741–2. https://doi.org/10.1016/j.anai.2018.07.034.
25. Kerse N, Buetow S, Mainous AG 3rd, et al. Physician-patient relationship and medication compliance: a primary care investigation. Ann Fam Med. 2004;2:455–61.
26. Pizzulli A, Perna S, Florack J, Pizzulli A, Giordani P, Tripodi S, et al. The impact of tele-monitoring on adherence to nasal corticosteroid treatment in children with seasonal allergic rhinoconjunctivitis. Clin Exp Allergy. 2014;44:1246–54.
27. Senna G, Lombardi C, Canonica GW, Passalacqua G. How adherent to sublingual immunotherapy prescriptions are patients? The manufacturers' viewpoint. J Allergy Clin Immunol. 2010;126:668–9.
28. Tripodi S, Comberiati P, Di Rienzo BA. A web-based tool for improving adherence to sublingual immunotherapy. Pediatr Allergy Immunol. 2014;25:611–2.

Chapter 7
Clinical Decision Support Systems for Allergic Diseases and Asthma

Paolo Maria Matricardi and Jean Bousquet

Contents

P. M. Matricardi (✉)
Department of Pediatric Respiratory Medicine, Immunology and Critical Care Medicine, Charité–Universitätsmedizin Berlin, a corporate member of Freie Universität Berlin and Humboldt–Universität zu Berlin, Berlin, Germany

Institute of Allergology, Charité—Universitätsmedizin Berlin, Corporate Member of Freie Universität Berlin and Humboldt-Universität zu Berlin, Berlin, Germany

Fraunhofer Institute for Translational Medicine and Pharmacology ITMP, Allergology and Immunology, Berlin, Germany
e-mail: paolo.matricardi@charite.de

J. Bousquet
Institute of Allergology, Charité—Universitätsmedizin Berlin, Corporate Member of Freie Universität Berlin and Humboldt-Universität zu Berlin, Berlin, Germany

Fraunhofer Institute for Translational Medicine and Pharmacology ITMP, Allergology and Immunology, Berlin, Germany

ARIA, Montpellier, France

P. M. Matricardi, S. Dramburg, *Digital Allergology*, Health Informatics,
https://doi.org/10.1007/978-3-031-71021-6_7

Abstract Clinical Decision Support Systems (CDSS) are "information systems designed to improve clinical decision making". We review here the benefits, challenges, and barriers to the use of CDSS in medicine and in particular clinical allergology. CDSS can be described and classified according to the nature of the CDSS information and algorithms, targets, timing, integration with existing systems, users, and other characteristics. Effectiveness, risks, and limitations of the use of CDSS must be always considered, and guidelines for use and adopters are essential to maximize benefits. MASK-Air® and AllergyMonitor®-@IT2020, two examples of electronic CDSS for allergic rhinitis, and many other CDSS dedicated to the management of patients with asthma, chronic urticaria, atopic dermatitis, and other allergic diseases are presented. Lastly, the perspectives of this rapidly evolving and expanding area of digital health for allergology are discussed.

7.1 Definitions and Historical Background

Many definitions have been formulated for Clinical Decision Support Systems (CDSS), albeit none is considered universally accepted, and more will probably come. However, the Agency for Healthcare Research and Quality, Rockville, MD proposed in 2010: *"Clinical decision support (CDS) provides timely information, usually at the point of care, to help inform decisions about a patient's care. CDS tools and systems help clinical teams by taking over some routine tasks, warning of potential problems, or providing suggestions for the clinical team and patient to consider"* [1]. *"CDS can be used on a variety of platforms (such as the Internet, personal computers, electronic medical record networks, handheld devices, or written materials)"*. A very popular and concise definition states that *"CDSS are information systems designed to improve clinical decision making"* [2]. A longer and more pragmatic definition proposed that *"a traditional CDSS is comprised of software designed to be a direct aid to clinical-decision making, in which the characteristics of an individual patient are matched to a computerized clinical knowledge base and patient-specific assessments or recommendations are then presented to the clinician for a decision"* [3].

While definitions differ, most experts agree that CDSS roots are at least half a century old [4]. The first attempts of the use of a computer to assist clinician were academic exercises, blamed by most clinicians as a threat to the doctor's freedom and autonomy and inferior to the doctor's competence, or welcomed by clinical scientists as seminal experiments to transform and improve disease management [5]. In a second phase, they slowly started to spread in hospitals and clinics, taking advantage of the introduction of computer systems in clinical care, and data acquisition from electronic clinical record forms [6]. Today, in the era of smartphones, tablets, wearables, and biometric monitoring devices, CDSS are progressively spreading across the general population, occasionally bypassing health systems and doctors to directly reach and target the patient [7].

The terminology CDSS coexists with that of computer-assisted diagnosis and treatment (CAD/CAT), contributing to the rapidly growing field of medicine using computer technology and telehealth to aid in the diagnosis and treatment of various diseases [8, 9].

7.2   Benefits, Challenges, and Barriers

CDSS offer many potential benefits. They can increase adherence to evidence-based medicine and reduce variation in clinical practice. Misdiagnosis may affect 800,000 patients annually in the USA [10]. They can also assist with information management to support clinicians' decision-making abilities, reduce their mental workload, and improve clinical workflows [11]. When well designed and implemented, CDSS can improve health care quality to increase efficiency and reduce health care costs [11].

However, many barriers to CDSS development and implementation exist. (i) The medical knowledge base is incomplete partly due to insufficient clinical evidence. (ii) Methodologies are still being developed. (iii) Often, their acceptance and use are tied to electronic medical records (EMRs), which are now becoming widely used. (iv) Low clinician demand for CDSS is another important barrier. (v) Clinicians may feel that they reduce their autonomy. (vi) Alert fatigue may reduce the impact after prolonged use. (vii) Reimbursement strategies do not usually exist and the use of some CDSS may be time consuming. (vii) Legal problems always need to be included.

7.3   Basic Structure and Classification

In most CDSS, information obtained from an individual patient is matched with the information already computerized to be used by software algorithms producing patient-specific outputs such as reports or recommendations. Information is acquired either manually or preferably imported from electronic clinical record forms, and the output is produced either electronically and/or on paper for traditional archiviation [12].

Software algorithms may follow rules (e.g., in the IF_THEN format) programmed by the developer, or their suggested decision is modeled through artificial intelligence (AI) supervised and unsupervised procedures, such as machine learning (ML). Whatever the approach, algorithms are applied to the clinical information of the individual patient and generate an output given to the end user through a communication tool (e.g., mobile application, front-end of electronic health records [EHRs], websites) [13]. In some CDSS, additional information (e.g., epidemiological, environmental) can also be provided to reinforce the knowledge base and the

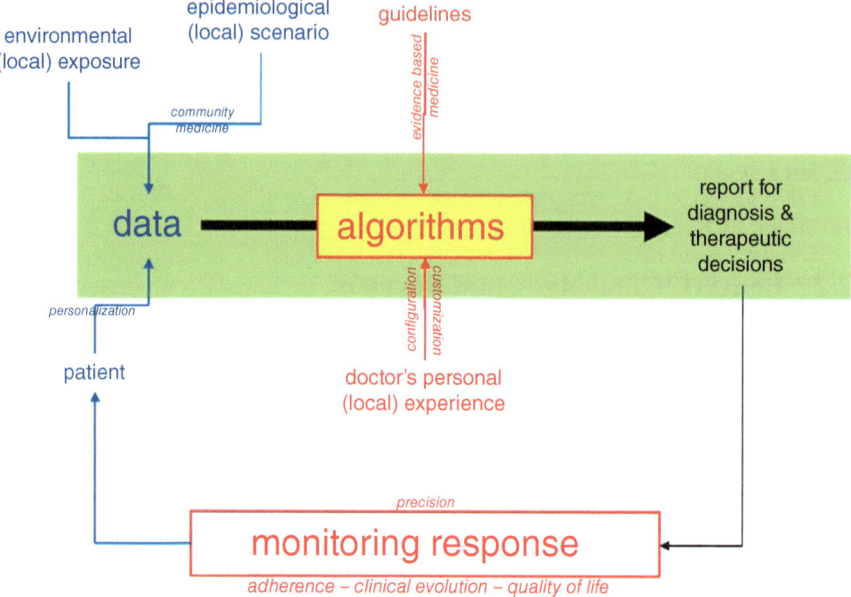

Fig. 7.1 General concepts of a clinical decision support system. Three elements compose a CDSS: (**a**) data—from the patient and also from the environment (to which the patient is exposed and from the community in which he/she is living); (**b**) algorithm-mathematical formulas (simple or complex) that take the data and generate reports; and (**c**) reports—can be delivered as a written report, a suggestion of further diagnostic examinations, a therapeutic plan to the operator (i.e., the doctor) as a suggestion to be considered for his/her actual diagnostic or therapeutic decision. [From Ref. 73, with permission]

context surrounding and influencing the value of the information coming from the individual patient (Fig. 7.1).

This topic is still not a chapter in most textbooks of medicine, and the attempts of classifying CDSS' complex and highly diversified galaxy are in their infancy. The following paragraphs, partially based on the outstanding work of experts [6, 12], offer just some examples of features diversity within an incomplete list of domains. An extended description of characteristics, advantages, and limitations of individual types of CDSS listed here falls beyond the scope of the present text and have been thoroughly illustrated elsewhere [6].

(a) **Nature of the information and algorithms**—The way background information is acquired and elaborated is being used to divide CDSS in "knowledge-based" and "non-knowledge-based" [6].

    (i) In the knowledge-based type, the available information is a set of available data acquired from literature, practice, or patient-directed evidence, and then it is interconnected with associations and rules or algorithms.

    (ii) The non-knowledge-based category, while having a similar structure as the knowledge-based one, takes advantage of machine learning approaches, i.e., software who can learn from acquired data and generate mathematical algorithms that can be applied to the patient's data to generate outcomes. Machine learning can adopt many different strategies, ranging from artificial neural networks, support vector machines, and others.

(iii) Interestingly, some CDSS can use both knowledge and not-knowledge based approaches.

(b) **Target**—The primary goal of CDSS is to improve healthcare delivery by helping doctors taking clinical real-time decisions directly at the point of care [7]. These decisions are normally based on the information acquired by the doctor during training, continuing education, and own routine clinical practice. In addition, doctors can spend time to acquire additional information, specific for the case, from the literature, databanks, and other web-based sources. However, the amount of retrieved information is almost invariably a small proportion of the one available, the latter being constantly growing in our technological world. In addition, health data obtained by the health care systems per individual patients are also rapidly growing, a trend reinforced by -omics approaches, genetic tests, mobile health (mHealth) apps and electronic diaries (e-Diaries) [14], complex diagnostics (e.g., protein microarrays), remote patient monitoring via wearables, and so on [15]. In other words, the amount of data that a single doctor should examine in a few minutes is increasing, up to a point that a hallmark of personalized precision medicine is so invasive and overwhelming to become in extreme cases a counterproductive cause of "imprecision medicine."

With this shared background, CDSS differ in the way they aim at improving healthcare delivery improvement, by helping doctor's adherence to international or national guidelines and evidence-based procedures [16], supporting early diagnosis, reducing errors, facilitating screening procedures in primary healthcare (PHC) [17], contributing to quick and right decision making in acute situations in the emergency room [18], assisting self-management in patients with chronic conditions [19], improving workflow in the clinical setting [20], alerting when critical values are reached and risks are raised beyond a preestablished threshold so that intervention is needed [21], reminding when preventive health tasks are overdue [22], and providing advice for drug prescription [23] and cost reduction [24].

(c) **Timing**—CDSS can operate before, during, or after a diagnosis is done. They can be useful to elaborate a diagnostic strategy requiring a rational sequence of interconnected diagnostic steps, each one being influenced by the outcome of the previous one [25]. For example, as point-of-care devices, they can be helpful in the emergency room to quickly evaluate the patient and make a diagnosis [18]. Alternatively, CDSS can be useful in interpreting data acquired through an e-Diary after the diagnosis is done and the response to therapy is examined [12, 26].

(d) **Integration with existing systems**—CDSS differ in the way the patient's data are acquired. While some require direct input from the patient or health care personnel [27], most interact with the electronic health record [28]. The second scenario is the preferred one as it is time-saving, less redundant and preventing errors deriving by data manually imputed.

(e) **User**—CDSS users may be very heterogeneous, including the PHC doctor [17, 29], the emergency room doctor [18], the health care allied personnel [30], the laboratory [31], the pharmacist [32], or the patient themselves [33].

7.4 Effectiveness, Risks, and Limitations

The effectiveness of CDSS has been examined by several trials, and a certain number of meta-analyses have been published. Trials are so heterogenous in their nature, target, population, and design that effectiveness can be, in our opinion, measured only on a case-by-case basis.

However, some characteristics of CDSS seem to be associated with a certain degree of effectiveness, including automatic electronic prompts versus user activation of the system [34], integration into the clinical workflow versus a separate application or software, synchronous support at the point of care versus prior to or after the patient encounter, and production of recommendations for care as opposite to assessments only [35]. It has therefore been suggested that an effective system should be above all user-friendly so to minimize clinicians' effort to receive and act on system recommendations. Moreover, it seems that the involvement of the local health care professional in the design of support tools is also factor relevant for success [35].

Nevertheless, a few systematic reviews have also concluded that a beneficial impact and cost-effectiveness of CDSS have still to be demonstrated [36].

Similarly, a more recent meta-analysis, retrieving 5340 articles and recruiting only eight studies on CDSS embedded in electronic clinical health records, found inconclusive evidence in support of this methodology, mostly due to methodological biases and study heterogeneity [37]. A conclusion by the authors of this study was that further research is needed to provide evidence on the intervention effect and concerning the interaction of healthcare setting features and the characteristics and implementation processes of CDSS in clinical practice [37].

Interestingly, systematic reviews of randomized controlled trials have thoroughly assessed the effectiveness of CDSS in different areas and found that, while a beneficial impact on the process of medical care was shown in 52–64% of the studies, patient outcomes were improving in only 15–31% of trials investigating also this essential target [2]. The six metanalyses focused on trials (i) informing the ordering of diagnostic tests [38], (ii) prescription and management of drugs [39], (iii) monitoring and dosing of narrow therapeutic index drugs [40], (iv) guiding primary prevention and screening [41], (v) managing chronic disease [42], and (vi) providing acute care [43].

This lack of evidence about clinical efficacy of CDSS may be due to their intrinsic limitations that may affect the design, implementation, and even their use in the routine clinical practice. Weaknesses, disadvantages, risks, and limitations may concern privacy and data protection, user-friendliness, data acquisition and accuracy, algorithms precision and their generalizability, patient or user's acceptance, clarity of reporting, and readiness to consider suggestions. In addition, stand-alone CDSS can disrupt clinician's workflow, their alert systems may generate the so-called alert fatigue, their routine use may induce excess reliance and trust, reducing diagnostic skills and generating a sort of "CDSS addiction or dependence" [6].

7.5 Guidelines for Users, and Adopters

As illustrated above, CDSS are tools also targeted to better implement evidence-based guidelines, whose effectiveness should be evaluated and validated with a rigorous scientific approach in trials and metanalyses. Before that, the validation process should include iterative qualitative and quantitative assessment early in the software development cycle [3]. It is also essential that their validation is not only produced by the developers, but also by third parties with independent studies [2]. Validation is, however, not sufficient to guarantee correct implementation by users. The users' level of understanding, preparation, awareness, training, and experience around CDSS methodology are important factors for successful implementation. Although physicians are slowly developing tolerance and interest in the use of CDSS, the skepticisms and resistance of the earliest times are still predominant today, especially when the non-knowledge based category is considered [12]. It seems that doctor's digital literacy is a condition for earlier and proper use of CDSS, and direct participation of the general practitioners (GP) and other users in their development should be always considered [44]. End user participation, reliability, and accountability are relevant points to be considered when targeting a widespread adoption of any digital solution [45]. The effectiveness of CDSS must be tested by using its informatic version in a real-life scenario. In addition, an interesting approach to preliminary validation tests may involve specialists and GPs, through a step-by-step procedure [14].

7.6 Examples of Electronic CDSS in Rhinitis

7.6.1 MASK-Air®: A CDSS for Therapeutic Control of Allergic Rhinitis

In 2015, a first e-CDSS was proposed for AR diagnosis using intradermal skin tests [46]. Since then, although many digital devices are dedicated to allergic rhinitis, only few have been used in studies published in peer-reviewed international journals [47]. A very large collaborative network is focused on rhinitis and its treatment, accumulating evidence through the worldwide use of *MASK-Air* (*MASK* stands for

Mobile Airways Sentinel Network). Nowadays, MASK-Air® is by far the world-wide most used digital platform for the management of allergic rhinitis (AR) [48, 49] (Fig. 7.2). The unmet need targeted by MASK-Air® is quite simple; although pollen-induced allergic rhinitis affects worldwide many hundreds million people, the connection between a physician's prescriptions and the patient's behavior for its treatment is poor [50]. Drugs are prescribed for the entire season independently from the presence of absence of exposure to the culprit pollen and the consequent allergic symptoms. Not surprisingly, most patients take their drugs just on-demand and guidelines are not followed [50]. Astonishingly, when allergists are patients themselves, they tend to self-medication procedures and do not follow the very same prescriptions they usually recommend to their patients [51]. Shared decision-making helps patients to take on own responsibilities and transform them into active participant in their health preservation and management [52].

Generated by the Allergy and its Impact on Asthma (ARIA) consortium, MASK-Air® is a CDSS supporting screening, diagnostic precision, early optimization of therapy, and user-friendly monitoring of AR [53]. The development process of MASK-Air® involved a key opinion leader consensus on specific treatment recommendations [54] and relied upon profound expertise in symptom data collection through mobile health technology integrating the CDSS [55].

In parallel with MASK-Air®, the ARIA consortium is planning the production of a CDSS targeted to the integration in the care pathways of AR of community pharmacies, crucial players in the above-mentioned self-management approach to this disease [56, 57]. CDSS use demonstrated that German pharmacists don't acquire the information required to diagnose AR, so that the self-medication process often leads to wrong medication [58]. The implementation of a CDSS targeted to the pharmacist successfully addressed this gap in the pharmacist's diagnostic role and effectively improved selectivity and appropriateness in drug delivery to the patient [59]. Next step will be facilitating the monitoring of patient's symptom control and adjusting symptomatic treatment accordingly [59]. This innovative approach deserves evaluation and validation in real-life scenarios.

7.6.2 @llergyMonitor and @IT-2020: e-Diary and CDSS for seasonal AR and AIT Prescription

Seasonal Allergic Rhinitis (SAR) is mostly provoked by pollen and sometimes by fungal spores seasonally dispersed in the outdoor air [60]. This disease is very heterogeneous in terms of sensitization profiles and clinical manifestations, being simple in cold climates and very complex in temperate zones. Accordingly, while, for example, in Sweden birch is the dominating, almost exclusive cause of pollen allergy, in Southern European countries a long list of pollen species may be involved [61]. This geographical diversity in pollen allergic patients imposes localized diagnostic guidelines and makes a correct diagnosis very difficult in polysensitized

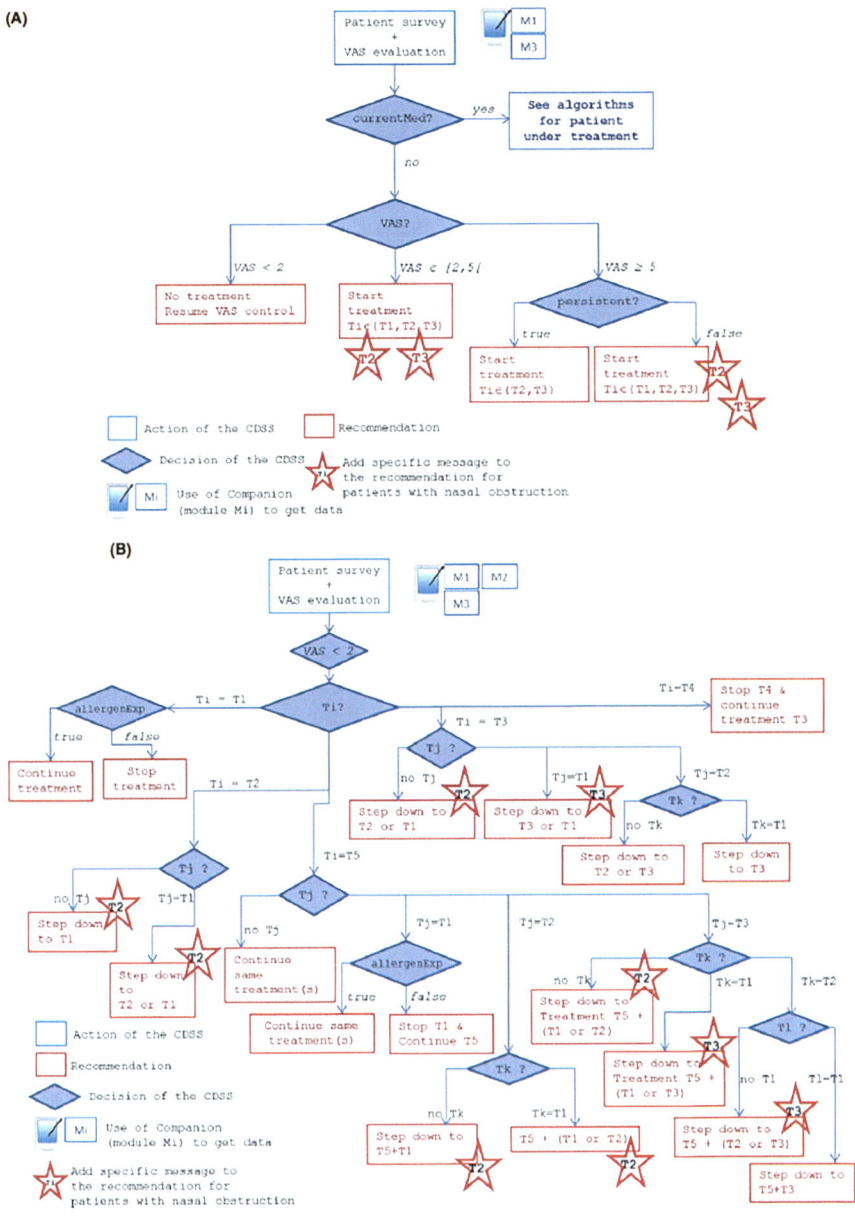

Fig. 7.2 Decision processes underlying treatment recommendations for (**a**) patients not currently on any AR medication, (**b**) patients with well-controlled AR (i.e., VAS score < 2/10 cm), AR, allergic rhinitis; VAS, visual analogue scale; M1, module 1; M2, module 2; M3, module 3; Ti, class of current treatment (in case of polypharmacy, Ti = maximum class). Tj, Tk and Tl, medications added to Ti, order of class $l < k < j < i$. T1, antihistamine (oral, intranasal, and eye drops), leukotriene receptor antagonist, cromone (intranasal and eye drops); T2, intranasal corticosteroid (INCS); T3, INCS + Azelastine; T4 add short course of oral corticosteroids; T5, consider referral and allergen-specific immunotherapy [49]

patients living in temperate climatic zones [62]. Several apps on pollen exposure and seasonal allergic rhinitis have been developed, and only three of them have been the object of several scientific studies in many countries in Europe [45]: Pollen [63], MASK-Air [48], and AllergyMonitor [64]. Among different tools, these apps contain e-Diaries facilitating monitoring of allergic symptoms (nasal, ocular, bronchial) typical of respiratory allergies. Through internationally standardized questions, patients record symptoms and medication intake on a daily basis, while information on local pollen concentrations is also acquired from aerobiological pollen stations [63, 64]. Patient's adherence to daily compilation of these type of e-Diaries was quite high in the context of a blended approach, with a valuable interaction between the prescribing doctor and the patient [65]. AllergyMonitor aims at multiple targets, including improving disease awareness and adherence to daily therapy with nasal corticosteroids in children with grass pollen allergy [66], prospectively measuring disease severity [67], discriminating the culprit allergen in polysensitized patients [68], and predicting a positive nasal allergen provocation test [69].

The @IT-2020 project started in 2015 and aimed at developing a CDSS facilitating correct diagnosis of pollen allergy, which must be based on a thorough clinical history and the definition of the patient's sensitization profile, completed in most polysensitized patients by component resolved diagnosis, i.e., IgE assays for allergenic molecules [65, 70, 71]. Importantly, diagnostic procedures are based on international guidelines including ARIA, GINA (Global Initiative for Asthma), and EAACI (European Academy of Allergy and Clinical Immunology) guidelines for SPT, molecular IgE assays, and pollen season definitions [64]. A correct identification of the culprit pollen in polysensitized patients is a diagnostic goal essential for the precise prescription of allergen immunotherapy [71, 72]. Accordingly, within the @IT-2020 concept, a CDSS aiming at supporting precise AIT prescription for SAR should not only incorporate and elaborate information from these preliminary diagnostic steps (clinical history, skin tests, molecular tests), but also integrate them with prospective information acquired by the e-Diaries [73] (Fig. 7.3). The MASK-Air further expanded this concept, proposing the use of e-Diaries not only for a correct stratification of the patients to be treated with allergen immunotherapy, but also to decide its cessation [74].

The usability and impact of @IT2020-CDSS for SAR on doctor's AIT prescription decisions have been preliminarily tested in a theoretical experiment performed with allergists and other doctors [14]. After educational training on the @IT2020-CDSS algorithm, 46 doctors (18 allergy specialists, AS, and 28 GP in Rome and in Pordenone, Italy) expressed their hypothetical AIT prescription for 10 clinical index cases. Decisions based on different stages of the algorithm were recorded step-by-step. The usability and perceived impact of the algorithm were also evaluated. The combined use of CRD (Component Resolved Diagnosis) and an e-Diary increased the hypothetical AIT prescriptions, both among AS and GP. AIT prescription for pollen and alternaria allergy, based on anamnesis and SPT was heterogeneous but converged toward a consensus by integrating CRD and e-Diary information. Doctors considered the algorithm useful and recognized its potential in enhancing traditional diagnostics. The implementation of CRD and e-Diary in the @IT2020-CDSS

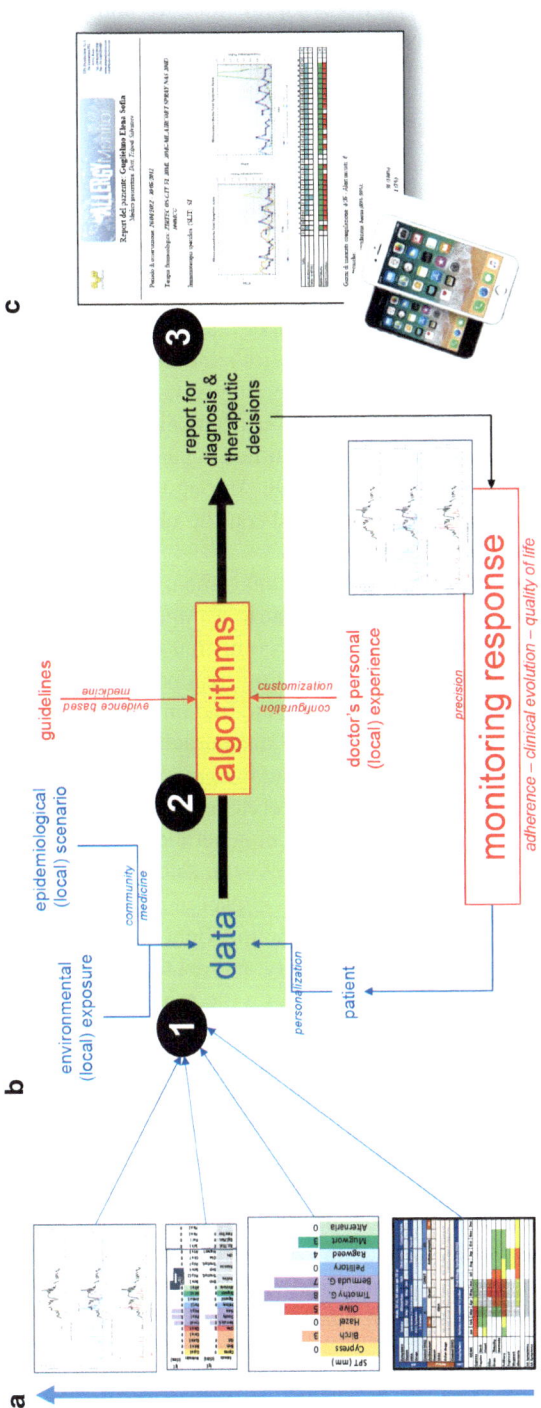

Fig. 7.3 General concepts of a clinical decision support system applied to @IT-2020. Three elements compose @IT-2020: (1) data—from clinical history, skin prick tests, IgE tests for extracts and molecules, and e-Diary monitoring of symptoms, medication, and QoL parameters during the pollen season, integrated by environmental information (daily pollen counts); (2) algorithm-mathematical formulas (simple or complex) that take the data and generating reports; and (3) clinical reports, synthesizing prescriptions, adherence to compilation and medication, side effects, symptoms, and quality of life

algorithm improved consensus on AIT prescription for SAR among AS and GP. The potential usefulness of such a system for etiological diagnosis of SAR and AIT prescription in real-world clinical practice deserves further investigation [45, 75] (Fig. 7.4).

7.7   Examples of Electronic CDSS in Asthma

Asthma is a chronic condition, so heterogeneous in its clinical manifestations and mechanisms to be considered a syndrome, rather than a single disease entity [76]. Accordingly, diagnostic procedures, classification, and therapeutic approaches are equally complex and diversified [77]. Not surprisingly, many patient needs are still unmet [78] and guidelines implementation is far from being optimal in the clinical routine [79]. Given this situation, digital tools aimed at guiding asthma management are growing both in number and attention [80]. Among them, studies focusing on CDSS for asthma management have already been the object of a few systematic reviews [81–83].

One of the first CDSS studies in asthma management evaluated its accuracy to support assessment and management of pediatric asthma in a subspecialty clinic [84]. The system performed quite accurately compared to clinicians in assessing asthma control, but was inaccurate in suggesting treatment. One systemic review [81], performed in 2014, screened 5787 articles to find only eight eligible trials, six of which at risk of bias. Outcomes were rather discouraging, showing low usage of the implemented systems due to poor workflow integration or to negative end user beliefs, low compliance with the advice offered, and increased prescription of inhaled steroid [81]. Authors stated that "current generation of CDSS is unlikely to result in improvements of outcomes for patients with asthma" [81]. Another, more recent systematic review found evidence of an impact of electronic alerts in reducing excessive prescription of SABA (Short Acting Beta Agonists), a category of drugs whose abuse is linked to asthma severity and death [82]. Three studies had low risk of bias: one reported a positive effect on the primary outcome of interest, excessive SABA prescribing; another reported positive effects on the ratio of inhaled corticosteroid (ICS)-SABA prescribing, and asthma control; a third reported no effect on outcomes of interest [82]. A review showed poor quality of the four trials examined and suggested a need for increased focus on the methods of conducting and reporting RCT trials of different decision support systems in asthma care, as well as in other conditions [83]. A more recent, broad systematic review aimed to evaluate the impact of CDSS on assessment and disease-specific management of breathlessness and associated diseases in real-world clinical settings [85]. In 18 studies focusing on asthma, those with children reported a positive impact on the proportion diagnosed with asthma but a mixed impact on exacerbations, symptom days, and influenza vaccination rates post-implementation. Other positive outcomes included an improved adherence to guidelines on spirometry, asthma action plans, peak-flow measurements, and oxygen saturation measurement. In adults, a poor

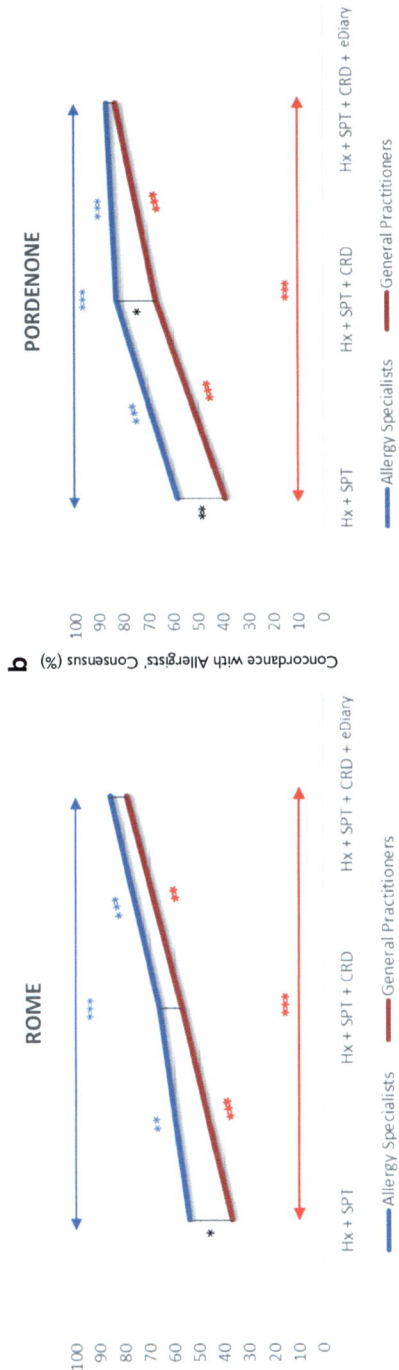

Fig. 7.4 Concordance (%) of the "hypothetical" prescription of allergen immunotherapy with the most prevalent final decision among allergy specialists for each medical category (allergy specialists and general practitioners) at each of the three diagnostic steps proposed in the CDSS @IT-2020 in Rome (a) and Pordenone (b). CRD, component resolved diagnostics; e-Diary, electronic clinical diary; Hx, clinical history; SWE, sensitization to whole extract. *$p < 0.05$, **$p < 0.01$, ***$p < 0.001$. Reproduced with slight modifications from [14] with permission

specificity in diagnosing asthma in one study was compensated by improved guideline adherence, peak-flow measurements, ICS prescription, and use of asthma action plans in other studies. Last, improved symptoms, Asthma Quality of Life Questionnaire (AQLQ) score, forced expiratory volume one second (FEV-1) value, airway hyperresponsiveness, and reduced exacerbations were also observed, while the outcomes regarding hospitalization rates were mixed [85].

Some additional sketches on individual studies may provide a few examples of CDSS strategies currently pursued in asthma management and proposed reasons for their success or failure. The initial impact of implementing CDSS software in the form of a computer-guided consultation in PHC has been recently investigated in deprived areas of Greater Manchester [86]. This study encouragingly concluded that an end-to-end digital service solution not only is feasible for asthma within primary care but also that its adoption increases implementation of guideline-level management, impacts on healthcare inequality, helps identifying "high risk" asthma patients, and guiding proper therapy escalation and de-escalation [86]. Another study showed low use of a CDSS for asthma by 490 patients visited over one year by 121 Canadian clinicians, with the system opened only in 205 of 1033 (19.8%) visits and an asthma action plan created in 121 of 1033 (11.7%) visits [87]. According to the authors, workflows and cultures across clinics, physician beliefs regarding asthma diagnosis, and relevance of the clinical complaint influenced uptake [87]. "AsthmaTuner", a self-management system collecting lung function and symptom data via Bluetooth spirometer and patient app, respectively, provides automated treatment recommendations for patients and an interface for health professionals and, compared to usual care, improved symptom control among patients with uncontrolled asthma [88].

This mixed scenario of lights and shadows on the effectiveness of CDSS for asthma care has been recently thoroughly reviewed [89]. While lack of use and poor documentation of objective measures of lung function seem to be the major barriers to their effectiveness, future initiatives should focus on digital asthma surveillance systems, aimed not only at supporting adherence to best-practice guidelines of asthma diagnosis but also at prompting use of objective methods to confirm an asthma diagnosis within the electronic health records [89].

7.8 CDSS for Chronic Urticaria, Atopic Dermatitis, Food, and Drug Allergies, and for Allergy Screening in Primary Care

Unlike respiratory allergies, skin, venom, food, and drug allergies have rarely been the focus of CDSS. However, large projects have produced interesting outcomes and will likely pave the way for further promising developments.

7.8.1 Dermatology

Allergy is a relevant area in dermatology, given the high and growing burden of chronic urticaria (CU) and atopic dermatitis (AD). Over 20 years ago, a Korean group had developed a knowledge model for chronic urticaria assessment and integrated it into a CDSS for clinical practice [90]. However, this project has not produced further publications in the following years. More recently, a self-evaluation digital platform for patients with CU has been developed by the worldwide network UCARE [91]. This CRUSE app (Chronic Urticaria Self Evaluation) [92] supports CU patients to monitor their own disease thanks to the wide adoption of patient-reported outcomes measures (PROMs) and assist in the attempts of controlling disease exacerbations. Interestingly, CU patients were involved in the development of the platform and have shown a significant interest in its use [93], further confirming that this digital tool is matching an unmet need [94]. Several digital health tools, including web searches and social media platforms, wearable biosensors, mobile apps, 3D full body scanners, and optical coherence tomography have been developed to help diagnosis and monitoring of patients with atopic dermatitis [95]. However, to our knowledge, none of these tools have been so far integrated in a CDSS. Similarly, a practical algorithm to assist management of AD patients at point of care has been elaborated [96], but no information on its integration in a CDSS is retrievable. Recently, a mixed reality interactive shared decision-making game has been developed and successfully used by a small group of pediatric patients with AD as a tool to improve awareness and self-management [97].

7.8.2 Food allergy

The literature on CDSS for food allergy is scarce. In the USA, guidelines for the management of food allergy in childhood have been consolidated in five steps to create a CDSS for the PHC setting. A pilot testing in four practices highlighted the need of educating the health care provider in using such a novel tool [98].

7.8.3 Drug allergy

A recent systematic review identified 17 drug allergy alert systems (DAAS), of which 9 commercially available, that have been developed so far to reduce preventable adverse drug events [99]. The overall outcome of this review was quite discouraging, being the DAAS very heterogeneous and failing their target in most cases, mainly because of non-exact match at drug prescribing and a high override rate (patients had already tolerated the drug or taken without allergic reactions). Interestingly, opioids, monoclonal antibodies, non-antibiotic sulfonamides, statins, and NSAIDs had higher override, while contrast media, salicylate analgesics, and antibiotics override were lower [99]. Indeed, alert "overrides" is a well-known and recognized problem in this area of digital allergology [100]. Recently, machine learning has been applied to hospital HERs to identify, classify, and alert of allergy to anesthetic drugs before surgery [101]. In that preliminary study, developers conclude that their CDSS was able to support physicians' decision-making and increased safety for patients undergoing surgery [101]. Similarly, apps have been successfully used in a hospital setting [102] and in PHC [103] to de-label allergy to penicillin or other antibiotics.

7.8.4   Primary care

CDSS have been developed for allergy screening and early diagnosis in a PHC setting. One of these was not very precise in predicting the recommendations of allergists, however, it was useful to improve the allergy diagnostic precision of GPs regarding allergies, who also positively judged their impact in daily clinical practice, although their decision-making on medication and referral remained unaffected [104].

7.9   Perspectives

The growing interest and initiatives in digital health are producing a growing number of attempts to develop and use CDSS in the management of allergic diseases. While some projects seem to be quite slow, but broad and solid enough in their scientific premises, others are faster but more exposed to failure. A general, clear conclusion is that allergists, PHC doctors, and the patients themselves must be involved in the developing process of support tools in order to increase chances of acceptance by the end users. Validation studies of developed CDSS are frequently lacking or, when performed, either biased being performed by the developers themselves or failing to meet their expectations. Overall, the way to successful implementation of a Clincial Decision Support System in the daily practice is still long and users exposed to available tools should be protected by regulatory agencies and a proper application of certification procedures.

Disclosure of Potential Conflict of Interest   None.

References

1. Clinical decision support. Agency for Healthcare Research and Quality, Rockville, MD; 2019.   https://www.ahrq.gov/cpi/about/otherwebsites/clinical-decision-support/index. html#:~:text=Clinical%20decision%20support%20(CDS)%20provides,team%20and%20 patient%20to%20consider.
2. Roshanov PS, Fernandes N, Wilczynski JM, Hemens BJ, You JJ, Handler SM, Nieuwlaat R, Souza NM, Beyene J, Van Spall HG, Garg AX, Haynes RB. Features of effective computerised clinical decision support systems: meta-regression of 162 randomised trials. BMJ. 2013;346:f657. https://doi.org/10.1136/bmj.f657.
3. Sim I, Gorman P, Greenes RA, Haynes RB, Kaplan B, Lehmann H, Tang PC. Clinical decision support systems for the practice of evidence-based medicine. J Am Med Inform Assoc. 2001;8(6):527–34. https://doi.org/10.1136/jamia.2001.0080527.
4. Power D. Decision support systems: a historical overview. In: Handbook on decision support systems 1. International handbooks information system. Berlin, Heidelberg: Springer; 2008.
5. Shortliffe EH, Buchanan BG. Artificial intelligence. N Engl J Med. 1980;302(26):1482.
6. Sutton RT, Pincock D, Baumgart DC, Sadowski DC, Fedorak RN, Kroeker KI. An overview of clinical decision support systems: benefits, risks, and strategies for success. NPJ Digit Med. 2020;3:17. https://doi.org/10.1038/s41746-020-0221-y.
7. Dias D. Wearable health devices—vital sign monitoring, systems and technologies; 2018. https://doi.org/10.3390/s18082414.
8. Hamid N, Portnoy JM, Pandya A. Computer-assisted clinical diagnosis and treatment. Curr Allergy Asthma Rep. 2023;23(9):509–17.
9. Pfaar O, Demoly P, Gerth van Wijk R, Bonini S, Bousquet J, Canonica GW, et al. Recommendations for the standardization of clinical outcomes used in allergen immunotherapy trials for allergic rhinoconjunctivitis: an EAACI position paper. Allergy. 2014;69(7):854–67.
10. Harris E. Misdiagnosis might harm up to 800,000 US patients annually. JAMA. 2023;330(7):586.
11. Challenges and Barriers to Clinical Decision Support (CDS) Design and Implementation Experienced in the Agency for Healthcare Research and Quality CDS Demonstrations. https://digital.ahrq.gov/sites/default/files/docs/page/CDS_challenges_and_barriers.pdf? editor 2010.
12. Berner ES, editor. Clinical decision support systems. Theory and practice. 3rd ed. Springer Nature; 2016.
13. Deo RC. Machine learning in medicine. Circulation. 2015;132:1920–30.
14. Arasi S, Castelli S, Di Fraia M, Villalta D, Tripodi S, Perna S, et al. @IT-2020: an innovative algorithm for allergen immunotherapy prescription in seasonal allergic rhinitis. Clin Exp Allergy. 2021;51(6):821–8. https://doi.org/10.1111/cea.13867.
15. Tang HHF, Sly PD, Holt PG, Holt KE, Inouye M. Systems biology and big data in asthma and allergy: recent discoveries and emerging challenges. Eur Respir J. 2020;55(1):1900844. https://doi.org/10.1183/13993003.00844-2019.
16. Kwok R, Dinh M, Dinh D, Chu M. Improving adherence to asthma clinical guidelines and discharge documentation from emergency departments: implementation of a dynamic and integrated electronic decision support system. Emerg Med Australas. 2009;21(1):31–7. https://doi.org/10.1111/j.1742-6723.2008.01149.x.
17. van Venrooij LT, Rusu V, Vermeiren RRJM, Koposov RA, Skokauskas N, Crone MR. Clinical decision support methods for children and youths with mental health disorders in primary care. Fam Pract. 2022;39(6):1135–43. https://doi.org/10.1093/fampra/cmac051. Erratum in: Fam Pract 2022 Jul 29; PMID: 35656854; PMCID: PMC9680662
18. Khan NU, Khan UR, Ahmed N, Ali A, Raheem A, Soomar SM, Waheed S, Kerai SM, Baig MA, Salman S, Saleem SG, Jamali S, Razzak JA. Improvement in the diagnosis and practices of emergency healthcare providers for heat emergencies after HEAT (heat emergency aware-

ness & treatment) an educational intervention: a multicenter quasi-experimental study. BMC Emerg Med. 2023;23(1):12. https://doi.org/10.1186/s12873-022-00768-5.

19. Liu K, Xie Z, Or CK. Effectiveness of Mobile App-assisted self-care interventions for improving patient outcomes in type 2 diabetes and/or hypertension: systematic review and meta-analysis of randomized controlled trials. JMIR Mhealth Uhealth. 2020;8(8):e15779. https://doi.org/10.2196/15779. Erratum in: JMIR Mhealth Uhealth 2020 Aug 19;8(8):e23600. PMID: 32459654; PMCID: PMC7435643

20. Olakotan OO, Yusof MM. Evaluating the alert appropriateness of clinical decision support systems in supporting clinical workflow. J Biomed Inform. 2020;106:103453. https://doi.org/10.1016/j.jbi.2020.103453.

21. Caballero-Ruiz E, García-Sáez G, Rigla M, Villaplana M, Pons B, Hernando ME. A web-based clinical decision support system for gestational diabetes: automatic diet prescription and detection of insulin needs. Int J Med Inform. 2017;102:35–49. https://doi.org/10.1016/j.ijmedinf.2017.02.014.

22. Njie GJ, Proia KK, Thota AB, Finnie RKC, Hopkins DP, Banks SM, Callahan DB, Pronk NP, Rask KJ, Lackland DT, Kottke TE, Community Preventive Services Task Force. Clinical decision support systems and prevention: a community guide cardiovascular disease systematic review. Am J Prev Med. 2015;49(5):784–95. https://doi.org/10.1016/j.amepre.2015.04.006.

23. Armando LG, Miglio G, de Cosmo P, Cena C. Clinical decision support systems to improve drug prescription and therapy optimisation in clinical practice: a scoping review. BMJ Health Care Inform. 2023;30(1):e100683. https://doi.org/10.1136/bmjhci-2022-100683.

24. Chen W, Howard K, Gorham G, O'Bryan CM, Coffey P, Balasubramanya B, Abeyaratne A, Cass A. Design, effectiveness, and economic outcomes of contemporary chronic disease clinical decision support systems: a systematic review and meta-analysis. J Am Med Inform Assoc. 2022;29(10):1757–72. https://doi.org/10.1093/jamia/ocac110.

25. Schmidt HG, Mamede S. Improving diagnostic decision support through deliberate reflection: a proposal. Diagnosis (Berl). 2022;10(1):38–42. https://doi.org/10.1515/dx-2022-0062. Osheroff, J. et al. Improving Outcomes with Clinical Decision Support: An Implementer's Guide. (HIMSS Publishing, 2012)

26. Nimri R, Battelino T, Laffel LM, Slover RH, Schatz D, Weinzimer SA, Dovc K, Danne T, Phillip M, NextDREAM Consortium. Insulin dose optimization using an automated artificial intelligence-based decision support system in youths with type 1 diabetes. Nat Med. 2020;26(9):1380–4. https://doi.org/10.1038/s41591-020-1045-7.

27. Berner ES, Kasiraman RK, Yu F, Ray MN, Houston TK. Data quality in the outpatient setting: impact on clinical decision support systems. AMIA Annu Symp Proc. 2005;2005:41–5.

28. Thayer JG, Miller JM, Fiks AG, Tague L, Grundmeier RW. Assessing the safety of custom web-based clinical decision support systems in electronic health records: a case study. Appl Clin Inform. 2019;10(2):237–46. https://doi.org/10.1055/s-0039-1683985.

29. Jeffries M, Salema NE, Laing L, Shamsuddin A, Sheikh A, Avery A, Chuter A, Waring J, Keers RN. The implementation, use and sustainability of a clinical decision support system for medication optimisation in primary care: a qualitative evaluation. PLoS One. 2021;16(5):e0250946. https://doi.org/10.1371/journal.pone.0250946.

30. Thompson C, Mebrahtu T, Skyrme S, Bloor K, Andre D, Keenan AM, Ledward A, Yang H, Randell R. The effects of computerised decision support systems on nursing and allied health professional performance and patient outcomes: a systematic review and user contextualisation. Health Soc Care Deliv Res. 2023:1–85. https://doi.org/10.3310/GRNM5147.

31. Walter Costa MB, Wernsdorfer M, Kehrer A, Voigt M, Cundius C, Federbusch M, Eckelt F, Remmler J, Schmidt M, Pehnke S, Gärtner C, Wehner M, Isermann B, Richter H, Telle J, Kaiser T. The clinical decision support system AMPEL for laboratory diagnostics: implementation and technical evaluation. JMIR Med Inform. 2021;9(6):e20407. https://doi.org/10.2196/20407.

32. Cuvelier E, Robert L, Musy E, Rousselière C, Marcilly R, Gautier S, Odou P, Beuscart JB, Décaudin B. The clinical pharmacist's role in enhancing the relevance of a clinical decision support system. Int J Med Inform. 2021;155:104568. https://doi.org/10.1016/j.ijmedinf.2021.104568.

33. Wiwatkunupakarn N, Aramrat C, Pliannuom S, Buawangpong N, Pinyopornpanish K, Nantsupawat N, Mallinson PAC, Kinra S, Angkurawaranon C. The integration of clinical decision support systems into telemedicine for patients with multimorbidity in primary care settings: scoping review. J Med Internet Res. 2023;25:e45944. https://doi.org/10.2196/45944.

34. Garg AX, Adhikari NK, McDonald H, Rosas-Arellano MP, Devereaux PJ, Beyene J, Sam J, Haynes RB. Effects of computerized clinical decision support systems on practitioner performance and patient outcomes: a systematic review. JAMA. 2005;293(10):1223–38. https://doi.org/10.1001/jama.293.10.1223.

35. Kawamoto K, Houlihan CA, Balas EA, Lobach DF. Improving clinical practice using clinical decision support systems: a systematic review of trials to identify features critical to success. BMJ. 2005;330(7494):765. https://doi.org/10.1136/bmj.38398.500764.8F.

36. Black AD, Car J, Pagliari C, Anandan C, Cresswell K, Bokun T, McKinstry B, Procter R, Majeed A, Sheikh A. The impact of eHealth on the quality and safety of health care: a systematic overview. PLoS Med. 2011;8(1):e1000387. https://doi.org/10.1371/journal.pmed.1000387.

37. El Asmar ML, Dharmayat KI, Vallejo-Vaz AJ, Irwin R, Mastellos N. Effect of computerised, knowledge-based, clinical decision support systems on patient-reported and clinical outcomes of patients with chronic disease managed in primary care settings: a systematic review. BMJ Open. 2021;11(12):e054659. https://doi.org/10.1136/bmjopen-2021-054659.

38. Roshanov PS, You JJ, Dhaliwal J, Koff D, Mackay JA, Weise-Kelly L, et al. Can computerized clinical decision support systems improve practitioners' diagnostic test ordering behavior? A decision-maker-researcher partnership systematic review. Implement Sci. 2011;6:88.

39. Hemens BJ, Holbrook AM, Tonkin M, Mackay JA, Weise-Kelly L, Navarro T, et al. Computerized clinical decision support systems for drug prescribing and management: a decision-maker-researcher partnership systematic review. Implement Sci. 2011;6:89.

40. Nieuwlaat R, Connolly S, Mackay JA, Weise-Kelly L, Navarro T, Wilczynski NL, et al. Computerized clinical decision support systems for therapeutic drug monitoring and dosing: a decision-maker-researcher partnership systematic review. Implement Sci. 2011;6:90.

41. Souza NM, Sebaldt RJ, Mackay JA, Prorok J, Weise-Kelly L, Navarro T, et al. Computerized clinical decision support systems for primary preventive care: a decision-maker-researcher partnership systematic review of effects on process of care and patient outcomes. Implement Sci. 2011;6:87.

42. Roshanov PS, Misra S, Gerstein HC, Garg AX, Sebaldt RJ, Mackay JA, et al. Computerized clinical decision support systems for chronic disease management: a decision-maker-researcher partnership systematic review. Implement Sci. 2011;6:92.

43. Sahota N, Lloyd R, Ramakrishna A, Mackay J, Prorok J, Weise-Kelly L, et al. Computerized clinical decision support systems for acute care management: a decision-maker-researcher partnership systematic review of effects on process of care and patient outcomes. Implement Sci. 2011;6:91.

44. Ford E, Edelman N, Somers L, Shrewsbury D, Lopez Levy M, van Marwijk H, Curcin V, Porat T. Barriers and facilitators to the adoption of electronic clinical decision support systems: a qualitative interview study with UK general practitioners. BMC Med Inform Decis Mak. 2021;21(1):193. https://doi.org/10.1186/s12911-021-01557-z.

45. Rudin RS, Fischer SH, Shi Y, et al. Trends in the use of clinical decision support by health system-affiliated ambulatory clinics in the United States, 2014–2016. Am J Account Care. 2019;7(4):4–10.

46. Jabez Christopher J, Khanna Nehemiah H, Kannan A. A clinical decision support system for diagnosis of Allergic Rhinitis based on intradermal skin tests. Comput Biol Med. 2015;65:76–84.

47. Antó A, Sousa-Pinto B, Czarlewski W, Pfaar O, Bosnic-Anticevich S, Klimek L, Matricardi P, Tripodi S, Fonseca JA, Antó JM, Bousquet J. Automatic market research of mobile health apps for the self-management of allergic rhinitis. Clin Exp Allergy. 2022;52(10):1195–207. https://doi.org/10.1111/cea.14135.

48. Bousquet J, Caimmi DP, Bedbrook A, Bewick M, Hellings PW, Devillier P, Arnavielhe S, et al. Pilot study of mobile phone technology in allergic rhinitis in European countries: the MASK-rhinitis study. Allergy. 2017;72(6):857–65. https://doi.org/10.1111/all.13125.

49. Courbis AL, Murray RB, Arnavielhe S, Caimmi D, Bedbrook A, Van Eerd M, et al. Electronic clinical decision support system for allergic rhinitis management: MASK e-CDSS. Clin Exp Allergy. 2018;48(12):1640–53.

50. Sousa-Pinto B, Sa-Sousa A, Vieira RJ, et al. Behavioral patterns in allergic rhinitis medication in Europe: a study using MASK-air® real-world data. Allergy. 2022;77(9):2699–711. https://doi.org/10.1111/all.15275.

51. Bousquet J, Murray R, Price D, et al. The allergic allergist behaves like a patient. Ann Allergy Asthma Immunol. 2018;121(6):741–2. https://doi.org/10.1016/j.anai.2018.07.034.

52. Petersen C. Use of patient-generated health data for shared decision-making in the clinical environment: ready for prime time. Mhealth. 2021;7:39. https://doi.org/10.21037/mhealth.2020.03.05.

53. Bousquet J. Electronic clinical decision support system (eCDSS) in the management of asthma: from theory to practice. Eur Respir J. 2019;53(4):1900339. https://doi.org/10.1183/13993003.00339-2019.

54. Bousquet J, Arnavielhe S, Bedbrook A, et al. The Allergic Rhinitis and its Impact on Asthma (ARIA) score of allergic rhinitis using mobile technology correlates with quality of life: the MASK study. Allergy. 2018;73(2):505–10. https://doi.org/10.1111/all.13307.

55. Bédard A, Basagaña X, Anto JM, et al. Mobile technology offers novel insights into the control and treatment of allergic rhinitis: the MASK study. J Allergy Clin Immunol. 2019;144(1):135–43. https://doi.org/10.1016/j.jaci.2019.01.053.

56. Tan R, Cvetkovski B, Kritikos V, Price D, Yan K, Smith P, Bosnic-Anticevich S. Identifying the hidden burden of allergic rhinitis (AR) in community pharmacy: a global phenomenon. Asthma Res Pract. 2017;3(1):8.

57. Tan R, Cvetkovski B, Kritikos V, et al. Management of allergic rhinitis in the community pharmacy: identifying the reasons behind medication self-selection. Pharm Pract (Granada). 2018;16(3):1332. https://doi.org/10.18549/PharmPract.2018.03.1332.

58. Bertsche T, Nachbar M, Fiederling J, et al. Assessment of a computerised decision support system for allergic rhino-conjunctivitis counselling in German pharmacy. Int J Clin Pharm. 2012;34(1):17–22. https://doi.org/10.1007/s11096-011-9584-0.

59. Lourenço O, Bosnic-Anticevich S, Costa E, et al. Managing allergic rhinitis in the pharmacy: an ARIA guide for implementation in practice. Pharmacy (Basel). 2020;8(2):E85. https://doi.org/10.3390/pharmacy8020085.

60. Dondi A, Tripodi S, Panetta V, et al. Pollen-induced allergic rhinitis in 1360 Italian children: comorbidities and determinants of severity. Pediatr Allergy Immunol. 2013;24(8):742–51. https://doi.org/10.1111/pai.12136.

61. D'Amato G, Spieksma FT, Liccardi G, Jäger S, Russo M, Kontou-Fili K, Nikkels H, Wüthrich B, Bonini S. Pollen-related allergy in Europe. Allergy. 1998;53(6):567–78. https://doi.org/10.1111/j.1398-9995.1998.tb03932.x.

62. Valenta R, Twaroch T, Swoboda I. Component-resolved diagnosis to optimize allergen-specific immunotherapy in the Mediterranean area. J Investig Allergol Clin Immunol. 2007;17(Suppl. 1):36–40.

63. Kmenta M, Zetter R, Berger U, Bastl K. Pollen information consumption as an indicator of pollen allergy burden. Wien Klin Wochenschr. 2016;128(1–2):59–67. https://doi.org/10.1007/s00508-015-0855-y.

64. Tripodi S, Giannone A, Sfika I, Pelosi S, Dramburg S, Bianchi A, et al. Digital technologies for an improved management of respiratory allergic diseases: 10 years of clinical studies using an online platform for patients and physicians. Ital J Pediatr. 2020;46(1):105. https://doi.org/10.1186/s13052-020-00870-z.

65. Di Fraia M, Tripodi S, Arasi S, et al. Adherence to prescribed E-Diary recording by patients with seasonal allergic rhinitis: observational study. J Med Internet Res. 2020;22(3):e16642. https://doi.org/10.2196/16642.
66. Pizzulli A, Perna S, Florack J, Pizzulli A, Giordani P, Tripodi S, Pelosi S, Matricardi PM. The impact of telemonitoring on adherence to nasal corticosteroid treatment in children with seasonal allergic rhinoconjunctivitis. Clin Exp Allergy. 2014;44(10):1246–54. https://doi.org/10.1111/cea.12386.
67. Dramburg S, Perna S, Di Fraia M, Tripodi S, Arasi S, Castelli S, et al. Prospective (e-diary) vs retrospective (ARIA) measures of severity in allergic rhinoconjunctivitis: an observational compatibility study. Allergy. 2023;78(2):550–3. https://doi.org/10.1111/all.15499.
68. Bianchi A, Tsilochristou O, Gabrielli F, Tripodi S, Matricardi PM. The smartphone: a novel diagnostic tool in pollen allergy? J Investig Allergol Clin Immunol. 2016;26(3):204–7. https://doi.org/10.18176/jiaci.0060.
69. Barreto M, Tripodi S, Arasi S, Landi M, Montesano M, Pelosi S, et al. Factors predicting the outcome of allergen-specific nasal provocation test in children with grass pollen allergic rhinitis. Front Allergy. 2023;4:1186353. https://doi.org/10.3389/falgy.2023.1186353.
70. Roberts G, Pfaar O, Akdis CA, Ansotegui IJ, Durham SR, Gerth van Wijk R, et al. EAACI Guidelines on allergen immunotherapy: allergic rhinoconjunctivitis. Allergy. 2018;73(4):765–98. https://doi.org/10.1111/all.13317.
71. Dramburg S, Hilger C, Santos AF, de Las Vecillas L, Aalberse RC, Acevedo N, et al. EAACI molecular allergology user's guide 2.0. Pediatr Allergy Immunol. 2023;34(Suppl. 28):e13854. https://doi.org/10.1111/pai.13854.
72. Matricardi PM, Dramburg S, Potapova E, Skevaki C, Renz H. Molecular diagnosis for allergen immunotherapy. J Allergy Clin Immunol. 2019;143(3):831–43. https://doi.org/10.1016/j.jaci.2018.12.1021.
73. Matricardi PM, Potapova E, Forchert L, Dramburg S, Tripodi S. Digital allergology: towards a clinical decision support system for allergen immunotherapy. Pediatr Allergy Immunol. 2020;31(Suppl. 24):61–4. https://doi.org/10.1111/pai.13165.
74. Bousquet J, Jutel M, Pfaar O, Fonseca JA, Agache I, Czarlewski W, et al. The role of mobile health technologies in stratifying patients for AIT and its cessation: the ARIA-EAACI perspective. J Allergy Clin Immunol Pract. 2021;9(5):1805–12. https://doi.org/10.1016/j.jaip.2021.02.035.
75. Dramburg S, Marchante Fernández M, Potapova E, Matricardi PM. The potential of clinical decision support systems for prevention, diagnosis, and monitoring of allergic diseases. Front Immunol. 2020;11:2116. https://doi.org/10.3389/fimmu.2020.02116.
76. Lancet T. A plea to abandon asthma as a disease concept. Lancet. 2006;368(9537):705. https://doi.org/10.1016/S0140-6736(06)69257-X.
77. Papi A, Brightling C, Pedersen SE, Reddel HK. Asthma Lancet. 2018;391(10122):783–800. https://doi.org/10.1016/S0140-6736(17)33311-1.
78. Papadopoulos NG, Čustović A, Cabana MD, Dell SD, Deschildre A, Hedlin G, Hossny E, Le Souëf P, Matricardi PM, Nieto A, Phipatanakul W, Pitrez PM, Pohunek P, Gavornikova M, Jaumont X, Price DB. Pediatric asthma: an unmet need for more effective, focused treatments. Pediatr Allergy Immunol. 2019;30(1):7–16. https://doi.org/10.1111/pai.12990.
79. Chapman KR, Boulet LP, Rea RM, Franssen E. Suboptimal asthma control: prevalence, detection and consequences in general practice. Eur Respir J. 2008;31(2):320–5.
80. Huang X, Matricardi PM. Allergy and asthma care in the mobile phone era. Clin Rev Allergy Immunol. 2019;56(2):161–73. https://doi.org/10.1007/s12016-016-8542-y.
81. Matui P, Wyatt JC, Pinnock H, Sheikh A, McLean S. Computer decision support systems for asthma: a systematic review. NPJ Prim Care Respir Med. 2014;24:14005. https://doi.org/10.1038/npjpcrm.2014.5.
82. McKibben S, De Simoni A, Bush A, Thomas M, Griffiths C. The use of electronic alerts in primary care computer systems to identify the excessive prescription of short-acting beta$_2$-agonists for people with asthma: a systematic review. NPJ Prim Care Respir Med. 2018;28(1):14. https://doi.org/10.1038/s41533-018-0080-z.

83. Augestad KM, Berntsen G, Lassen K, Bellika JG, Wootton R, Lindsetmo RO, Study Group of Research Quality in Medical Informatics and Decision Support (SQUID). Standards for reporting randomized controlled trials in medical informatics: a systematic review of CONSORT adherence in RCTs on clinical decision support. J Am Med Inform Assoc. 2012;19(1):13–21. https://doi.org/10.1136/amiajnl-2011-000411.

84. Hoeksema LJ, Bazzy-Asaad A, Lomotan EA, Edmonds DE, Ramirez-Garnica G, Shiffman RN, et al. Accuracy of a computerized clinical decision-support system for asthma assessment and management. J Am Med Inform Assoc. 2011;18(3):243–50.

85. Sunjaya AP, Ansari S, Jenkins CR. A systematic review on the effectiveness and impact of clinical decision support systems for breathlessness. NPJ Prim Care Respir Med. 2022;32(1):29. https://doi.org/10.1038/s41533-022-00291-x.

86. Chakrabarti B, Kane B, Barrow C, Stonebanks J, Reed L, Pearson MG, Davies L, Osborne M, England P, Litchfield D, McKnight E, Angus RM. The feasibility and impact of implementing a computer-guided consultation to target health inequality in Asthma. NPJ Prim Care Respir Med. 2023;33(1):6. https://doi.org/10.1038/s41533-023-00329-8.

87. Lam Shin Cheung J, Paolucci N, Price C, Sykes J, Gupta S, Canadian Respiratory Research Network. A system uptake analysis and GUIDES checklist evaluation of the electronic asthma management system: a point-of-care computerized clinical decision support system. J Am Med Inform Assoc. 2020;27(5):726–37. https://doi.org/10.1093/jamia/ocaa019.

88. Ljungberg H, Carleborg A, Gerber H, Ofverstrom C, Wolodarski J, Menshi F, et al. Clinical effect on uncontrolled asthma using a novel digital automated self-management solution: a physician-blinded randomised controlled crossover trial. Eur Respir J. 2019;54(5)

89. Moloney M, Digby G, MacKinnon M, Morra A, Barber D, Queenan J, Gupta S, To T. Lougheed MD, Primary care asthma surveillance: a review of knowledge translation tools and strategies for.quality improvement. Allergy Asthma Clin Immunol. 19(1):3.

90. Kwak M, Han SB, Kim G, Choi J, Chun J, Lee K, et al. The knowledge modeling for chronic urticaria assessment in clinical decision support system with PDA. In: AMIA 2003 symposium proceedings. p. 902.

91. Maurer M, Kolkhir P, Ramanauskaite A, Cherrez-Ojeda I. Digital health and chronic urticaria. In: Matricardi PM, Dramburg S, editors. Digital allergology: from theory to practice. Springer.

92. https://cruse-control.com

93. Cherrez-Ojeda I, Vanegas E, Cherrez A, Felix M, Weller K, Magerl M, et al. Chronic urticaria patients are interested in apps to monitor their disease activity and control: a UCARE CURICT analysis. Clin Transl Allergy. 2021;11(10):e12089.

94. Anto A, Maurer R, Gimenez-Arnau A, Cherrez-Ojeda I, Hawro T, Magerl M, et al. Automatic screening of self-evaluation apps for urticaria and angioedema shows a high unmet need. Allergy. 2021;76(12):3810–3.

95. Sitaru S. Digital health and atopic dermatitis. In: Matricardi PM, Dramburg S, editors. Digital allergology: from theory to practice. Springer.

96. Luger T, Adaskevich U, Anfilova M, Dou X, Murashkin NN, Namazova-Baranova L, et al. Practical algorithm to inform clinical decision-making in the topical treatment of atopic dermatitis. J Dermatol. 2021;48(8):1139–48. https://doi.org/10.1111/1346-8138.15921.

97. Chang LS, Kuo HC, Suen JJ, Yang PH, Hou CP, Sun HR, Lee ZM, Huang YH. Multimedia mixed reality interactive shared decision-making game in children with moderate to severe atopic dermatitis, a pilot study. Children (Basel). 2023;10(3):574. https://doi.org/10.3390/children10030574.

98. Otto AK, Dyer AA, Warren CM, Walkner M, Smith BM, Gupta RS. The development of a clinical decision support system for the management of pediatric food allergy. Clin Pediatr (Phila). 2017;56(6):571–8. https://doi.org/10.1177/0009922816669097.

99. Luri M, Leache L, Gastaminza G, Idoate A, Ortega A. A systematic review of drug allergy alert systems. Int J Med Inform. 2022;159:104673. https://doi.org/10.1016/j.ijmedinf.2021.104673.

100. Nanji KC, Seger DL, Slight SP, et al. Medication-related clinical decision support alert over-rides in inpatients. J Am Med Inform Assoc. 2018;25(5):476–81. https://doi.org/10.1093/jamia/ocx115.
101. Berge GT, Granmo OC, Tveit TO, Munkvold BE, Ruthjersen AL, Sharma J. Machine learning-driven clinical decision support system for concept-based searching: a field trial in a Norwegian hospital. BMC Med Inform Decis Mak. 2023;23(1):5. https://doi.org/10.1186/s12911-023-02101-x.
102. Blumenthal KG, Wickner PG, Hurwitz S, et al. Tackling inpatient penicillin allergies: assessing tools for antimicrobial stewardship. J Allergy Clin Immunol. 2017;140(1):154–61. https://doi.org/10.1016/j.jaci.2017.02.005.
103. Allen HI, Vazquez-Ortiz M, Murphy AW, Moylett EM. De-labeling penicillin-allergic children in outpatients using telemedicine: potential to replicate in primary care. J Allergy Clin Immunol Pract. 2020;8(5):1750–2. https://doi.org/10.1016/j.jaip.2019.12.034.
104. Flokstra-de Blok BM, van der Molen T, Christoffers WA, et al. Development of an allergy management support system in primary care. J Asthma Allergy. 2017;10:57–65. https://doi.org/10.2147/JAA.S123260.

Chapter 8
Databanks and Expert Systems in Allergomics: Scientific and Clinical Implications

Ronald van Ree

Contents

Abstract Existing allergen databases serve several different purposes. Some are primarily designed to facilitate bioinformatics sequence comparisons of novel food proteins with established allergens, in the frame of allergenicity risk assessment. Others are more comprehensive repositories that provide broader information about allergens, including biochemical and structural data, B- and T-cell epitope data, and clinical and epidemiological data. Various bioinformatic and machine learning tools are being provided to address allergenicity, both for predicting potential cross-reactivity of novel proteins with existing allergens and for predicting their de novo sensitizing potential, i.e., whether they may become new allergens. This chapter provides an overview of the most important allergen databases and discusses the opportunities they provide to service various stakeholders with interest in allergen molecules and allergic diseases. Overall, bringing comprehensive multifaceted allergen information together and applying machine learning and artificial intelli-

R. van Ree (✉)
Departments of Experimental Immunology and of Otorhinolaryngology, Amsterdam University Medical Centers, Amsterdam, The Netherlands
e-mail: r.vanree@amsterdamumc.nl

© The Author(s), under exclusive license to Springer Nature Switzerland AG 2025
P. M. Matricardi, S. Dramburg, *Digital Allergology*, Health Informatics,
https://doi.org/10.1007/978-3-031-71021-6_8

gence approaches may in the future refine the process of allergenicity risk assessment and provide better insights into the molecular basis of cross-reactivity. Whether these developments will also help to answer what turns proteins into allergens remains to be seen, but it is very likely that this cannot be answered with molecular information on proteins only, knowing that exogenous factors play an important role in the process of sensitization.

Databases with information on allergens exist in many flavors, differing in format depending on the applications they intend to service (Fig. 8.1) [1, 2]. The aims of the various databases range from regulating conformity in allergen nomenclature, providing a resource for allergenicity risk assessment of genetically modified crops, novel food proteins, and novel foods, to databases that aim to provide comprehensive scientific information on allergens for interested stakeholders, ranging from clinicians and patients to basic and translational scientists from academia and industry. In this chapter, we will discuss the most important databases along these lines.

8.1 Allergen Nomenclature Database

One could say that the mother of allergen databases is the one established under the auspices of the World Health Organization (WHO) and the International Union of Immunological Societies (IUIS), the Allergen Nomenclature database [3]. This database lists all proteins that have received an official allergen name recognized by the WHO/IUIS Allergen Nomenclature Subcommittee [4–7]. This committee, a panel of academic allergen experts, evaluates applications for possible new

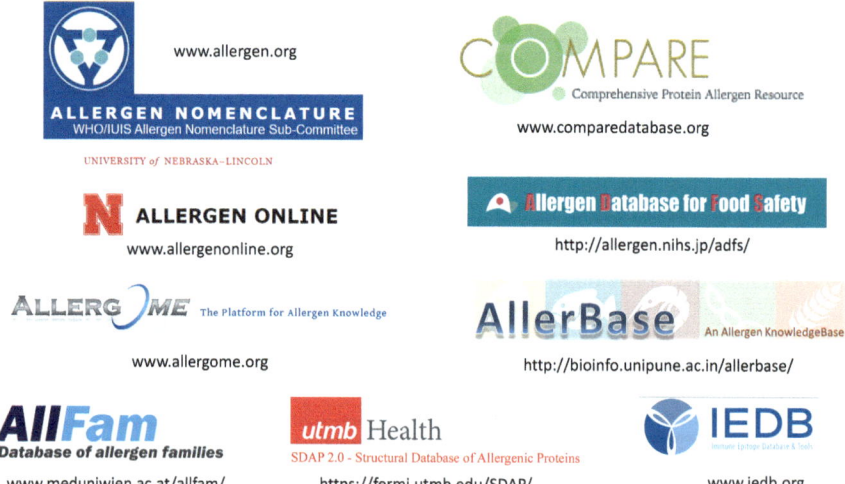

Fig. 8.1 Logos and internet addresses of the most important allergen databases

allergens, brought to its attention by means of a (now online) application form submitted by researchers. An accepted new allergen will receive its official name following a nomenclature system that was developed in the early eighties, adopted by the WHO in 1986 [8] and revised in 1994 [9]. The system, based on Linnaean binominal nomenclature, was originally proposed by a group of prominent allergy researchers, David Marsh, Henning Löwenstein, Thomas Platts-Mills, Te Piao King, and Larry Goodfriend. The main function of this database is to make sure that only proteins with a minimal sound degree of evidence supporting their IgE binding properties receive an official allergen name, and that the whole allergy field uses the same name for such IgE binding proteins. Overall, the system functions quite well, especially since journals in the field (are supposed to) demand proof that a new allergen name is indeed recognized by the committee. This prevents different proteins from entering the public domain under the same allergen name. Since designations are frequently also given out without the committee getting access to a full draft paper, the peer review of the soundness of the claim is suboptimal. Although the database receives some financial support from non-profit organizations IUIS, the European Academy of Allergy and Clinical Immunology (EAACI), and the American Academy of Allergy Asthma and Immunology (AAAAI), its continuity is largely dependent on the voluntary efforts of the members of the WHO/IUIS Allergen Nomenclature Subcommittee.

8.2   Allergome

In 2003, the Allergome database was released [10]. The driving force behind Allergome was (and is) Adriano Mari who maintains the database via a company he founded, Allergen Data Laboratories. Allergome is by far the most comprehensive allergen database around. It provides information on allergen sources, offers links to the WHO/IUIS database, to taxonomic databases, to UniProt and PDB, and it provides allergological and epidemiological data. Moreover, Allergome also provides a quite comprehensive list of literature references associated with each listed molecule. In addition, several different bioinformatic tools are available, including sequence alignment and reference search tools. Its comprehensiveness and user-friendly design have made Allergome a database that is widely used by different stakeholders. On the other hand, it is important to realize that the database also lists homologs of allergens that are likely or possibly allergens but that have not been identified as such, including some from sources that are not known to be allergenic. Although these entries can be recognized by a label "in silico," this practice has been criticized. The same is true for the fact that Allergome has sometimes provided WHO/IUIS-like names to entries that have not (yet) been listed in the WHO/IUIS Allergen Nomenclature Database. Despite these criticisms, Allergome remains a very informative and versatile resource for people with interest in allergens.

8.3   Allergenicity Risk Assessment: AOL, COMPARE, ADFS

An important driver behind the creation of allergen databases has been the allergenicity risk assessment of potential transgenes to be introduced into crops, resulting in genetically modified (GM) crops and GM foods [11]. Ideally, allergenicity risk assessment would include both aspects of allergenicity of proteins, i.e., their capacity to induce IgE de novo (sensitization), and their capacity to bind already existing IgE based on cross-reactivity, possibly leading to symptoms (elicitation). Predicting sensitization potential of proteins that lack structural homology with established allergens was very difficult, if not impossible. In other words, we do not (yet?) have tools to predict whether a novel protein can "start a new allergen family." Databases created for allergenicity risk assessment have therefore focused on evaluating the risk of cross-reactivity with established allergens. The database pioneering in this field has been Allergen Online (AOL), established in 2005 and hosted by the Food Allergy Research and Resource Program at the University of Nebraska, under the leadership of Rick Goodman [12]. Its main function was (and still is) to offer a resource where mainly agricultural biotech (AgBiotech) companies can perform bioinformatic searches comparing a candidate transgene against all the sequences of allergens in the database. The aim is to evaluate whether there is a relevant risk that a protein resembles an existing allergen sufficiently enough to be recognized by specific IgE based on cross-reactivity, and consequently may cause allergic reactions in patients sensitive to the existing allergen. As for the nomenclature database, the process of updating is performed by an independent academic expert panel, but the maintenance of the AOL database has always been financially supported by commercial parties that are dependent on the database for their allergenicity risk assessment, mainly AgBiotech companies. More recently, non-AgBiotech companies such as novel food companies and enzyme producers for food industry increasingly turn to using the database for their allergenicity risk assessment as well. In parallel with AOL, also in 2005, a Japanese allergen database for allergenicity risk assessment, the Allergen Database for Food Safety (ADFS), was established [13, 14]. It uses AOL as its resource for allergens, supplemented with literature search, but it is not clear how potential new allergens from literature are exactly being evaluated. In 2016, a new initiative led to the creation of a third allergen database for bioinformatic allergenicity risk assessment, the Comprehensive Protein Allergen Resource (COMPARE) [15]. The COMPARE database also took the AOL list of allergens (version 16) as its starting point, to then independently further develop their own algorithms to update on a yearly basis. Like AOL, COMPARE has an independent academic expert panel that evaluates new candidate sequences on a yearly basis. The database is hosted by the Health and Environmental Sciences Institute in Washington DC, a tripartite (academia, industry, and regulators) nonprofit organization that receives financial support from industry to maintain and yearly update the database.

Although no comprehensive data is available on database use, AOL has long been to be the most used allergen database for allergenicity risk assessment and dossiers submitted to regulatory authorities around the world. Since its introduction in 2017, COMPARE is now increasingly being used as well. AOL and COMPARE largely contain the same list of allergens but differences do exist. Some can simply be explained by the time window used for annual updates, but the exact algorithms used for searching potential new allergens also differ. The COMPARE website is quite transparent concerning the algorithms used, and the evaluation reports of the expert panel are publicly accessible. For AOL, the publicly available information on the algorithms is perhaps less detailed and the evaluation reports are not accessible. In recent years, mass spectrometry (MS) based proteomic approaches to characterize allergen sources have resulted in a high number of publications that report new allergens but with only partial evidence-based sequence information. This has led to another difference between COMPARE and AOL. COMPARE decided to only list the peptides (of ≥ 10 amino acids) identified by MS as new entries, because the full sequence is usually not covered by the combined peptides and therefore strictly speaking not supported by experimental evidence. Since the latest update in 2023, COMPARE now groups peptides from the same allergen together with a link to the full sequence for convenience of the user. AOL lists the full sequence, originating from a protein database like UniProt that matches the combined peptides. This explains why the number of entries in COMPARE is increasingly becoming higher than those in AOL.

AOL, ADFS, and COMPARE have primarily been established for facilitating bioinformatic searches as an integral part of the weight-of-evidence approach for allergenicity risk assessment, according to the guidelines of FAO/WHO and CODEX Alimentarius Commission [11, 16]. Apart from the bioinformatic search, the weight-of-evidence approach includes among other an evaluation of susceptibility to pepsin digestion and the source of the protein and its history of safe use (or not). The requirements for the bioinformatics part of the assessment have been the topic of a lot of discussion [17–24]. Currently, in the regulatory environment most emphasis is given to performing a search using an 80-mer sliding window to scan the whole sequence of a candidate transgene against the allergen database. Any hit of $\geq 35\%$ identity is considered a potential risk, and regulatory authorities may ask for serum screening with sera that contain IgE against the source with which the hit was found, preferably but not necessarily against the actual allergen. The latter may prove very difficult if it concerns a (sometimes very) minor allergen. The 35% threshold is very conservative anyway, knowing that cross-reactivity is rarely seen below 50% full sequence identity [25]. Consequently, quite a high number of false-positive hits may occur [19, 21, 22]. Some authorities even require an 8-mer search, with any 100% 8-mer identity hit being considered a potential risk. It has been well established that 8-mer searches result in very high numbers of false-positive hits [20, 23], and therefore most authorities stick to the 80-mer sliding window. It has been proposed that using 1:1 FASTA and E-values on top of that can filter out false-positives from the 80-mer sliding window screen [19, 22, 24].

On top of the discussion about the methods and criteria used in bioinformatics searches, other ideas for further refinement are being considered. In the food allergy arena, it is well accepted that some allergens are more risky than other ones. For example, food allergens belonging to the PR-10 protein family are associated almost exclusively with mild or no symptoms, whereas legume, seed, and nut 2S albumins are an established risk factor for severe symptoms [26–32]. Although it is not fully clear what the explanation of the difference in clinical relevance is, resistance to gastro-intestinal digestion and abundance in the food are likely major contributors. From a risk assessment point of view, all of this is of course very relevant information, but it is not considered in the current system at all. A bioinformatics hit with a 2S albumin is certainly more of a red flag than a hit with a PR-10 allergen.

We also know much more about thresholds for reactions to major allergenic foods at a total protein level but have not translated that to a molecular level [33, 34]. Such translation could provide a threshold of exposure at molecular level that creates a risk. Obviously, expression of a transgene at trace amounts or at high levels will make a difference.

Apart from knowing more and more about the clinical relevance of individual food allergens, we are also gaining increasing insight into the 3D structure of allergens and the location of epitopes that are important for IgE recognition [35, 36]. It is not far-fetched to state that identity of a transgene concentrated around a known surface exposed major IgE epitope is of more relevance than identity with a more hidden sequence to which no IgE binding has been reported.

It will be a challenge to integrate all these elements into algorithms for risk assessment, but databases are available that host information about allergen structure and IgE epitopes [37, 38]. It is worthwhile to explore how information from these different databases can be linked. Developments in the field of machine learning and artificial intelligence may in the future facilitate their integration and refine the risk assessment process.

8.4 Allergen Structure and IgE Epitopes: AllFam, SDAP, IEDB, AllerBase

Two allergen databases focus on allergen structure, the AllFam database [39] and the Structural Database of Allergenic Proteins (SDAP) [37, 40]. The former one classifies allergens from the WHO/IUIS Allergen Nomenclature database into protein families, based on protein family definitions from the Protein Family database (Pfam) [41]. The SDAP database hosts available structural (i.e., crystal structures and NMR structures) as well as epitope data of allergens, mostly from those listed in the WHO/IUIS Allergen Nomenclature database. For both databases, the frequency of updating is quite unclear and irregular. The most comprehensive database with IgE epitopes is the Immune Epitope Database (IEDB) [42–45]. This database also contains a list of T-cell epitopes of allergens. IEDB entries are identified by biweekly PubMed literature and Protein Database (PDB) searches, reviewed by immunology experts, aiming at inclusion within eight weeks after publication. The information contained in AllFam, SDAP and IEDB, and their bioinformatics tools, offer promising opportunities to bring bioinformatics strategies for allergenicity risk assessment carried out via comprehensive allergen sequence databases like AOL and COMPARE to the next level.

In 2017, the establishment of another allergen database was reported, the AllerBase database [38]. AllerBase takes the WHO/IUIS Nomenclature database as starting point and is updated weekly based on literature searches, but it is not completely clear how new candidate sequences are evaluated before acceptance for entry into the database. Besides listing allergen sequences, where available, AllerBase also includes information about IgE epitopes, cross-reactivity, 3D structures, and IgE antibodies.

8.5   Novel Foods: Whole Genome Screening

There is growing interest in novel foods that can replace (mammalian and avian) meat and seafood as a dietary source of protein. Essentially, novel foods are foods that have not been consumed on a regular basis before and therefore have no history of safe consumption. This can of course vary in different parts of the world. Examples of novel foods are insects, fungal protein-based and algae-based foods, and in vitro cultured meat. Not unexpectedly, insects have been shown to contain proteins that are homologous with known invertebrate allergens such as tropomyosins and arginine kinases, acknowledged as major allergens in crustaceans and mollusks [46]. In the European Union (EU), insect-based foods therefore now need to be labeled with a warning for patients with allergy to such sea foods. In general, regulatory authorities in the EU request that novel foods undergo an allergenicity risk assessment very much like GM crops. Where GM crops are foods with a long history of consumption (e.g., soy and corn) containing one novel (transgenic) protein, novel foods are whole new foods. In the EU, the consequence is that essentially the whole genome of a novel food needs to be screened against allergen databases like AOL or COMPARE. It comes as no surprise that this can result in quite significant lists of hits using the conservative (false-positive prone) 80-mer sliding window search, due to the presence of evolutionary conserved proteins that have been identified as allergens in some organisms [17]. These hits frequently also display a high degree of identity to human homologs, making a significant allergenicity risk unlikely. Moreover, such bioinformatics hits often relate to minor allergens for which evidence of allergenicity is weak, and suitable sera for cross-reactivity screening are very hard to find. The regulatory approach of whole genome screening therefore is a significant hurdle that complicates market admission of novel foods. One could argue that only significant homology of proteins in novel foods to food allergens with established convincing clinical relevance, such as seed storage proteins like 2S albumins and 7S and 11S globulins, invertebrate tropomyosins, fish parvalbumins, fruit and nut lipid transfer proteins, and gibberellin-regulated proteins, is to be considered a potential risk that needs to be further assessed and that may require labeling of the novel food. On the other hand, the presence of proteins in a novel food with homology to highly conserved allergens, either associated with mild local symptoms only, such as PR-10 proteins and profilins, or for which very weak evidence for clinical relevance is available, may then be judged to be of limited immediate risk for allergic patients and not require labeling of the novel food. A categorization of allergens in databases like AOL and COMPARE according to their clinical relevance would facilitate such an approach.

8.6   Allergen Databases: What Makes a Protein an Allergen?

A question that has fascinated allergy researchers already for a long time is whether allergenic proteins share common properties that explain why they became allergens. Because allergens have only been identified in a limited number of protein families [3, 39, 47], the thought that specific biochemical and/or biophysical characteristics drive allergenicity may sound logical at first sight. On the other hand, it is hard to imagine overarching properties for a very diverse spectrum of allergenic protein families such as allergenic enzymes (e.g., cysteine and serine proteases), allergenic lipid binding proteins (e.g., lipocalins and lipid transfer proteins), allergenic calcium-binding proteins (e.g., parvalbumins and calmodulins), and allergenic seed storage proteins (e.g., 2S albumins and 7S and 11S globulins). Despite this obvious diversity, a variety of strategies has been put forward to develop algorithms that can predict allergenicity based on sequence information, especially since the onset of machine learning and artificial intelligence [48–60]. Before going into that, it is important to reflect a bit more on how allergenicity is defined. As already indicated in the paragraph on databases used for allergenicity risk assessment, there is the broader definition which says that any protein binding IgE is an allergen. This is the definition that is used for most, if not all allergen databases. If a sound demonstration of IgE binding to a protein is reported, its sequence is accepted for being added to the dataset. If a novel protein exhibits significant sequence identity to a listed allergen, cross-reactivity is possible. A more stringent definition of allergenicity is that an allergen is a protein that can de novo induce IgE antibodies, i.e., act as primary sensitizer. Probably the most prevalent food allergen belongs to the pathogenesis-related proteins of class 10 (PR-10). The primary sensitizer within this family of proteins is the PR-10 protein from birch pollen, Bet v 1 [61, 62]. The broad spectrum of cross-reactive food homologs such as Mal d 1 in apple, Pru p 1 in peach, Api g 1 in celery, and Ara h 8 in peanut are generally acknowledged to be incapable of acting as primary sensitizers. On the other hand, storage proteins in tree nuts (e.g., Cor a 9 and Cor a 14 in hazelnut, and Jug r 1 in walnut), legumes (e.g., Ara h 1, Ara h 2, and Ara h 3 in peanut), seeds (e.g., Ses i 1 in sesame seed), or lipid transfer protein in peach (Pru p 3) are each considered primary sensitizers [29, 63]. It is justified to assume that possible properties driving allergenicity differ between these two categories of allergenic proteins. Along the same lines, one could also question whether respiratory allergens and food allergens, with a different route of sensitization, are likely to have overlapping characteristics that would turn them into allergens. Sequences for all these proteins, primary and cross-reactive allergens, respiratory and food allergens, are combined in allergen databases. When attempting to predict allergenicity of novel proteins using algorithms developed by machine learning approaches on sequences of all allergens present in allergen databases, this heterogeneity should be considered. For such predictions, it is of course furthermore essential to have sequences of (likely) non-allergenic comparators. Different approaches have been applied for selection of the non-allergenic control dataset.

A tool called EVALLER aims to predict allergenicity based on a comparison of overlapping peptides of variable length, covering sequences of allergens and non-allergens, using a machine learning approach [54, 58]. Very simplified, the assumption is that peptides found in allergenic proteins but not in the related proteins from the non-allergenic dataset are the determinants for allergenicity. The allergen dataset was a mix of protein sequences selected from the WHO/IUIS Allergen Nomenclature database, AOL, SDAP, Protall (later renamed InformAll), and Allergome, after evaluating the quality of published proof for allergenicity. For the control dataset, the EVALLER developers chose a selection of proteins from the human proteome and that of three allergenic sources (two fungi, *Aspergillus fumigatus* and *Candida albicans*, and house dust mite, *Dermatophagoides pteronyssinus*) from which they removed all known allergen sequences. The choice of the human proteome appears to be sound because allergy human proteins is expected to be extremely rare because all proteins are being seen as "own, not foreign." One could however argue that the reason for not developing an (allergic) immune response is because the default is to develop tolerance / ignorance for non-foreign proteins, not their biochemical protein family characteristics. The proteome of allergenic sources can for another reason be criticized. Since 2007, when the EVALLER approach was published, e.g., 15 new allergens have been identified in *Dermatophagoides pteronyssinus* house dust mite, among which a major allergen Der p 23 [64], so the proteome used as non-allergenic dataset certainly was not devoid of allergens.

Another machine learning approach [52], focusing on molecular motifs representing IgE epitopes, used an allergen dataset derived from a combination of WHO/IUIS, Swiss-Prot, AOL and SDAP, and a non-allergen dataset derived from Swiss-Prot, using sequences from three organisms (tomato, celery, and pear), excluding any entries listing the word allergen or allergy, lipid transfer protein, cupin, chitinase, or profilin. This non-allergenic dataset can be criticized as well because there are many more allergenic protein families with representatives in these three foods which would have remained in the selection if they were not designated as allergen in Swiss-Prot.

J. Westerhout et al. reported on a Random Forest algorithm to predict allergenicity of novel proteins, based on their physicochemical and biochemical properties [60]. As allergen dataset, the COMPARE database was used. For the non-allergenic dataset, these authors took all sequences from UniProt, removing all human proteins, and all proteins listed as allergens that were not in COMPARE.

Recently, Japanese researchers reported a machine learning method, allerStat, that searches for amino acid subsequences that are statistically significantly over-represented in allergenic proteins [50]. They also used full-length sequences from the COMPARE database, complemented with unique sequences from the ADSF database, as allergenic dataset. As non-allergenic dataset, the authors chose the proteome of 20 common allergenic foods from which they removed known allergens, thereby assuming that the knowledge on their allergen spectrum is virtually complete. Knowing that with every yearly update, new allergens from one of more of these 20 foods are added, it is justified to have some doubt about the strength of this approach.

Overall, the different approaches in search for the ultimate algorithm to predict allergenicity use different datasets and different machine learning approaches. Whether any of these approaches will prove to be useful for allergenicity risk assessment, but also for better understanding of the process of sensitization, remains to be seen.

8.7   Can Sequence-Based Predictions Really Answer the Question of What Makes a Protein an Allergen?

Undoubtedly, the continuously growing datasets of protein and allergen sequences ("big data"), together with developments in machine learning and artificial intelligence, provide opportunities to search for answers to the enigma of allergenicity. Having said that, it may also turn out to be a mission impossible to predict whether a protein will become an allergen, i.e., will be capable of de novo induction of IgE antibodies, purely based on its amino acid sequence. The process of sensitization is complex and influenced by many factors other than just the patterns in the amino acid sequence and/or physicochemical and biochemical properties of the protein (Fig. 8.2). First, there is the route of exposure, i.e., the inhalant, the oral or the dermal route. The oral route involves exposure to digestive enzymes, which is absent for the other two routes. In general, the oral route is more skewed toward tolerance (we all must eat and tolerate foreign food protein), whereas the inhalant and dermal routes are more dedicated to preventing pathogens from successfully invading the host. Oral exposure to food proteins is orders of magnitude higher than to inhaled indoor or outdoor allergen sources. For food protein, it is now quite established that the skin is an important route of exposure [65], whereas compared to consumption, exposure is again orders of magnitude lower. The importance of the level of exposure is further illustrated by the observation that most major allergens are major protein components within aqueous allergen extracts, like seed, legume, and nut storage proteins, the major birch pollen allergen Bet v 1, the major house dust mite allergens Der p 1 and Der p 2, and so on. There are exceptions like the lipid transfer protein in peach, but here its concentrated presence in the peel of the fruit may facilitate sensitization via the skin. Exposure to allergenic proteins never happens in isolation. In food, allergens are usually consumed in the context

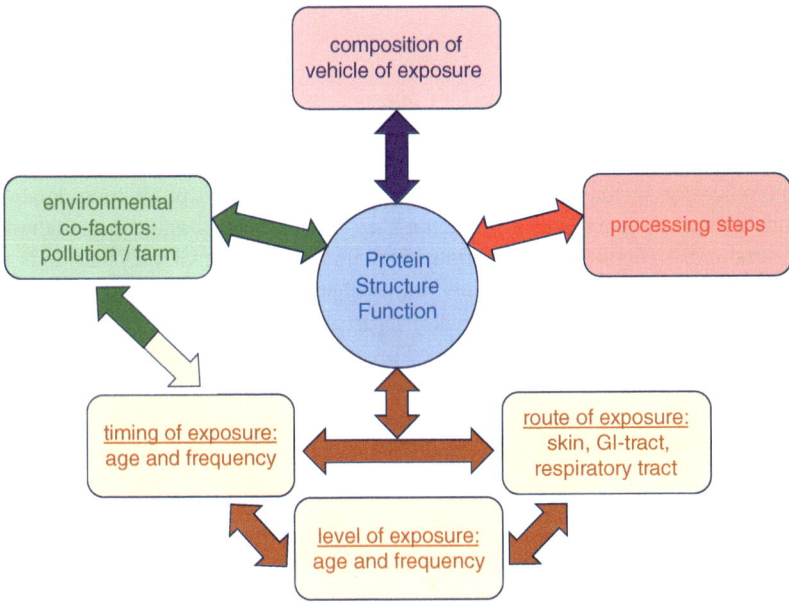

Fig. 8.2 The multifactorial process of sensitizationThe process of sensitization is a function of endogenous structural and functional properties of the (potentially allergenic) protein and a series of interplaying exogenous factors that influence the interaction of the protein with the immune system. The complexity makes it unlikely that algorithms based on the primary structure of a protein alone can predict allergenicity.

of composite and/or processed foods. Some food allergens have been shown to become more allergenic upon processing, others less [46, 66–70]. Boiled peanuts are less allergenic than roasted peanuts, although they contain the same primary sequences of their storage proteins [71]. On the other hand, PR-10 food allergens lose their allergenicity upon processing. Also, environmental allergens are not inhaled in pure form but as part of complex structures such as pollen or house dust mite fecal particles. Moreover, other co-factors, not part of the allergenic source organism, have been shown to stimulate (e.g., diesel exhaust particles) [72] or prevent (e.g., bacterial/fungal components in farmer's environment) sensitization [73]. Some inhaled or skin-exposed proteins only behave as allergens if exposure is high or frequent, like for occupational allergens [74]. Timing of exposure also matters. High exposure at a very young age can prevent sensitization to e.g., peanut and egg [75]. Taking all this together, it seems very unlikely that algorithms purely based on amino acid sequences of proteins will be able to reliably predict whether a novel protein will become an allergen. A stronger case can probably be made for reliably predicting cross-reactivity between acknowledged allergens and novel proteins, using sequence-based prediction tools, machine learning, and computer modeling.

8.8   Conclusion

Allergen databases are a rich source of information that can assist with allergenicity risk assessment of novel foods, and the study of the process of sensitization, but also with the development of molecular approaches for allergy diagnostics and allergen immunotherapy. Increasing the variety of information stored in allergen databases, beyond listing allergen names with their amino acid sequences, and complementing it with structural and epitope information, and with data on clinical relevance and exposure thresholds leading to symptoms, may enhance their predictive potential, with respect to grading the risk of cross-reactivity in already sensitized patients. The complex process of sensitization is influenced by many protein-associated factors (amino acid sequence, biochemical function, physicochemical properties, exposure timing, route and level, type of processing) and exogenous protein-independent factors (environmental co-factors). This makes the prediction of new allergens very difficult if not impossible, even with state-of-the-art machine learning and artificial intelligence.

References

1. Radauer C. Navigating through the jungle of allergens: features and applications of allergen databases. Int Arch Allergy Immunol. 2017;173(1):1–11.
2. Radauer C, Breiteneder H. Allergen databases—a critical evaluation. Allergy. 2019;74(11):2057–60.
3. Chapman MD, Pomés A, Breiteneder H, Ferreira F. Nomenclature and structural biology of allergens. J Allergy Clin Immunol. 2007;119(2):414–20.
4. Chan SK, Pomés A, Hilger C, Davies JM, Mueller G, Kuehn A, et al. Keeping allergen names clear and defined. Front Immunol. 2019;10:2600.
5. Goodman RE, Breiteneder H. The WHO/IUIS allergen nomenclature. Allergy. 2019;74(3):429–31.
6. Pomés A, Davies JM, Gadermaier G, Hilger C, Holzhauser T, Lidholm J, et al. WHO/IUIS Allergen nomenclature: providing a common language. Mol Immunol. 2018;100:3–13.
7. Radauer C, Nandy A, Ferreira F, Goodman RE, Larsen JN, Lidholm J, et al. Update of the WHO/IUIS allergen nomenclature database based on analysis of allergen sequences. Allergy. 2014;69(4):413–9.
8. Marsh DG, Goodfriend L, King TP, Lowenstein H, Platts-Mills TA. Allergen nomenclature. Bull World Health Organ. 1986;64(5):767–74.
9. King TP, Hoffman D, Løwenstein H, Marsh DG, Platts-Mills TA, Thomas W. Allergen nomenclature. Allergy. 1995;50(9):765–74.
10. Mari A, Scala E, Palazzo P, Ridolfi S, Zennaro D, Carabella G. Bioinformatics applied to allergy: allergen databases, from collecting sequence information to data integration. The Allergome platform as a model. Cell Immunol. 2006;244(2):97–100.
11. Goodman RE, Vieths S, Sampson HA, Hill D, Ebisawa M, Taylor SL, et al. Allergenicity assessment of genetically modified crops—what makes sense? Nat Biotechnol. 2008;26(1):73–81.
12. Goodman RE, Ebisawa M, Ferreira F, Sampson HA, van Ree R, Vieths S, et al. AllergenOnline: a peer-reviewed, curated allergen database to assess novel food proteins for potential cross-reactivity. Mol Nutr Food Res. 2016;60(5):1183–98.
13. Nakamura R, Teshima R, Takagi K, Sawada J. Development of Allergen Database for Food Safety (ADFS): an integrated database to search allergens and predict allergenicity. Kokuritsu Iyakuhin Shokuhin Eisei Kenkyusho Hokoku. 2005;123:32–6.

14. Nakamura R, Nakamura R, Teshima R. Major revision of the allergen database for food safety (ADFS) and validation of the motif-based allergenicity prediction tool. Kokuritsu Iyakuhin Shokuhin Eisei Kenkyusho Hokoku. 2009;127:44–9.
15. van Ree R, Sapiter Ballerda D, Berin MC, Beuf L, Chang A, Gadermaier G, et al. The COMPARE database: a public resource for allergen identification, adapted for continuous improvement. Front Allergy. 2021;2:700533.
16. Ladics GS, Selgrade MK. Identifying food proteins with allergenic potential: evolution of approaches to safety assessment and research to provide additional tools. Regul Toxicol Pharmacol. 2009;54(Suppl. 3):S2–6.
17. Abdelmoteleb M, Zhang C, Furey B, Kozubal M, Griffiths H, Champeaud M, et al. Evaluating potential risks of food allergy of novel food sources based on comparison of proteins predicted from genomes and compared to www.AllergenOnline.org. Food Chem Toxicol. 2021;147:111888.
18. Goodman RE. Practical and predictive bioinformatics methods for the identification of potentially cross-reactive protein matches. Mol Nutr Food Res. 2006;50(7):655–60.
19. Herman RA, Song P. Validation of bioinformatic approaches for predicting allergen cross reactivity. Food Chem Toxicol. 2019;132:110656.
20. Herman RA, Song P. Allergen false-detection using official bioinformatic algorithms. GM Crops Food. 2020;11(2):93–6.
21. Ladics GS, Bannon GA, Silvanovich A, Cressman RF. Comparison of conventional FASTA identity searches with the 80 amino acid sliding window FASTA search for the elucidation of potential identities to known allergens. Mol Nutr Food Res. 2007;51(8):985–98.
22. Silvanovich A, Bannon G, McClain S. The use of E-scores to determine the quality of protein alignments. Regul Toxicol Pharmacol. 2009;54(Suppl. 3):S26–31.
23. Silvanovich A, Nemeth MA, Song P, Herman R, Tagliani L, Bannon GA. The value of short amino acid sequence matches for prediction of protein allergenicity. Toxicol Sci. 2006;90(1):252–8.
24. Song P, Herman R, Kumpatla S. 1:1 FASTA update: Using the power of E-values in FASTA to detect potential allergen cross-reactivity. Toxicol Rep. 2015;2:1145–8.
25. Aalberse RC. Structural biology of allergens. J Allergy Clin Immunol. 2000;106(2):228–38.
26. Asarnoj A, Nilsson C, Lidholm J, Glaumann S, Östblom E, Hedlin G, et al. Peanut component Ara h 8 sensitization and tolerance to peanut. J Allergy Clin Immunol. 2012;130(2):468–72.
27. Datema MR, Lyons SA, Fernández-Rivas M, Ballmer-Weber B, Knulst AC, Asero R, et al. Estimating the risk of severe peanut allergy using clinical background and IgE sensitization profiles. Front Allergy. 2021;2:670789.
28. Datema MR, van Ree R, Asero R, Barreales L, Belohlavkova S, de Blay F, et al. Component-resolved diagnosis and beyond: multivariable regression models to predict severity of hazelnut allergy. Allergy. 2018;73(3):549–59.
29. Dreskin SC, Koppelman SJ, Andorf S, Nadeau KC, Kalra A, Braun W, et al. The importance of the 2S albumins for allergenicity and cross-reactivity of peanuts, tree nuts, and sesame seeds. J Allergy Clin Immunol. 2021;147(4):1154–63.
30. Fernández-Rivas M, Bolhaar S, González-Mancebo E, Asero R, van Leeuwen A, Bohle B, et al. Apple allergy across Europe: how allergen sensitization profiles determine the clinical expression of allergies to plant foods. J Allergy Clin Immunol. 2006;118(2):481–8.
31. Kallen EJJ, Revers A, Fernández-Rivas M, Asero R, Ballmer-Weber B, Barreales L, et al. A European-Japanese study on peach allergy: IgE to Pru p 7 associates with severity. Allergy. 2023;78(9):2497–509.
32. Lyons SA, Datema MR, Le TM, Asero R, Barreales L, Belohlavkova S, et al. Walnut allergy across Europe: distribution of allergen sensitization patterns and prediction of severity. J Allergy Clin Immunol Pract. 2021;9(1):225–35.e10.
33. Ballmer-Weber BK, Fernandez-Rivas M, Beyer K, Defernez M, Sperrin M, Mackie AR, et al. How much is too much? Threshold dose distributions for 5 food allergens. J Allergy Clin Immunol. 2015;135(4):964–71.

34. Houben GF, Baumert JL, Blom WM, Kruizinga AG, Meima MY, Remington BC, et al. Full range of population eliciting dose values for 14 priority allergenic foods and recommendations for use in risk characterization. Food Chem Toxicol. 2020;146:111831.
35. Ivanciuc O, Schein CH, Garcia T, Oezguen N, Negi SS, Braun W. Structural analysis of linear and conformational epitopes of allergens. Regul Toxicol Pharmacol. 2009;54(Suppl. 3):S11–9.
36. Oezguen N, Zhou B, Negi SS, Ivanciuc O, Schein CH, Labesse G, et al. Comprehensive 3D-modeling of allergenic proteins and amino acid composition of potential conformational IgE epitopes. Mol Immunol. 2008;45(14):3740–7.
37. Ivanciuc O, Schein CH, Braun W. SDAP: database and computational tools for allergenic proteins. Nucleic Acids Res. 2003;31(1):359–62.
38. Kadam K, Karbhal R, Jayaraman VK, Sawant S, Kulkarni-Kale U. AllerBase: a comprehensive allergen knowledgebase. Database (Oxford) 2017;2017.
39. Radauer C, Bublin M, Wagner S, Mari A, Breiteneder H. Allergens are distributed into few protein families and possess a restricted number of biochemical functions. J Allergy Clin Immunol. 2008;121(4):847–52.
40. Schein CH, Negi SS, Braun W. Still SDAPing along: 20 years of the structural database of allergenic proteins. Front Allergy. 2022;3:863172.
41. Finn RD, Bateman A, Clements J, Coggill P, Eberhardt RY, Eddy SR, et al. Pfam: the protein families database. Nucleic Acids Res. 2014;42:D222–30.
42. Fleri W, Vaughan K, Salimi N, Vita R, Peters B, Sette A. The immune epitope database: how data are entered and retrieved. J Immunol Res. 2017;2017:5974574.
43. Martini S, Nielsen M, Peters B, Sette A. The immune epitope database and analysis resource program 2003–2018: reflections and outlook. Immunogenetics. 2020;72(1–2):57–76.
44. Vaughan K, Peters B, Larche M, Pomes A, Broide D, Sette A. Strategies to query and display allergy-derived epitope data from the immune epitope database. Int Arch Allergy Immunol. 2013;160(4):334–45.
45. Vita R, Mahajan S, Overton JA, Dhanda SK, Martini S, Cantrell JR, et al. The Immune Epitope Database (IEDB): 2018 update. Nucleic Acids Res. 2019;47(D1):D339–d43.
46. Zhao J, Timira V, Ahmed I, Chen Y, Wang H, Zhang Z, et al. Crustacean shellfish allergens: influence of food processing and their detection strategies. Crit Rev Food Sci Nutr. 2022;1-29
47. Breiteneder H, Radauer C. A classification of plant food allergens. J Allergy Clin Immunol. 2004;113(5):821–30.
48. Dall'Antonia F, Keller W. SPADE web service for prediction of allergen IgE epitopes. Nucleic Acids Res. 2019;47(W1):W496–w501.
49. Fiers MW, Kleter GA, Nijland H, Peijnenburg AA, Nap JP, van Ham RC. Allermatch, a webtool for the prediction of potential allergenicity according to current FAO/WHO Codex alimentarius guidelines. BMC Bioinformatics. 2004;5:133.
50. Goto K, Tamehiro N, Yoshida T, Hanada H, Sakuma T, Adachi R, et al. Novel machine learning method allerStat identifies statistically significant allergen-specific patterns in protein sequences. J Biol Chem. 2023;299(6):104733.
51. Krutz NL, Kimber I, Winget J, Nguyen MN, Limviphuvadh V, Maurer-Stroh S, et al. Application of AllerCatPro 2.0 for protein safety assessments of consumer products. Front. Allergy. 2023;4:1209495.
52. Kumar KK, Shelokar PS. An SVM method using evolutionary information for the identification of allergenic proteins. Bioinformation. 2008;2(6):253–6.
53. Li KB, Issac P, Krishnan A. Predicting allergenic proteins using wavelet transform. Bioinformatics. 2004;20(16):2572–8.
54. Martinez Barrio A, Soeria-Atmadja D, Nistér A, Gustafsson MG, Hammerling U, Bongcam-Rudloff E. EVALLER: a web server for in silico assessment of potential protein allergenicity. Nucleic Acids Res. 2007;35(Web Server issue):W694-700
55. Maurer-Stroh S, Krutz NL, Kern PS, Gunalan V, Nguyen MN, Limviphuvadh V, et al. AllerCatPro-prediction of protein allergenicity potential from the protein sequence. Bioinformatics. 2019;35(17):3020–7.

56. Negi SS, Braun W. Cross-react: a new structural bioinformatics method for predicting allergen cross-reactivity. Bioinformatics. 2017;33(7):1014–20.
57. Nguyen MN, Krutz NL, Limviphuvadh V, Lopata AL, Gerberick GF, Maurer-Stroh S. AllerCatPro 2.0: a web server for predicting protein allergenicity potential. Nucleic Acids Res. 2022;50(W1):W36–w43.
58. Soeria-Atmadja D, Lundell T, Gustafsson MG, Hammerling U. Computational detection of allergenic proteins attains a new level of accuracy with in silico variable-length peptide extraction and machine learning. Nucleic Acids Res. 2006;34(13):3779–93.
59. Stadler MB, Stadler BM. Allergenicity prediction by protein sequence. FASEB J. 2003;17(9):1141–3.
60. Westerhout J, Krone T, Snippe A, Babé L, McClain S, Ladics GS, et al. Allergenicity prediction of novel and modified proteins: not a mission impossible! development of a random forest allergenicity prediction model. Regul Toxicol Pharmacol. 2019;107:104422.
61. Breiteneder H, Kraft D. The History and science of the major birch pollen allergen bet v 1. Biomol Ther. 2023;13(7)
62. Hoffmann-Sommergruber K, Demoly P, Crameri R, Breiteneder H, Ebner C, Da Camara L, Machado M, et al. IgE reactivity to Api g 1, a major celery allergen, in a Central European population is based on primary sensitization by Bet v 1. J Allergy Clin Immunol. 1999;104(2 Pt 1):478–84.
63. Asero R, Brusca I, Cecchi L, Pignatti P, Pravettoni V, Scala E, et al. Why lipid transfer protein allergy is not a pollen-food syndrome: novel data and literature review. Eur Ann Allergy Clin Immunol. 2022;54(5):198–206.
64. Weghofer M, Grote M, Resch Y, Casset A, Kneidinger M, Kopec J, et al. Identification of Der p 23, a peritrophin-like protein, as a new major Dermatophagoides pteronyssinus allergen associated with the peritrophic matrix of mite fecal pellets. J Immunol. 2013;190(7):3059–67.
65. Brough HA, Nadeau KC, Sindher SB, Alkotob SS, Chan S, Bahnson HT, et al. Epicutaneous sensitization in the development of food allergy: what is the evidence and how can this be prevented? Allergy. 2020;75(9):2185–205.
66. Cabanillas B, Novak N. Effects of daily food processing on allergenicity. Crit Rev Food Sci Nutr. 2019;59(1):31–42.
67. Costa J, Bavaro SL, Benedé S, Diaz-Perales A, Bueno-Diaz C, Gelencser E, et al. Are physicochemical properties shaping the allergenic potency of plant allergens? Clin Rev Allergy Immunol. 2022;62(1):37–63.
68. Costa J, Villa C, Verhoeckx K, Cirkovic-Velickovic T, Schrama D, Roncada P, et al. Are physicochemical properties shaping the allergenic potency of animal allergens? Clin Rev Allergy Immunol. 2022;62(1):1–36.
69. Haidar E, Lakkis J, Karam M, Koubaa M, Louka N, Debs E. Peanut allergenicity: an insight into its mitigation using thermomechanical processing. Food Secur. 2023;12(6)
70. Masthoff LJ, Hoff R, Verhoeckx KC, van Os-Medendorp H, Michelsen-Huisman A, Baumert JL, et al. A systematic review of the effect of thermal processing on the allergenicity of tree nuts. Allergy. 2013;68(8):983–93.
71. Turner PJ, Mehr S, Sayers R, Wong M, Shamji MH, Campbell DE, et al. Loss of allergenic proteins during boiling explains tolerance to boiled peanut in peanut allergy. J Allergy Clin Immunol. 2014;134(3):751–3.
72. Bartra J, Mullol J, del Cuvillo A, Dávila I, Ferrer M, Jáuregui I, et al. Air pollution and allergens. J Investig Allergol Clin Immunol. 2007;17(Suppl. 2):3–8.
73. Wlasiuk G, Vercelli D. The farm effect, or: when, what and how a farming environment protects from asthma and allergic disease. Curr Opin Allergy Clin Immunol. 2012;12(5):461–6.
74. Larsen AI, Cederkvist L, Lykke AM, Wagner P, Johnsen CR, Poulsen LK. Allergy development in adulthood: an occupational cohort study of the manufacturing of industrial enzymes. J Allergy Clin Immunol Pract. 2020;8(1):210–8.
75. Logan K, Bahnson HT, Ylescupidez A, Beyer K, Bellach J, Campbell DE, et al. Early introduction of peanut reduces peanut allergy across risk groups in pooled and causal inference analyses. Allergy. 2023;78(5):1307–18.

Chapter 9
Digital Health and Asthma

Cristina Jácome, Ana Margarida Pereira, Bernardo Sousa Pinto, and João Almeida Fonseca

Contents

C. Jácome
Department of Community Medicine, Information and Health Decision Sciences, Center
for Health Technology and Services Research (CINTESIS) @ RiSE, MEDCIDS, Faculty
of Medicine of the University of Porto, Porto, Portugal

A. M. Pereira · J. A. Fonseca (✉)
Department of Community Medicine, Information and Health Decision Sciences, Center
for Health Technology and Services Research (CINTESIS) @ RiSE, MEDCIDS, Faculty
of Medicine of the University of Porto, Porto, Portugal

Allergy Unit CUF Porto Hospital & Instituto, Porto, Portugal

Patient Centred Innovation and Technology, Centro de Investigação em Tecnologias e
Serviços de Saúde, Centre for Health Technology and Services Research, University of Porto,
Porto, Portugal

B. Sousa Pinto
Department of Community Medicine, Information and Health Decision Sciences, Center
for Health Technology and Services Research (CINTESIS) @ RiSE, MEDCIDS, Faculty
of Medicine of the University of Porto, Porto, Portugal

Patient Centred Innovation and Technology, Centro de Investigação em Tecnologias e
Serviços de Saúde, Centre for Health Technology and Services Research, University of Porto,
Porto, Portugal

P. M. Matricardi, S. Dramburg, *Digital Allergology*, Health Informatics,
https://doi.org/10.1007/978-3-031-71021-6_9

135

Abstract This chapter starts by introducing the current unmet needs in asthma care and the potential role of digital health in revolutionizing how patients with asthma are managed. We will specifically approach the use of digital solutions in asthma to (i) improve surveillance at a population level, (ii) improve diagnosis and stratification at an individual level, and (iii) promote better management, namely through the use of mHealth, electronic patient-reported outcome measures (ePROMs), clinical decision support system (CDSS), and disease registries. In the end, we propose a digital health-integrated asthma care pathway aiming to achieve better patient-centered outcomes and reduce healthcare access inequalities.

9.1   Introduction

Asthma is one of the most common non-communicable diseases worldwide, affecting 262 million people [1]. The variable intensity of symptoms and airflow obstruction are key features of asthma [2]. This intra-individual variability demonstrates the crucial role of regular monitoring to identify the "**window of opportunity,**" a period of symptoms worsening that can promptly activate interventions and adjustments in treatment plans to prevent deterioration [3–6]. Adding to the intra-individual variability, asthma also has considerable inter-individual heterogeneity in its presentation, severity, and response to treatment [7, 8]. All these asthma specificities contribute to the complexity of asthma diagnosis and management in clinical practice.

Long-term goals for asthma management are to achieve good **control**, maintain normal lung function, reduce exacerbations, and minimize the impact on daily activities and quality of life [2]. Although asthma care has substantially improved over the years, inadequate asthma control remains a reality [9]. This is of great concern for all patients, but mainly for those with difficult-to-control and severe asthma. This minority group largely contributes to poor outcomes, including frequent emergency room visits, hospitalizations, and higher healthcare costs.

Multiple factors can cause the lack of asthma control. Among the most relevant are the overestimation of the level of asthma control by patients, poor assessment of asthma control by physicians, low adherence to treatment (including poor inhaler technique), the existence of complex multimorbidity patterns, and co-occurrence of different phenotypes (Table 9.1).

These unmet health needs can no longer be accepted and require novel care pathways to tackle them. Such pathways may benefit from digital health, which refers to the convergence of health care, informatics, and data science. **Digital health** is driving a revolution in asthma healthcare delivery [12]. It has a broad scope, including mobile health (mHealth), health information technologies (IT), wearable devices, telehealth and telemedicine, and personalized medicine through the use of algorithms, clinical decision support systems (CDSS), and digital biomarkers [12]. In asthma, it may be used to support disease identification, classification, and personalized care to ensure more adequate therapeutic management and patient

Table 9.1 Summary of current unmet needs in asthma care [10, 11]

Under- and misdiagnosis
Unsatisfactory disease awareness and overestimation of the level of asthma control by patients
Poor assessment of asthma control by the physician/healthcare providers
Management of comorbidities that vary across the life cycle with increasing complexity
Physician's noncompliance with guidelines and lack of action plans
Poor adherence of patients to treatments
Poor inhaler technique
Inadequate knowledge about self-management
Not matching treatment to the phenotypes
Insufficient capacity of randomized clinical trials to account for asthma heterogeneity and to represent real life
Incapacity of controlling some patients despite optimal pharmacotherapy and biologics (especially non-T2 phenotypes)
Inequalities in access to specialized asthma care

follow-up [11]. Moreover, it can be used to tackle the difficulties associated with dealing with the diverse aspects of asthma multimorbidity [13, 14]. Areas in rapid transformation include asthma diagnosis and stratification, remote monitoring and early warning tools, prediction of treatment response/decision support, and medication adherence. Advances are being driven by clinical research and real-world data (infodemiology methods, patient-generated data, disease registries) [15, 16], boosting multi-disciplinarity and **personalization**.

In this chapter, we will describe and provide examples of digital solutions contributing to revolutionizing how patients with asthma are managed. We will discuss the use of digital health tools in asthma to (i) improve surveillance at a population level, (ii) improve diagnosis and stratification at an individual level, and (iii) promote better, personalized asthma management. Finally, we will propose a digital health-integrated asthma care pathway including these innovative solutions.

9.2   Digital Health to Improve Asthma Surveillance at a Population Level

Digital health tools can provide information regarding asthma incidence, prevalence, burden, and exacerbation forecasts [15, 16]. "Classic" surveillance approaches can be complemented with data from other sources, such as those coming from internet users' activity measured with tools such as Google Trends (GTs) and analysis of social media data [16, 17]. This use of internet data, including the assessment of what is published online and what users search on the internet, with the ultimate aim of informing public health and public policy, is called **infodemiology**. [17] GTs are frequently used in infodemiology studies [18], informing on the relative volume of searches concerning a keyword (or set of keywords) entered into the Google search engine. The volume of online searches is expected to reflect the interest of internet users on a particular topic. In some cases, the volume of searches may, at least partially, reflect the incidence or burden of such disease [19]. However, GTs for the search term "asthma" appear to have limited usefulness as the available data suggests that it is strongly influenced by media coverage [16, 19]. Nevertheless, the weekly volume of online searches on "common cold"—a major risk factor for asthma exacerbations—was strongly correlated with English primary care surveillance data on asthma [16]. Moreover, it was correlated with the frequency of asthma hospitalizations in Portugal, Spain, Brazil, Norway, and Finland [20]. Models built to predict the weekly number of asthma exacerbations for one year based on hospitalizations and GTs data from the three previous years presented good forecasting capability [20]. These results suggest that the volume of online searches on "common cold" may be helpful as a tool to forecast increases in asthma exacerbations and health services use, particularly if complemented with other data, such as pollen and air quality levels (both from outdoor and indoor spaces, if available) and surveillance data on viral infections. More traditional data, such as those coming from electronic health records (EHR), can also be used complementarily, as already done to forecast influenza outbreaks [21]. Combining data from different sources and technologies may help develop digital surveillance-supporting tools in asthma, including those targeting early warning for exacerbations.

9.3   Digital Health to Improve Asthma Diagnosis and Stratification at an Individual Level

Asthma over- and underdiagnosis is frequent and is associated with inappropriate treatment and potential harm to the patient [22]. Performing a correct and timely diagnosis of asthma when no objective tests are readily available, either in a clinical or research setting, is challenging. To tackle this difficulty, several **scores and prediction tools** have been developed to identify patients with possible/probable asthma (e.g., A2 and GALEN scores for adults [23], Asthma Predictive Index for preschoolers) [24, 25]. These tools can be included in digital solutions to support more accurate identification of patients with possible undiagnosed asthma. As an example, the A2 and GALEN scores were implemented in the AIRDOC app [26]. The A2/GALEN scores can be answered spontaneously by the patient or be suggested based on the presence of specific characteristics, such as allergic rhinitis, which is an indication for asthma screening [27]. In the case of a positive screening, the patient is advised to contact the physician and, if necessary, proceed with further diagnostic assessment. The effectiveness of this approach is still to be validated in clinical studies.

These occasional reporting approaches are prone to information bias, [28] which might limit their usefulness. Making use of the increasing computational power, ease of use, and widespread penetration of smartphones, several mobile apps have been designed to collect patient data on a daily basis (e.g., MASK-air [29],

InspirerMundi) [30]. Although this daily direct patient data is usually collected as part of a monitoring strategy for individuals who already have an asthma diagnosis, a recent study has shown that it has the potential to give valuable information regarding asthma under- or overdiagnosis. In this study, MASK-air data was used to identify **clusters** of asthma patients and respective control patterns based on the presence of self-reported asthma, asthma medication use, and asthma symptoms [31]. The cluster related to possible asthma underdiagnosis accounted for around 10% of the app users [31]. These results suggest that the prospective collection of symptoms and medication use through an app can help clarify asthma diagnosis. Future implementation of clustering algorithms could be used to identify the patients that most benefit from a clinical evaluation targeting asthma diagnosis.

9.4 Digital Health for a Better, Personalized Asthma Management

Several digital health tools are available to improve the care of patients with asthma. These tools go from short message service (SMS)-based dose reminders [32] to telemedicine interventions [33] and multidimensional interactive mobile apps [26, 34, 35]. A review found that all these digital health interventions were well-received and accepted by patients, caregivers, and clinicians [36]. Nevertheless, they had varying degrees of success. The authors suggested that to be successful, digital tools for asthma monitoring and treatment personalization should combine accurate and objective measurement of adherence and of other clinical parameters with careful consideration of ease of use, clear communication of measured data, personalization, and patient engagement aspects [36]. Moreover, tools including CDSS should be based on the best available scientific evidence [37, 38]. In the following subsections, we will describe several tools, either currently available or under active development, that aim to promote a better management of patients with asthma while trying to answer those current challenges.

9.4.1 Patient Objective Monitoring Using mHealth

mHealth tools can be used to record, track, report, and share health data, deliver individually tailored disease education, promote positive health-related behaviors, and facilitate evidence-based care [35, 39]. Preliminary studies have shown the potential of mHealth tools to compare patients' reported symptoms associated with different medication schemes, to clarify patients' behaviors toward medication use/adherence, and to assess the impact on work productivity [40–43]. In asthma, their use is supported by the fact that around two-thirds of patients report being interested in using apps as part of their care [44].

Asthma mHealth includes not only standalone apps to be used in smartphones/ tablets but also connected external devices. External devices can help assess adherence to treatments (e.g., smart inhalers), monitor lung function (e.g., digital spirometers), and evaluate other physiological, health, and environmental measures that might be relevant in asthma care (e.g., oxygen saturation with digital oximeters, physical activity with activity trackers, air quality with indoor particulate sensors) [35]. However, the wide usage of external devices is bothersome, costly, and relies on the manufacturer's proprietary systems. The smartphone's embedded **sensors** may be a suitable alternative for many of the usages of external devices [45]. The smartphone's camera allows adherence measurement (objective verification of inhaler usage) based on real-time video capture of the inhaler's dosage counter, image processing techniques, and machine learning tools [46]. The Inspirers Inhaler Dosage Counter Detection Tool (available in the InspirerMundi app) was considered feasible and acceptable to monitor inhaler adherence in 107 real-world patients with asthma [30]. A tool to monitor pill intake using digital image processing, which analyzes blister images to detect missing and remaining pills, was developed and is being integrated into mHealth solutions [47].

Another embedded sensor, the smartphone's microphone, can be used to record cough, voice, breathing, and lung auscultation sounds that can be automatically analyzed to give information on a patient's respiratory status. Several studies targeting asthma and other respiratory disorders have described the use of apps to detect cough [48, 49], to support specific respiratory disease diagnoses based on cough patterns [48, 50], and to monitor clinical evolution and disease deterioration [51, 52] using changes in cough frequency and characteristics. The ResAppDx app, including an automated cough analysis algorithm, has shown good diagnostic accuracy (vs. clinical diagnosis) for asthma, pneumonia, lower respiratory tract disease, croup, and bronchiolitis in a study including 585 pediatric patients [50]. Another study, including 79 adults with asthma, found that nocturnal cough could detect weeks with asthma control deterioration and may have prognostic value for the early detection of asthma attacks [52]. Besides cough, analyzing voice, breathing, and forced expiratory maneuver sounds have been used to estimate lung function, showing promising results [53–55]. We tested the feasibility of smartphone auscultation in both children ($n = 92$) and adults ($n = 42$) during medical appointments, also with promising results. The auscultation with different smartphone built-in microphones was able to record lung sounds with quality and capture adventitious sounds [56].

Ultimately, sensor-collected data can be combined with data from other sources, such as georeferenced environmental factors and self-reported data (e.g., patient-reported outcome measures (PROM) and questionnaires).

9.4.2   The Path from PROMs to Digital Biomarkers

There are several PROMs assessing asthma control, such as the Asthma Control Test (ACT) [57], the Asthma Control Questionnaire (ACQ) [58], and the Control of Allergic Rhinitis and Asthma Test (CARAT) [59, 60]. These PROMs differ, among others, in their scope, recall period, and development and validation processes. CARAT's measurement properties were recently evaluated in a first-of-its-kind meta-analysis, confirming good internal consistency, reliability, construct validity, and responsiveness. This meta-analysis of measurement properties has set a higher level of evidence for asthma and/or allergic rhinitis control questionnaires, as the remaining PROMs have not been assessed using such an approach [61].

Some of the aforementioned PROMs have been implemented in digital tools. CARAT, which has been validated for digital use [62], is available in MASK-air (among other apps), where, even though assessing different timeframes, it has been shown to display moderate correlation with the visual analogue scale (VAS) evaluating daily asthma symptoms and with the percent of work/activities impairment due to allergies [63]. Besides these "traditional" PROMs, digital apps may also include specific tools to assess asthma symptoms or control, and they can also be used to develop new tools. A new score, **e-DASTHMA**, has recently been developed using MASK-air data [64]. It is a data-driven digital biomarker assessing daily asthma control and considering both symptoms and medication use [64]. It has been validated using MASK-air and INSPIRERS data and displayed moderate-high validity, high reliability, and moderate responsiveness [64].

The digital implementation of these PROMs, scales, and scores makes them more readily available for patients, allowing easier reporting and sharing with their physicians with automatic processing and enhanced data visualization. In asthma, they can be used in a strategy similar to the one used in diabetes (where daily glycemia data is complemented with periodic glycated hemoglobin assessment), with e-DASTHMA assessing short-term control and CARAT long-term control [64, 65]. This strategy has also been proposed for allergic rhinitis [65, 66]. These digital biomarkers can potentially improve patient monitoring, outcome prediction, and rapid assessment of exacerbations. Moreover, this digital biomarker-based strategy is being proposed to help monitor treatments effectiveness, with a particular relevance in severe asthma, where it can be used for deciding on biologics initiation/change, the definition of early stopping rules, and patient follow-up [65]. Finally, **electronic PROMs** (ePROMs) and **digital biomarkers** can, and should be, used as part of CDSS to support asthma management.

9.4.3 CDSS and Digital Prediction Tools to Further Support Patient Self-management

CDSS aid clinical decision-making by matching the characteristics of an individual patient with a computerized clinical knowledge base to provide patient-specific assessments or recommendations that are then presented to the clinician and/or the patient for a decision [38]. An effective CDSS should use the best scientific evidence to provide personalized information, adequately filtered and presented at appropriate times, ultimately leading to enhanced healthcare delivery [37, 38, 67]. In allergic diseases diagnosis, the possibility of implementing and using CDSS has been identified as a strength of mHealth, and the increasing amount of available scientific information, together with the increasing complexity of care personalization, is further raising the need for such systems [68]. In asthma, however, their relevance and impact are still to be thoroughly demonstrated. A systematic review on CDSS for healthcare professionals (HCP) managing asthma patients concluded that the current generation of CDSS was rarely used and that advice was not followed, making it unlikely that CDSS may lead to improved outcomes for asthma patients [69]. Another review on CDSS for HCP and/or asthma patients found that CDSS can improve asthma management processes and clinical outcomes, especially if it comprises multiple components (e.g., reminders and education) and promotes collaborative care (i.e., targeting both patients and physicians) [70]. Nevertheless, the effects of the CDSS on user workload, patient safety, costs, and patient and provider satisfaction remain understudied [70–72].

Recently, the increasing imbalance between healthcare capacity and demand, alongside the challenges posed by the COVID-19 pandemic, has created new opportunities for CDSS development in asthma care [73]. Some promising concepts have been described. MyAirCoach system combines an inhaler adapter, an indoor air-quality monitor, a physical activity tracker, a portable spirometer, a fraction exhaled nitric oxide device, and an app [74]. The CDSS architecture and outcomes of the first prototype implementation have been published [75]. A pragmatic randomized controlled trial showed improved asthma control and quality of life and fewer severe exacerbations in the group using MyAirCoach [74]. Nevertheless, it was only tested in a small number of patients, and there is a lack of long-term data. Another CDSS is the LungHealth asthma computer-guided consultation (CGC), which supports accurate guideline-based staging of asthma treatment and control with software prompting guideline-standard asthma management. Its use in primary care was associated with a change in treatment in over 40% of asthma patients, with 82% escalating therapy. Although this increase in the implementation of guideline-based asthma treatment might improve patient outcomes while addressing healthcare inequalities, there is still no data regarding the real clinical consequences of implementing these changes [73]. The AIRDOC app also integrates a CDSS to support **self-management** of patients with chronic obstructive respiratory disease, using self-reported data and objective monitoring tools (e.g., smartphone auscultation and respiratory function) to provide coaching and individualized management recommendations [26]. The app architecture [26], privacy and security features [76], the CDSS knowledge base development [77], and the design of the clinical portal that will allow sharing of data with HCP [78] have been described. The structured process of knowledge base development, based on guideline recommendations and performed by a team of healthcare, data science, and IT professionals, intends to assure that this CDSS is based on the best available evidence [77], strengthening its potential effectiveness [37, 38]. This approach was initially validated using anonymized data from previous studies but still needs to be tested in real-life settings [77]. Finally, **digital prediction tools** with the potential to identify the risk of asthma exacerbations and issuing warnings are being developed (e.g., MASK-POLLAR approach [79], ProAir Digihaler-based predictive Machine Learning Tool) [80].

9.4.4 Disease Registries to Gather Relevant Data from Asthma Patients

Patient **disease registries** are organized systems that use observational methods to collect uniform data for a population defined by a particular disease [81]. They are powerful tools to evaluate disease outcomes in real-life settings and are considered one of the most cost-effective ways of collecting patient information and longitudinal follow-up data, especially in low-prevalence diseases [81, 82]. They can be used for several purposes, like describing the natural history of a disease, determining the clinical and cost-effectiveness of different management approaches, assessing the safety or harm of treatments, measuring or improving the quality of care, and supporting public health surveillance and disease control [81].

The prevalence of asthma worldwide is estimated to be around 5% [83] (ranging between 1% and 29% in different countries [2]), with only about 5% to 10% of the total population with asthma [84] presenting a severe form of the disease. Nevertheless, this subset of patients presents high treatment, psychological, and socioeconomic burdens and is responsible for more than 60% of asthma-related healthcare costs [85]. This makes the study of patients with severe asthma strikingly relevant. However, as **severe asthma** is present in only a small portion of the patients with asthma, and considering its high heterogeneity, only extensive collaborations (e.g., severe asthma registries) can provide robust evidence to advance severe asthma care. Reflecting the importance given to collecting data from sufficient participants to perform pooled analyses that may contribute to improving disease phenotyping and patient management, GINA recommends including severe asthma patients in disease registries as an intrinsic component of asthma care [2].

There are several severe asthma registries worldwide. For example, the **Portuguese Severe Asthma Registry** (Registo de Asma Grave, RAG; asmagrave. pt) is open to all physicians treating severe asthma patients [86]. RAG includes features such as an automatic assessment of patients' eligibility and security and interoperability features to enable data sharing while preserving patient confidentiality. It allows prospective clinical data collection, promotes standardized care and collaborative clinical research, and aims to inform evidence-based healthcare policies for severe asthma [86]. Recently, it was linked with CARATm, an app for patients with difficult-to-control/severe asthma [87]. The app allows for collecting self-reported clinical data, including asthma symptoms, medication use and side effects, exacerbations, and absenteeism. App data integration in RAG helps reduce healthcare professional burden, as the physician will only need to confirm the data already in the registry.

RAG collaborates and shares data with the International Severe Asthma Registry (ISAR) and the Severe Heterogeneous Asthma Research collaboration, Patient-centered (SHARP). ISAR is a global initiative where national registries share their data for research purposes [88]. It collects patient-level, anonymous, longitudinal, real-life, standardized, high-quality data from more than 25 countries worldwide. SHARP is a Pan-European network of registries and severe asthma centers that work together to perform registry-based real-world research [89]. The model of the SHARP Central Registry has been harmonized with the international Observational Medical Outcomes Partnership (OMOP) [90] common data model that allows federated analyses with other OMOP-harmonized severe asthma registries. ISAR and SHARP are currently performing over 30 research projects, most of which include data from RAG and several other national severe asthma registries.

9.5   A Digital Health-Integrated Asthma Care Pathway

The previous sections described how digital health can have a relevant role throughout the whole journey of the patient with asthma and explored some of its potentialities: helping in the correct asthma diagnosis [26, 31], measuring medication adherence [30, 35, 47], estimating lung function and respiratory status with smartphone sensors [52–56], allowing the application of digital biomarker-based strategies (including through CDSS) in patient monitoring and management [64, 65], improving the assessment of the risk of exacerbations and issuing warnings [79, 91], and gathering relevant data from asthma patients in disease registries [86, 88, 89]. Moreover, it can support phenotypic characterization and treatment personalization, including severe asthma [31, 42, 65], can ease the identification and help minimize short-acting β-agonist (SABA)/oral corticosteroid (OCS) overuse [92, 93], and promote shared-decision-making [94, 95].

Considering all these potential advantages of digital health tools for asthma diagnosis and management, an integrated asthma care pathway combining technological and organizational solutions may contribute to overcoming some of the limitations of current healthcare models [96]. In fact, healthcare systems struggle with the imbalance between capacity and demand, which appears to be associated with geographical/regional inequities. That is, traditional healthcare models appear to be particularly failing in more remote areas, where there is a lower offer of health services. As an example, a preliminary study performed in Portugal and Spain observed the frequency of asthma hospitalizations to be particularly high in some of the regions with the lowest population density and highest aging index [97].

In this context, we propose a digital health-integrated pathway (Fig. 9.1) aiming to (i) achieve better asthma control and quality of life, (ii) improve healthcare sustainability by reducing the need for unplanned outpatient visits, emergency department visits, and hospitalizations, and (iii) tackle existing inequities in asthma care. The proposed integrated pathway requires a network of institutions involved in supporting and treating asthma patients, including not only primary care and hospital care institutions but also community pharmacies, social care, and other community organizations. This network should be capable of (i) identifying more critically ill patients, (ii) providing closer/intensive care to these patients, and (iii) integrating digital solutions centered on the patient and their

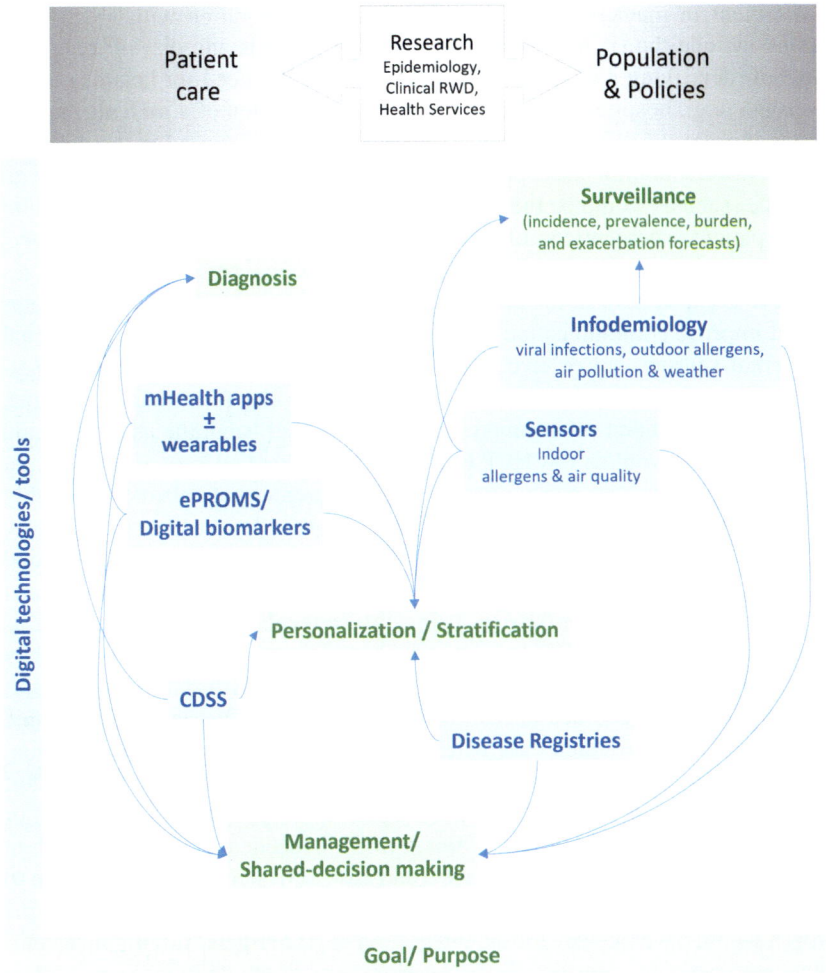

Fig. 9.1 Proposed approach for a digital health-integrated asthma care pathway that will target both better patient care and improved population and health policies, supported by the best evidence from different types of research. mHealth apps, using internal and external smartphone sensors (including wearables), applying ePROMS/digital biomarkers, and implementing CDSS will be central in patient care, contributing to improved asthma diagnosis, promotion of shared decision-making, and personalized medicine. Disease registries will support individual patient care while informing clinical research and policies. Infodemiology will be essential to asthma surveillance but can also be used to support patient management and personalized care, namely through exacerbation forecasts. Indoor sensors (e.g., for allergen and air quality) can be used by individual patients or at public places (e.g., schools or public buildings) to promote personalized patient management further and improve disease surveillance (for example, informing exacerbation forecasts)*CDSS* clinical decision support system, *ePROMS* electronic patient-reported outcome measures, *RWD* real-world data

empowerment in managing the disease in close collaboration with HCP. Such solutions include the (i) routine use of electronic records and disease registries capable of identifying patients with a potentially greater need for healthcare services usage (e.g., hospital admissions) and (ii) the inclusion of a **mHealth application** that assesses ePROMS/digital biomarkers and can be used in the patient's daily life to self-monitor and improve their asthma control. An application with that profile (such as would be the case of MASK-air [13] or AIRDOC [26]) could increase patients' perceptions of their disease, improve therapeutic adherence, constitute a vehicle through which patients would receive personalized messages to improve control, help in the early detection of situations of asthma deterioration, and improve communication with HCP. This app could be linked to internal and external sensors and receive data from other sources (e.g., infodemiology-based data, surveillance on air quality and pollen levels) to further personalize care and support guided self-management. On the other hand, the use of specific **disease registries** would allow HCP to collect information on a set of key relevant variables (including those needed for the identification of patients most probably requiring further assessment and treatment) in a standardized and structured way irrespective of their work setting or location. For this pathway, the application and the disease registries would need to be adequately integrated with each other and with electronic health records (e.g., using **interoperability standards** such as FHIR [98] or openEHR [99] and common data models such as those developed by OMOP [90, 100]). Therefore, data entered by the patients in the mobile health application could be recorded in real time in the disease registries and electronic health records. The provided data would be presented in **dashboards**, allowing HCP to monitor patients' asthma control between appointments and send alert messages if necessary (for example, during periods of poorer disease control or less adherence to therapy). When an appointment is needed, **telemedicine** might facilitate access and reduce patient travels and costs. Physicians also seem open to using it to recruit and assess patients in clinical research [101]. Finally, this approach would pave the way for the integration of (i) **artificial intelligence** components automatically detecting early deteriorations of the daily monitoring data reported by the patient in the mHealth application, (ii) CDSS components targeting both physicians and patients and strengthening collaborative care and shared decision-making.

In short, this strategy proposes adopting integrated digital health tools supported by the best evidence with real-world data and health technology assessment studies to deploy next-generation care pathways within a care network involving hospital-based care, community-based care, and social services. Such digital-based strategies should be able to provide data-driven, personalized, efficient, and interconnected care to asthma patients, especially to those with more severe disease, and deliver better asthma control with minimal need for acute care episodes. Such digital-based change management has a high potential to overcome limitations of access to healthcare, reducing inequalities in asthma care and ultimately improving the overall quality of care and patient experience.

References

1. Safiri S, Carson-Chahhoud K, Karamzad N, Sullman MJM, Nejadghaderi SA, Taghizadieh A, et al. Prevalence, deaths, and disability-adjusted life-years due to asthma and its attributable risk factors in 204 countries and territories, 1990–2019. Chest. 2022;161(2):318–29. https://doi.org/10.1016/j.chest.2021.09.042.
2. Global initiative for asthma: global strategy for asthma management and prevention. https://ginasthma.org/wp-content/uploads/2023/05/GINA-2023-Full-Report-2023-WMS.pdf; 2023. Access 06/2023.
3. Buhl R, Kuna P, Peters MJ, Andersson TL, Naya IP, Peterson S, et al. The effect of budesonide/formoterol maintenance and reliever therapy on the risk of severe asthma exacerbations following episodes of high reliever use: an exploratory analysis of two randomised, controlled studies with comparisons to standard therapy. Respir Res. 2012;13(1):59. https://doi.org/10.1186/1465-9921-13-59.
4. Chipps BE, Albers FC, Reilly L, Johnsson E, Cappelletti C, Papi A. Efficacy and safety of as-needed albuterol/budesonide versus albuterol in adults and children aged ≥4 years with moderate-to-severe asthma: rationale and design of the randomised, double-blind, active-controlled MANDALA study. BMJ Open Respir Res. 2021;8(1) https://doi.org/10.1136/bmjresp-2021-001077.
5. O'Byrne PM, FitzGerald JM, Bateman ED, Barnes PJ, Zhong N, Keen C, et al. Inhaled combined budesonide-formoterol as needed in mild asthma. N Engl J Med. 2018;378(20):1865–76. https://doi.org/10.1056/NEJMoa1715274.
6. Lugogo N, Skolnik N, Jiang Y. A paradigm shift for asthma care. J Fam Pract. 2022;71(Suppl. 6):S1–s10. https://doi.org/10.12788/jfp.0437.
7. Lui JK, Lutchen KR. The role of heterogeneity in asthma: a structure-to-function perspective. Clin Transl Med. 2017;6(1):29. https://doi.org/10.1186/s40169-017-0159-0.
8. Carr TF, Bleecker E. Asthma heterogeneity and severity. World Allergy Organ J. 2016;9(1):41. https://doi.org/10.1186/s40413-016-0131-2.
9. Larsson K, Kankaanranta H, Janson C, Lehtimäki L, Ställberg B, Løkke A, et al. Bringing asthma care into the twenty-first century. NPJ Prim Care Respir Med. 2020;30(1):25. https://doi.org/10.1038/s41533-020-0182-2.
10. Busse WW, Kraft M. Current unmet needs and potential solutions to uncontrolled asthma. Eur Respir Rev. 2022;31(163) https://doi.org/10.1183/16000617.0176-2021.
11. Caminati M, Vaia R, Furci F, Guarnieri G, Senna G. Uncontrolled asthma: unmet needs in the management of patients. J Asthma Allergy. 2021;14:457–66. https://doi.org/10.2147/jaa.S260604.
12. US Food and Drug Administration: What is digital health? https://www.fda.gov/medical-devices/digital-health-center-excellence/what-digital-health Accessed 06/2023.
13. Bousquet J, Anto JM, Sousa-Pinto B, Czarlewski W, Bedbrook A, Haahtela T, et al. Digitally-enabled, patient-centred care in rhinitis and asthma multimorbidity: The ARIA-MASK-air(®) approach. Clin Transl Allergy. 2023;13(1):e12215. https://doi.org/10.1002/clt2.12215.
14. Varkonyi-Sepp J, Freeman A, Ainsworth B, Kadalayil LP, Haitchi HM, Kurukulaaratchy RJ. Multimorbidity in difficult asthma: the need for personalised and non-pharmacological approaches to address a difficult breathing syndrome. J Pers Med. 2022;12(9) https://doi.org/10.3390/jpm12091435.
15. Moloney M, Digby G, MacKinnon M, Morra A, Barber D, Queenan J, et al. Primary care asthma surveillance: a review of knowledge translation tools and strategies for quality improvement. Allergy Asthma Clin Immunol. 2023;19(1):3. https://doi.org/10.1186/s13223-022-00755-2.
16. Sousa-Pinto B, Antó JM, Sheikh A, de Lusignan S, Haahtela T, Fonseca JA, et al. Comparison of epidemiologic surveillance and Google Trends data on asthma and allergic rhinitis in England. Allergy. 2022;77(2):675–8. https://doi.org/10.1111/all.15139.

17. Eysenbach G. Infodemiology and infoveillance: framework for an emerging set of public health informatics methods to analyze search, communication and publication behavior on the Internet. J Med Internet Res. 2009;11(1):e11. https://doi.org/10.2196/jmir.1157.
18. Mavragani A, Ochoa G. Google Trends in infodemiology and infoveillance: methodology framework. JMIR Public Health Surveill. 2019;5(2):e13439. https://doi.org/10.2196/13439.
19. Sousa-Pinto B, Heffler E, Antó A, Czarlewski W, Bedbrook A, Gemicioglu B, et al. Anomalous asthma and chronic obstructive pulmonary disease Google Trends patterns during the COVID-19 pandemic. Clin Transl Allergy. 2020;10(1):47. https://doi.org/10.1186/s13601-020-00352-9.
20. Sousa-Pinto B, Halonen JI, Antó A, Jormanainen V, Czarlewski W, Bedbrook A, et al. Prediction of asthma hospitalizations for the common cold using Google Trends: infodemiology study. J Med Internet Res. 2021;23(7):e27044. https://doi.org/10.2196/27044.
21. Lu FS, Hou S, Baltrusaitis K, Shah M, Leskovec J, Sosic R, et al. Accurate influenza monitoring and forecasting using novel internet data streams: a case study in the Boston Metropolis. JMIR Public Health Surveill. 2018;4(1):e4. https://doi.org/10.2196/publichealth.8950.
22. Kavanagh J, Jackson DJ, Kent BD. Over- and under-diagnosis in asthma. Breathe (Sheff). 2019;15(1):e20–e7. https://doi.org/10.1183/20734735.0362-2018.
23. Sá-Sousa A, Pereira AM, Almeida R, Araújo L, Couto M, Jacinto T, et al. Adult asthma scores-development and validation of multivariable scores to identify asthma in surveys. J Allergy Clin Immunol Pract. 2019;7(1):183–90.e6. https://doi.org/10.1016/j.jaip.2018.06.024.
24. Castro-Rodriguez JA, Forno E, Padilla O, Casanello P, Krause BJ, Borzutzky A. The asthma predictive index as a surrogate diagnostic tool in preschoolers: analysis of a longitudinal birth cohort. Pediatr Pulmonol. 2021;56(10):3183–8. https://doi.org/10.1002/ppul.25592.
25. Castro-Rodríguez JA, Holberg CJ, Wright AL, Martinez FD. A clinical index to define risk of asthma in young children with recurrent wheezing. Am J Respir Crit Care Med. 2000;162(4 Pt 1):1403–6. https://doi.org/10.1164/ajrccm.162.4.9912111.
26. Almeida R, Jácome C, Martinho D, Vieira Marques P, Jacinto T, Ferreira A, et al. AIRDOC: Smart mobile application for individualized support and monitoring of respiratory function and sounds of patients with chronic obstructive disease. In: 12th IADIS International Conference e-Health 2020, EH 2020, part of the 14th Multi Conference on Computer Science and Information Systems, MCCSIS 2020: IADIS; 2020. p. 78–88.
27. Bousquet J, Khaltaev N, Cruz AA, Denburg J, Fokkens WJ, Togias A, et al. Allergic Rhinitis and its Impact on Asthma (ARIA) 2008 update (in collaboration with the World Health Organization, GA(2)LEN and AllerGen). Allergy. 2008;63(Suppl. 86):8–160. https://doi.org/10.1111/j.1398-9995.2007.01620.x.
28. Mirabelli MC, Beavers SF, Flanders WD, Chatterjee AB. Reliability in reporting asthma history and age at asthma onset. J Asthma. 2014;51(9):956–63. https://doi.org/10.3109/02770903.2014.930480.
29. Bousquet J, Arnavielhe S, Bedbrook A, Bewick M, Laune D, Mathieu-Dupas E, et al. MASK 2017: ARIA digitally-enabled, integrated, person-centred care for rhinitis and asthma multimorbidity using real-world-evidence. Clin Transl Allergy. 2018;8:45. https://doi.org/10.1186/s13601-018-0227-6.
30. Jácome C, Almeida R, Pereira AM, Amaral R, Mendes S, Alves-Correia M, et al. Feasibility and acceptability of an asthma app to monitor medication adherence: mixed methods study. JMIR Mhealth Uhealth. 2021;9(5):e26442. https://doi.org/10.2196/26442.
31. Bousquet J, Sousa-Pinto B, Anto JM, Amaral R, Brussino L, Canonica GW, et al. Identification by cluster analysis of patients with asthma and nasal symptoms using the MASK-air® mHealth app. Pulmonology. 2023;29(4):292–305. https://doi.org/10.1016/j.pulmoe.2022.10.005.
32. Britto MT, Rohan JM, Dodds CM, Byczkowski TL. A randomized trial of user-controlled text messaging to improve asthma outcomes: a pilot study. Clin Pediatr (Phila). 2017;56(14):1336–44. https://doi.org/10.1177/0009922816684857.

33. van den Wijngaart LS, Roukema J, Boehmer ALM, Brouwer ML, Hugen CAC, Niers LEM, et al. A virtual asthma clinic for children: fewer routine outpatient visits, same asthma control. Eur Respir J. 2017;50(4) https://doi.org/10.1183/13993003.00471-2017.
34. Davis SR, Peters D, Calvo RA, Sawyer SM, Foster JM, Smith LD. A consumer designed smartphone app for young people with asthma: pilot of engagement and acceptability. J Asthma. 2021;58(2):253–61. https://doi.org/10.1080/02770903.2019.1680997.
35. Kouri A, Gupta S. Mobile health for asthma. Chest Pulm. 2023;1(1):100002. https://doi.org/10.1016/j.chpulm.2023.100002.
36. Mosnaim G, Safioti G, Brown R, DePietro M, Szefler SJ, Lang DM, et al. Digital health technology in asthma: a comprehensive scoping review. J Allergy Clin Immunol Pract. 2021;9(6):2377–98. https://doi.org/10.1016/j.jaip.2021.02.028.
37. Purcell GP. What makes a good clinical decision support system. Br Med J. 2005;330(7494):740–1.
38. Sim I, Gorman P, Greenes RA, Haynes RB, Kaplan B, Lehmann H, et al. Clinical decision support systems for the practice of evidence-based medicine. J Am Med Inform Assoc. 2001;8(6):527–34. https://doi.org/10.1136/jamia.2001.0080527.
39. Roess A. The promise, growth, and reality of mobile health—another data-free zone. N Engl J Med. 2017;377(21):2010–1. https://doi.org/10.1056/NEJMp1713180.
40. Bédard A, Antó JM, Fonseca JA, Arnavielhe S, Bachert C, Bedbrook A, et al. Correlation between work impairment, scores of rhinitis severity and asthma using the MASK-air(®) App. Allergy. 2020;75(7):1672–88. https://doi.org/10.1111/all.14204.
41. WHO Global Observatory for eHealth. mHealth: new horizons for health through mobile technologies: second global survey on eHealth. https://apps.who.int/iris/handle/10665/44607; 2011.
42. Benfante A, Sousa-Pinto B, Pillitteri G, Battaglia S, Fonseca J, Bousquet J, et al. Applicability of the MASK-Air(®) app to severe asthma treated with biologic molecules: a pilot study. Int J Mol Sci. 2022;23(19) https://doi.org/10.3390/ijms231911470.
43. Sousa-Pinto B, Louis R, Anto JM, Amaral R, Sá-Sousa A, Czarlewski W, et al. Adherence to inhaled corticosteroids and long-acting β2-agonists in asthma: a MASK-air study. Pulmonology. 2023; https://doi.org/10.1016/j.pulmoe.2023.07.004.
44. Jácome C, Almeida R, Pereira AM, Araújo L, Correia MA, Pereira M, et al. Asthma app use and interest among patients with asthma: a multicenter study. J Investig Allergol Clin Immunol. 2020;30(2):137–40. https://doi.org/10.18176/jiaci.0456.
45. Majumder S, Deen MJ. Smartphone sensors for health monitoring and diagnosis. Sensors (Basel). 2019;19(9) https://doi.org/10.3390/s19092164.
46. Vieira-Marques P, Almeida R, Teixeira JF, Valente J, Jácome C, Cachim A, et al. InspirerMundi—remote monitoring of inhaled medication adherence through objective verification based on combined image processing techniques. Methods Inf Med. 2021;60(S 01):e9–e19. https://doi.org/10.1055/s-0041-1726277.
47. Holtkötter J, Amaral R, Almeida R, Jácome C, Cardoso R, Pereira A, et al. Development and validation of a digital image processing-based pill detection tool for an oral medication self-monitoring system. Sensors (Basel). 2022;22(8) https://doi.org/10.3390/s22082958.
48. Alqudaihi KS, Aslam N, Khan IU, Almuhaideb AM, Alsunaidi SJ, Ibrahim N, et al. Cough sound detection and diagnosis using artificial intelligence techniques: challenges and opportunities. IEEE Access. 2021;9:102327–44. https://doi.org/10.1109/access.2021.3097559.
49. Rahman MJ, Nemati E, Rahman M, Vatanparvar K, Nathan V, Kuang J. Efficient online cough detection with a minimal feature set using smartphones for automated assessment of pulmonary patients. In: Proceedings of the ninth international conference on ambient computing, applications, services and technologies (AMBIENT 2019), Porto, Portugal; 2019.
50. Porter P, Abeyratne U, Swarnkar V, Tan J, Ng T-w, Brisbane JM, et al. A prospective multicentre study testing the diagnostic accuracy of an automated cough sound centred analytic system for the identification of common respiratory disorders in children. Respir Res. 2019;20(1):81. https://doi.org/10.1186/s12931-019-1046-6.

51. Barata F, Cleres D, Tinschert P, Iris Shih CH, Rassouli F, Boesch M, et al. Nighttime continuous contactless smartphone-based cough monitoring for the ward: validation study. JMIR Form Res. 2023;7:e38439. https://doi.org/10.2196/38439.

52. Tinschert P, Rassouli F, Barata F, Steurer-Stey C, Fleisch E, Puhan MA, et al. Nocturnal cough and sleep quality to assess asthma control and predict attacks. J Asthma Allergy. 2020;13:669–78. https://doi.org/10.2147/jaa.S278155.

53. Teixeira JF, Teixeira LF, Fonseca J, Jacinto T. Automatic analysis of lung function based on smartphone recordings. In: Fred A, Gamboa H, Elias D, editors. Biomedical engineering systems and technologies. Cham: Springer International Publishing; 2015. p. 390–402.

54. Rahman MM, Ahmed T, Nemati E, Nathan V, Vatanparvar K, Blackstock E, et al. ExhaleSense: detecting high fidelity forced exhalations to estimate lung obstruction on smartphones. In: 2020 IEEE International Conference on Pervasive Computing and Communications (PerCom); 2020. p. 1–10.

55. Chun KS, Nathan V, Vatanparvar K, Nemati E, Rahman MM, Blackstock E, et al. Towards passive assessment of pulmonary function from natural speech recorded using a mobile phone. In: 2020 IEEE International Conference on Pervasive Computing and Communications (PerCom); 2020. p. 1–10.

56. Ferreira-Cardoso H, Jácome C, Silva S, Amorim A, Redondo MT, Fontoura-Matias J, et al. Lung auscultation using the smartphone-feasibility study in real-world clinical practice. Sensors (Basel). 2021;21(14) https://doi.org/10.3390/s21144931.

57. Nathan RA, Sorkness CA, Kosinski M, Schatz M, Li JT, Marcus P, et al. Development of the asthma control test: a survey for assessing asthma control. J Allergy Clin Immunol. 2004;113(1):59–65. https://doi.org/10.1016/j.jaci.2003.09.008.

58. Juniper EF, O'Byrne PM, Guyatt GH, Ferrie PJ, King DR. Development and validation of a questionnaire to measure asthma control. Eur Respir J. 1999;14(4):902–7. https://doi.org/10.1034/j.1399-3003.1999.14d29.x.

59. Nogueira-Silva L, Martins SV, Cruz-Correia R, Azevedo LF, Morais-Almeida M, Bugalho-Almeida A, et al. Control of allergic rhinitis and asthma test—a formal approach to the development of a measuring tool. Respir Res. 2009;10(1):52. https://doi.org/10.1186/1465-9921-10-52.

60. Fonseca JA, Nogueira-Silva L, Morais-Almeida M, Azevedo L, Sa-Sousa A, Branco-Ferreira M, et al. Validation of a questionnaire (CARAT10) to assess rhinitis and asthma in patients with asthma. Allergy. 2010;65(8):1042–8. https://doi.org/10.1111/j.1398-9995.2009.02310.x.

61. Vieira RJ, Sousa-Pinto B, Cardoso-Fernandes A, Jácome C, Portela D, Amaral R, et al. Control of allergic rhinitis and asthma test: a systematic review of measurement properties and COSMIN analysis. Clin Transl Allergy. 2022;12(9):e12194. https://doi.org/10.1002/clt2.12194.

62. Jácome C, Pereira R, Almeida R, Amaral R, Correia MA, Mendes S, et al. Validation of app and phone versions of the control of allergic rhinitis and asthma test (CARAT). J Investig Allergol Clin Immunol. 2021;31(3):270–3. https://doi.org/10.18176/jiaci.0640.

63. Sousa-Pinto B, Sá-Sousa A, Amaral R, Czarlewski W, Bedbrook A, Anto JM, et al. Assessment of the Control of Allergic Rhinitis and Asthma Test (CARAT) using MASK-air. J Allergy Clin Immunol Pract. 2022;10(1):343–5. https://doi.org/10.1016/j.jaip.2021.09.012.

64. Sousa-Pinto B, Jácome C, Pereira AM, Regateiro FS, Almeida R, Czarlewski W, et al. Development and validation of an electronic daily control score for asthma (e-DASTHMA): a real-world direct patient data study. Lancet Digit Health. 2023;5(4):e227–38. https://doi.org/10.1016/s2589-7500(23)00020-1.

65. Bousquet J, Shamji MH, Anto JM, Schünemann HJ, Canonica GW, Jutel M, et al. Patient-centered digital biomarkers for allergic respiratory diseases and asthma: the ARIA-EAACI approach—ARIA-EAACI Task Force Report. Allergy. 2023;78(7):1758–76. https://doi.org/10.1111/all.15740.

66. Sousa-Pinto B, Azevedo LF, Jutel M, Agache I, Canonica GW, Czarlewski W, et al. Development and validation of combined symptom-medication scores for allergic rhinitis. Allergy. 2022;77(7):2147–62. https://doi.org/10.1111/all.15199.

67. Osheroff JA, Teich JM, Middleton B, Steen EB, Wright A, Detmer DE. A roadmap for national action on clinical decision support. J Am Med Inform Assoc. 2007;14(2):141–5. https://doi.org/10.1197/jamia.M2334.
68. Pereira AM, Jácome C, Almeida R, Fonseca JA. How the smartphone is changing allergy diagnostics. Curr Allergy Asthma Rep. 2018;18(12):69. https://doi.org/10.1007/s11882-018-0824-4.
69. Matui P, Wyatt JC, Pinnock H, Sheikh A, McLean S. Computer decision support systems for asthma: a systematic review. NPJ Prim Care Respir Med. 2014;24:14005. https://doi.org/10.1038/npjpcrm.2014.5.
70. Fathima M, Peiris D, Naik-Panvelkar P, Saini B, Armour CL. Effectiveness of computerized clinical decision support systems for asthma and chronic obstructive pulmonary disease in primary care: a systematic review. BMC Pulm Med. 2014;14:189. https://doi.org/10.1186/1471-2466-14-189.
71. Dramburg S, Marchante Fernández M, Potapova E, Matricardi PM. The potential of clinical decision support systems for prevention, diagnosis, and monitoring of allergic diseases. Front Immunol. 2020;11:2116. https://doi.org/10.3389/fimmu.2020.02116.
72. Bousquet J. Electronic clinical decision support system (eCDSS) in the management of asthma: from theory to practice. Eur Respir J. 2019;53(4) https://doi.org/10.1183/13993003.00339-2019.
73. Chakrabarti B, Kane B, Barrow C, Stonebanks J, Reed L, Pearson MG, et al. The feasibility and impact of implementing a computer-guided consultation to target health inequality in Asthma. NPJ Prim Care Respir Med. 2023;33(1):6. https://doi.org/10.1038/s41533-023-00329-8.
74. Khusial RJ, Honkoop PJ, Usmani O, Soares M, Simpson A, Biddiscombe M, et al. Effectiveness of myAirCoach: a mHealth self-management system in asthma. J Allergy Clin Immunol Pract. 2020;8(6):1972–9.e8. https://doi.org/10.1016/j.jaip.2020.02.018.
75. Kocsis O, Lalos A, Arvanitis G, Moustakas K. Multi-model short-term prediction schema for mHealth empowering asthma self-management. Electron Notes Theor Comput Sci. 2019;343:3–17. https://doi.org/10.1016/j.entcs.2019.04.007.
76. Ferreira A, Almeida R, Almeida R, Jácome C, Fonseca J, Vieira-Marques P. mHealth to securely coach chronic patients; 2021. p. 805–13.
77. Pereira AM, Jácome C, Jacinto T, Amaral R, Pereira M, Sá-Sousa A, et al. Multidisciplinary development and initial validation of a clinical knowledge base on chronic respiratory diseases for mHealth decision support systems. J Med Internet Res. 2023;25:e45364.
78. Esteves A. Portal clínico—Uma visão integrada de múltiplas fontes de dados gerados por doentes respiratórios crónicos. FMUP—Faculdade de Medicina da Universidade do Porto; 2021.
79. Sofiev M, Palamarchuk Y, Bédard A, Basagana X, Anto JM, Kouznetsov R, et al. A demonstration project of Global Alliance against Chronic Respiratory Diseases: prediction of interactions between air pollution and allergen exposure-the Mobile Airways Sentinel NetworK-Impact of air POLLution on Asthma and Rhinitis approach. Chin Med J. 2020;133(13):1561–7. https://doi.org/10.1097/cm9.0000000000000916.
80. Lugogo NL, DePietro M, Reich M, Merchant R, Chrystyn H, Pleasants R, et al. A predictive machine learning tool for asthma exacerbations: results from a 12-week, open-label study using an electronic multi-dose dry powder inhaler with integrated sensors. J Asthma Allergy. 2022;15:1623–37. https://doi.org/10.2147/jaa.S377631.
81. Gliklich RE, Leavy MB, Dreyer NA: Registries for evaluating patient outcomes: a user's guide: 4th ed. https://effectivehealthcare.ahrq.gov/products/registries-guide-4th-edition/users-guide (Content last reviewed September 2020). Accessed July 09, 2023.
82. Hageman IC, van Rooij IALM, de Blaauw I, Trajanovska M, King SK. A systematic overview of rare disease patient registries: challenges in design, quality management, and maintenance. Orphanet J Rare Dis. 2023;18(1):106. https://doi.org/10.1186/s13023-023-02719-0.
83. Song P, Adeloye D, Salim H, Dos Santos JP, Campbell H, Sheikh A, et al. Global, regional, and national prevalence of asthma in 2019: a systematic analysis and modelling study. J Glob Health. 2022;12:04052. https://doi.org/10.7189/jogh.12.04052.

84. Chung KF, Wenzel SE, Brozek JL, Bush A, Castro M, Sterk PJ, et al. International ERS/ATS guidelines on definition, evaluation and treatment of severe asthma. Eur Respir J. 2014;43(2):343–73. https://doi.org/10.1183/09031936.00202013.
85. Wang E, Wechsler ME, Tran TN, Heaney LG, Jones RC, Menzies-Gow AN, et al. Characterization of severe asthma worldwide: data from the international severe asthma registry. Chest. 2020;157(4):790–804. https://doi.org/10.1016/j.chest.2019.10.053.
86. Sá-Sousa A, Fonseca JA, Pereira AM, Ferreira A, Arrobas A, Mendes A, et al. The Portuguese severe asthma registry: development, features, and data sharing policies. Biomed Res Int. 2018;2018:1495039. https://doi.org/10.1155/2018/1495039.
87. João C, Sá-Sousa A, Jácome C, Amaral C, Bernardo F, Valente J, et al. CARATm—uma aplicação móvel para recolha de dados auto-reportados no mundo real interoperável com o Registo Português de Asma Grave. Revista Portuguesa Imunoalergol. 2022;XXX(1):43.
88. Canonica GW, Alacqua M, Altraja A, Backer V, Bel E, Bjermer L, et al. International severe asthma registry: mission statement. Chest. 2020;157(4):805–14. https://doi.org/10.1016/j.chest.2019.10.051.
89. Bragt JJMHV, Hansen S, Djukanovic R, Bel EHD, Brinke AT, Wagers SS, et al. SHARP: enabling generation of real-world evidence on a pan-European scale to improve the lives of individuals with severe asthma. ERJ Open Res. 2021;7(2):00064–2021. https://doi.org/10.1183/23120541.00064-2021.
90. Stang PE, Ryan PB, Racoosin JA, Overhage JM, Hartzema AG, Reich C, et al. Advancing the science for active surveillance: rationale and design for the observational medical outcomes partnership. Ann Intern Med. 2010;153(9):600–6. https://doi.org/10.7326/0003-4819-153-9-201011020-00010.
91. Eikholt AA, Wiertz MBR, Hew M, Chan AHY, van Boven JFM. Electronic monitoring devices to support inhalation technique in patients with asthma: a narrative review. Curr Treat Options Allergy. 2023;10(1):28–52. https://doi.org/10.1007/s40521-023-00328-7.
92. Chan AHY, Pleasants RA, Dhand R, Tilley SL, Schworer SA, Costello RW, et al. Digital inhalers for asthma or chronic obstructive pulmonary disease: a scientific perspective. Pulm Ther. 2021;7(2):345–76. https://doi.org/10.1007/s41030-021-00167-4.
93. Maspero JF, Cruz AA, Beltran CFP, Ali Munive A, Montero-Arias F, Hernandez Pliego R, et al. The use of systemic corticosteroids in asthma management in Latin American countries. World Allergy Organ J. 2023;16(4):100760. https://doi.org/10.1016/j.waojou.2023.100760.
94. Lee DL, Hammond JW, Finkel K, Gardner DD, Nelson B, Baptist AP. An electronic shared decision-making app to improve asthma outcomes: a randomized controlled trial. J Allergy Clin Immunol Pract. 2023; https://doi.org/10.1016/j.jaip.2023.06.016.
95. Pereira AM, Jácome C, Amaral R, Jacinto T, Fonseca JA. Chapter 19: Real-time clinical decision support at the point of care. In: Agache I, Hellings P, editors. Implementing precision medicine in best practices of chronic airway diseases. Academic Press; 2019. p. 125–33.
96. Bousquet JJ, Schünemann HJ, Togias A, Erhola M, Hellings PW, Zuberbier T, et al. Next-generation ARIA care pathways for rhinitis and asthma: a model for multimorbid chronic diseases. Clin Transl Allergy. 2019;9:44. https://doi.org/10.1186/s13601-019-0279-2.
97. Vieira RJ, Sousa-Pinto B, Pereira AM, Cordeiro CR, Loureiro CC, Regateiro F, et al. Asthma hospitalizations: a call for a national strategy to fight health inequities. Pulmonology. 2023;29(3):179–83. https://doi.org/10.1016/j.pulmoe.2022.12.001.
98. HL7 Work Groups: HL7 FHIR: resource index. https://www.hl7.org/fhir/resourcelist.html; 2011+. Accessed 2023.
99. Ocean Informatics/Ocean Health Systems: OpenEHR Clinical Knowledge Manager. https://ckm.openehr.org/ckm/ (2007–2018). Access 2023.
100. Observational Health Data Sciences and Informatics: Standardized Data: The OMOP Common Data Model. https://www.ohdsi.org/data-standardization/ (2023). Access 2023.
101. Pereira AM, Almeida R, Amaral R, Alves-Correia M, Mendes S, Fonseca JA, et al. What do physicians think about the use of telemedicine to recruit and assess participants in mHealth-related clinical studies as a consequence of the COVID-19 pandemic? Telemed J E Health. 2022;28(9):1386–92. https://doi.org/10.1089/tmj.2021.0462.

Chapter 10
Digital Health Technologies in Young Children with Wheeze or Asthma

Yen Hoang Do, Paolo Maria Matricardi, Wojciech Feleszko, and Stephanie Dramburg

Contents

Abstract *Introduction*: Wheezing is a common condition affecting over 50% of children prior to their sixth birthday. Wheezing disorders can develop into asthma and both conditions, despite treatment, can generate a high disease-related morbid-

Y. H. Do (✉) · S. Dramburg
Department of Pediatric Respiratory Medicine, Immunology and Critical Care Medicine, Charité–Universitätsmedizin Berlin, a corporate member of Freie Universität Berlin and Humboldt–Universität zu Berlin, Berlin, Germany
e-mail: Hoang-yen.do@charite.de

P. M. Matricardi
Department of Pediatric Respiratory Medicine, Immunology and Critical Care Medicine, Charité–Universitätsmedizin Berlin, a corporate member of Freie Universität Berlin and Humboldt–Universität zu Berlin, Berlin, Germany

Institute of Allergology, Charité—Universitätsmedizin Berlin, Corporate Member of Freie Universität Berlin and Humboldt-Universität zu Berlin, Berlin, Germany

Fraunhofer Institute for Translational Medicine and Pharmacology ITMP, Allergology and Immunology, Berlin, Germany

W. Feleszko
Department of Pediatric Respiratory Diseases and Allergy, Medical University of Warsaw, Warsaw, Poland

© The Author(s), under exclusive license to Springer Nature Switzerland AG 2025
P. M. Matricardi, S. Dramburg, *Digital Allergology*, Health Informatics, https://doi.org/10.1007/978-3-031-71021-6_10

ity (ED visits, hospitalizations). Improved therapy adherence and self-management impact patient outcomes positively. While the interest in digital health solutions in the everyday life of wheezing and asthmatic children is growing, evidence regarding their effectiveness is unclear.

Objective: To summarize available information on digital health technologies for young children with wheeze and their potential role in the disease management of pediatric conditions.

Methods: A literature search on PubMed database was conducted, as well as an additional screening of 4 other publications for fitting reviews. The search terms "wheeze OR asthma, infants OR children, mobile OR digital" were used, as well as the "last 10 years" filter applied. Studies were included if they focused on a digital health intervention tested in children up to 12 years with an asthma or wheeze diagnosis.

Results: After full-text screening, 36 studies were included in the review, covering different categories of digital health interventions such as smart devices, telemedicine, Apps, gamification, and multi-component digital interventions in young children with wheeze.

Conclusion: Digital health interventions show substantial potential in various subcategories and settings of pediatric asthma and wheeze management. Future research focused on standardized disease outcomes, larger patient populations, and randomization is vital to make a widespread integration into routine clinical asthma or wheeze disease management possible.

10.1 Introduction

Wheezing is a common condition in preschool children [1, 2]. Studies have shown that up to 50% of children have had at least one wheezing episode prior to their sixth birthday. [3] Wheezing is described as a high-pitched whistle-like sound, caused by an expiratory flow limitation [4].

Asthma is a chronic respiratory disease, common in children and adults [5]. About 10% of children worldwide are affected by the condition [6]. Though both wheeze and asthma can appear in preschool-aged children, wheeze has a temporal pattern, with symptoms usually only appearing in discrete episodes and the child being well between those episodes. On the other hand, if the wheezing episodes start appearing frequently, usually as result of the viral infections and airway inflammation, which needs to be treated by corticosteroids, the child may be diagnosed with preschool asthma [7–9]. Since both wheeze and asthma have a highly variable clinical spectrum regarding pattern and symptoms, a clinical differentiation is difficult at times. Therefore, both conditions, common in young children, will be the topic of this review.

The management of wheezing and asthma is primarily aimed at respiratory symptom control, reduction of exacerbations, and improving quality of life [8].

However, despite treatment, wheezing and asthma are accompanied by a high disease-related morbidity, with an increased risk for emergency department visits and hospitalizations [3, 6, 7]. Both improved therapy adherence and guided self-management for respiratory diseases have shown to improve patient outcomes such as lung function parameters, hospitalization rates, and the number of unscheduled doctor's visits [5, 10]. Yet, to date many developed interventions are not broadly implemented in everyday practice [11–13]. Therefore, there is growing interest in the potential of digital health as a promising, fast-developing research area to enable more tailored self-management options and make a widespread adoption of digital health solutions into everyday life of children suffering from asthma or preschool wheeze possible [5, 6].

Observational studies and intervention trials to test the effectiveness of digital health solutions in children with wheeze and asthma are complex and still limited in number. Therefore, there are only few published reviews on digital technologies supporting the self-management of pediatric asthma and wheeze, since the highly varying technologies are often difficult to compare and evaluate. Consequently, the effectiveness of digital health interventions in the disease management has remained unclear [5, 14]. In this review, we summarize the published literature regarding digital health technologies for young children with wheeze and asthma and their potential role in the disease management of the pediatric conditions.

10.2 Methods

A literature search on the PubMed database was conducted on November 12, 2022. The following search term was used to perform the database search: "(wheeze OR asthma) AND (infants OR children) AND (mobile OR digital)." Additionally, four reviews with similar topics were screened for suitable references [5, 6, 14, 15]. After the initial search, 540 studies were left to be screened. To be included in the analysis, a study had to meet the following criteria: (1) include original research papers, clinical trials, case reports, (2) conducted in a study population with children up to 12 years, (3) participants having a wheezing or asthma diagnosis and, (4) a focus on a digital health intervention applicable among preschool children. After removing duplicate articles, titles and abstracts were screened on fulfillment of eligibility criteria. Articles not meeting inclusions criteria were excluded, leaving 49 articles for full-text screening. After full-text screening of the articles based on inclusion criteria, 32 studies left were included in the review focusing on digital health interventions across a variety of health care, community, and home settings. To focus on up-to-date interventions and recent telemedicine advances, the search results were limited to studies which have been published within the last 10 years (Fig. 10.1).

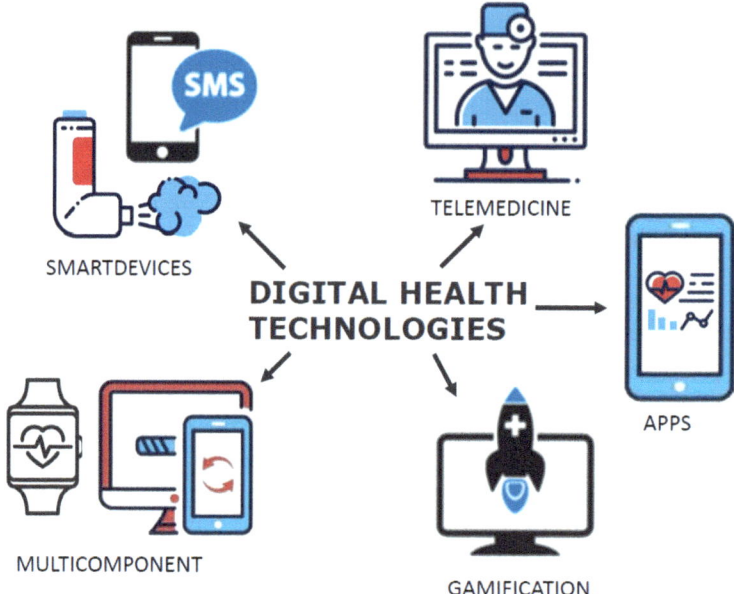

Fig. 10.1 Digital health technologies for young children with wheeze or asthma

10.3 Smart Devices

10.3.1 Smart Devices for Younger Children (<6 y)

Detection of pathological airway sounds - Especially for very young children, the assessment and treatment of respiratory symptoms are often difficult, since it is mainly based on the evaluation by parents/caretakers [4, 16], who may experience difficulties in differentiating wheezing from other breath sounds. A potential over- or underestimation of the symptom severity may consequently lead to an inadequate (non-)use of reliever medication by parents [17, 18]. To tackle this problem, portable smart devices have been developed to support healthcare professionals and parents in managing wheezing disorders in preschool children based on the recognition of abnormal respiratory sounds and cough [19–24].

For healthcare professionals, digital electronic stethoscopes, for example by Littman™ (3 M Health Care, USA) and Clinicloud™ (Clinicloud, Australia), have been compared to standard auscultation by a pediatrician in 20 children aged 5–9 years recruited at a children's Hospital in Melbourne, Australia [25], with results indicating that the digital stethoscopes were more sensitive in detecting wheeze in children than the experienced clinician performing classical auscultation. While studies on automatic sound recognition are currently advancing in adult healthcare [26–28], analyses among preschoolers are still limited in number. However, some digital stethoscopes (Clinicloud™ and Littman™) were recently specifically trained to detect pathologic pediatric breath sounds using an AI algorithm (StethoMe AI) with very high positive and negative percent agreements (PPA and NPA, 0.95 and 0.99, respectively) [29, 30]. These results suggest that AI can detect abnormal breath sounds with a reasonably high accuracy (Table 10.1).

With a focus on self-management, a portable wheeze detector (WheezeScan, OMRON Healthcare Co. Ltd., Japan) has been developed to support parents in the recognition of wheeze. The device uses a high-definition microphone to record and analyze respiratory sounds and detect wheezing sounds in preschool children [19]. After a successful validation with experienced clinicians [31], an exploratory single-armed pilot study among 20 German families with children aged 4–72 months suffering from doctor's diagnosed recurrent wheezing resulted in a good overall acceptance of the device. Further, the researchers observed an improvement in parental self-efficacy regarding the management of their child's condition [19]. A multicentric randomized controlled trial (RCT) is currently ongoing.

In addition to wheeze, cough is a common symptom of lower airway obstruction in children [32, 33]. As the objective assessment of cough frequency can be

Table 10.1 Smart devices developed for children with wheeze or asthma

Smart device	Function	Targeted age	Results	Reference
Digital stethoscopes by Littman and Clinicloud	The two digital stethoscope devices are able to detect pathological airway sounds such as wheeze and cough automatically	5–9 y	The digital stethoscope devices were able to describe the audiological characteristics of pathological airway sounds	Kevat et al. [25]
WheezeScan™ Detector	The Sensor-based detection device is able to detect wheezing and differentiate it from other airway sounds	<6 y	The detector has shown a high usability in testing	Dramburg et al. [19]
LEOSOUND™ Monitor	The device is able to detect acoustic airway events such as cough, over a long period of time (for e.g. overnight)	1–17 y	The monitor has received good general acceptance, as well as achieving a high sensitivity and specifity for wheezing and cough	Urban et al. [35]
Smart nebulizer	The smart nebulizer was able to connect to a mobile application through which the clinical specialist was able to remind the parent in case medication administration has been forgotten	<5 y	The device was able to improve the adherence rate to inhaled corticosteroids (ICS) significantly, reduce the number of ED visits, respiratory tract infections and medication usage	Zhou et al. [38]

(continued)

Table 10.1 (continued)

Smart device	Function	Targeted age	Results	Reference
Smart Inhalers – EMD with audiovisual reminders – e-MATIC study – Sensor-based EMD – Propeller Health™ – Digihaler™	Smart Inhalers have integrated or attached sensors, which allow the recording of administered medication. They are coupled with adherence reminders in form of text messages (SMS), audiovisual reminders, etc.	Varying, from 4–17 y	The inhalers had varying clinical outcomes such as increased adherence to medication [37, 38], improved asthma control and reduction in SABA-usage, but also a higher health care use [39] One smart inhaler [41] was able to measure inhalation parameters such as Peak Inspiratory Flow (PIV) and Inhaled Volume (inhV) in the tested children	Chan et al. [39], Vasbinder et al. [40], Gupta et al. [41], Merchant et al. [42], Chrystyn et al. [43]
Foxfit™	The system consists of a physical activity tracker connected to an app and a web-based dashboard accessible by the paediatric consultant	8–12 y	In the design study an evaluation plan to assess usability and feasibility of the app has been developed	Brons et al. [47]
Wearable breathing trainer	The wearable breathing trainer is able to improve dyfunctional breathing in children by measuring the breathing technique via sensors attached to the wearable trainer	6–12 y	In the design study the prototype for the breathing trainer has been developed. A validation study is still pending	Siering et al. [48]

EMD electronic monitoring device, *Apps* applications, *ICS* inhaled corticosteroids, *PIV* peak inspiratory flow, *inhV* inhaled volume

challenging, Kruizinga et al. developed and validated a smartphone-based algorithm differentiating cough from other ambient sounds with a sensitivity of 47.6% and a specificity of 99.8% in a pediatric population. Notwithstanding its relative low sensitivity value, the authors conclude that the algorithm is accurate enough to be used for a longitudinal follow-up, for example, in clinical care [34].

Another algorithm for cough and wheeze detection is used by the LEOSOUND™ system (Löwenstein Medical GmvH & Co, Germany), which allows the objective and automated measurement of nighttime symptoms by using a mobile portable electronic cough detector [35]. While the sensitivity and specificity of the device for cough detection were 89% and 99%, respectively, wheezing was detected even more accurately (98% sensitivity and specificity) [35].

Smart nebulizers - Many children suffering from wheezing disorders or asthma receive a combined prescription of anti-inflammatory treatment (e.g., inhalative corticosteroids) and reliever medication (e.g., short-acting-ß- agonists, SABA) [36, 37]. To increase the adherence to regular inhalative treatments, a smart nebulizing device has been tested by Zhou et al. in an RCT including 65 children under the age of 5 ys [38]. This device can wirelessly connect to a smart phone app, allowing the pediatrician to remind the parent of necessary nebulization in the case of missed administrations. After a study period of 12 weeks, the use of the smart nebulizer in the intervention group led to an improvement of various clinical outcomes such as wheezing, the number of visits to the emergency department (ED), and need for antibiotic therapy compared to standard therapy. In addition, the authors describe a significantly increased adherence to treatment in the intervention group (67.33% in smart nebulizing group vs 40.00% in conventional nebulizing group; $p < 0.05$) [38].

10.3.2 Smart Devices for Older Children (6–14 y)

While passive detectors are particularly useful for infants with limited abilities of cooperation, other technologies may prove suitable for older children according to the individual level of development and cooperation in performing specific actions such as breathing maneuvers. The fact that several devices have not yet been tested in children below age 6ys does not necessarily mean that this group of patients will not benefit from digital developments in the future. Therefore, we included also technologies tested among older age groups.

"**Smarthalers**"—An inhaler device featuring audiovisual reminders for medication intake has been tested in an RCT with 220 children aged 6–15 ys, attending a hospital's ED because of asthma exacerbations [39]. After a study period of 6 months, the electronic monitoring device not only led to a further reduction of asthma morbidity compared to conventional treatment (Δ(intervention-control) = 0.8; $p = 0.008$), but also to a significant increase of adherence to inhaled corticosteroids in children with asthma (median adherence 84% vs 30%, for children with and without digital support, respectively; $p < 0.0001$).

Similar positive effects have been shown in a 12-month RCT, including 209 children aged 4–11 ys using a smarthaler coupled with adherence reminders via a short message service (SMS) [40], as well as in a study with 127 children over 12 months [41], showing positive effects on asthma control among children (Δ(intervention-control) = 2.2; $p < 0.01$) using a digitally supported smarthaler. Interestingly, the intervention group of this RCT showed an increased health care use compared to control (incidence rate ratio(emergency department) = 2.2; SE = 0.5; $p < 0.01$; incidence rate ratio(hospital) = 3.4; $p < 0.01$).

A population health management platform combining a smarthaler, patient app, and physician's back-office (Propeller Health™, ResMed Inc., San Diego, USA) was tested in an RCT with 496 patients, including adult and pediatric (approx. 30%) patients (aged: 4–17 years) [42]. While the control group was supplied with sensors but had no access to remote feedback from a physician, the intervention group had access to the complete platform including remote monitoring and feedback features. The results showed a reduction in SABA-use compared to conventional treatment ($p < 0.001$) and consecutively an increase in SABA-free days (increase of 21% for the IG vs 17% for routine care, $p < 0.01$), but no significant reduction in asthma control. The authors add that a focus of remote monitoring is set on the precise identification of relevant triggers of exacerbations.

Finally, the multidose dry powder inhaler Digihaler™ (Teva Respiratory, USA) has been tested in 50 children diagnosed with asthma aged 4-17 years. The study group evaluated the device's capability to assess the effectiveness of the user's inhalation technique based on the Peak Inspiratory Flow (PIF) [43]. To this end, PIV and inhaled volume (inhV) were measured by both the Digihaler and an inhalation profile recorder. The results show a strong correlation between both devices (mean percentage difference of 0.16% for PIV, mean percentage difference of −6.11 for inhV), indicating that the "Digihaler"is not only able to record the time and dose of inhaled medication but may also be useful for measuring inhalation parameters such as PIV in children with asthma.

Smart devices promoting physical activity at home—While some of recently developed smart devices for children suffering from wheeze focus mainly on symptom and adherence monitoring, digital technologies are also suitable to support non-pharmacological interventions. Training exercises such as cycling, walking, or breathing exercises have shown to improve pulmonary function in children suffering from respiratory symptoms such as wheezing [44–46]. Focusing on this effect, digital health programs have endeavored to develop sensor-based smart devices able to promote physical activity at home.

An example is the app FoxFit™ (Digital Life, Netherlands), a blended intervention developed by Dutch pediatric pulmonologists in co-creation with children who have asthma aged 8–12 ys. The app can monitor physical activity via a sensor worn at the waist [47] and allows physician oversight of the activity data via a web-based dashboard. A tailored combination of behavior change principles, gamification, and attractive design aims to increase the user's physical activity. However, the clinical impact of the platform remains to be tested.

A different design to promote physical activity in children with obstructive airway diseases is a wearable breathing trainer, designed as a vest [48]. Its objective is to motivate children for breathing exercises to treat dysfunctional breathing. Combined with a mobile application, LED lights, and physical activity sensors for feedback, the prototype was positively evaluated by test users, but a validation study is still pending.

10.4   Telemedicine

The benefit of remote patient–doctor communication and feedback mechanisms for asthma and wheeze care has been shown in several studies mentioned above [39–43]. In addition, studies evaluated tools mainly focusing on doctor–parent/

patient communication over a distance, for example, live video calls, educational videos, and speech recognition support systems [49, 50].

Studies have shown that remote examination tools for off-site doctor's assessment allow the further improvement of treatment compliance and reduce visits to the emergency department [5, 8]. Remote clinical devices such as the multifunctional remote examination device (TytoCare Ltd., Israel, HigoSense Sp. z o.o., Poland) [51] are useful to obtain the patient's lung sound data, relevant for assessment of the patient's lung function [25, 52]. The aforementioned devices have also been compared with other stand-alone devices, permitting a higher rate of clinical diagnosis devices based on the data acquired from the remote device.

While telemedicine enables remote assessment by the doctor, it can also support parents by answering basic questions, reminding them of medication refills, and connecting them to a doctor if further assistance is needed. A system using speech recognition calls to deliver the functions mentioned above has been tested in an RCT with 1187 asthma-diagnosed children aged 3–12 [53]. After an observation time of 24 months, the novel telemedicine intervention improved medication adherence in the intervention group significantly compared to the control group (24-month mean adherence, 44.5% vs 35.5%, respectively, $p < 0.001$).

Healthcare delivery over a distance has been proposed as a useful intervention to provide care in more remote (usually rural) areas. Even though asthma prevalence seems similar between rural and urban populations [54, 55], a significantly increased disease-related morbidity has been observed in rural regions compared to urban areas [56]. Although telemedicine could support healthcare professionals in reaching out to underserved populations, only a few widely adapted telemedicine interventions enable remote access to doctor's consultations for asthma care.

Van Houten et al. conducted a study at a pediatric mobile clinic, which had experienced a high percentage of parents and their children not showing up for their appointments (no-show-rate), but with the newly implemented telehealth option parents had the possibility to attend the doctor's appointment with their child off-site [57]. After a study period of 10 months, the no-show rate decreased drastically from 36% to 7.98–18% per month and the telehealth option received much positive feedback, especially for its time efficiency and good usability.

In addition to synchronous remote attention, asynchronous techniques, such as the interpretation of video recordings, have been evaluated regarding their potential to increase adherence to treatment in non-clinical settings such as the home or school environment [58, 59]. In a study by Shields et al., healthcare professionals evaluated inhalation techniques based on recorded videos of children using inhalers and gave tips for improvement via phone calls [60]. After a study period of 12 weeks, no significant change in spirometry results could be observed. Still, all children had adopted an effective inhaler technique, gave positive feedback on the Mobile Direct Observation of Therapy (MDOT)- telehealth option, and showed improved Asthma Control Test scores (improved ACT scores from 13.1 to mean 17.8; $p = 0.007$).

Several studies have evaluated concepts of healthcare delivery in a school setting with positive results regarding symptom control and risk for ED visits/hospitalization [61, 62].

In summary, telehealth options offer a wide variety of support systems and could improve health access for children who have asthma by enabling remote doctor assessment, therapy control, and asthma education, without a trip to the doctor's office being necessary.

10.5 Apps

Since smartphones have become daily companions for the majority of the world's population [63], the development, and use of smartphone applications are continuously on the rise [64], tailored health applications for patients who have asthma being no exception to that rule [11, 62, 65, 66].

Asthma symptom diaries—Studies have shown that the reliable recording of patient self-reported outcomes such as respiratory symptoms and medication intake are an important component of monitoring wheeze and asthma control [36]. Administering outcome measures electronically via digital asthma diaries has many advantages, such as higher response rates and data quality [67].

A recently developed electronic asthma symptom diary has been tested by Clark et al. in 44 children aged 6–11 ys and their caregivers [68]. The electronic diary can record self-reported measures of the child such as daytime and nighttime asthma symptoms, impact on daily activity, nighttime awakening, and rescue medication use. Most participants found the ePASD items comprehensive and easy to understand.

Another asthma symptom diary app, targeting children between the age of 6 and 16, offers three distinct, age-related versions of the app, one for younger children affected by asthma, one for older children, and one for the caregiver [69]. The finished product consists of an asthma symptom diary app as well as a corresponding online platform, allowing the monitoring of the patient's symptom by the attending pediatrician based on real-time data sent from the mobile application. The app has been tested on its usability by 85 children and parents and has achieved a high usability in all versions (>93 points on a scale from 0 to 100 points).

Adherence reminders and educational apps—Although the use of inhaled corticosteroids in children with obstructive airway diseases has been associated with reduced airway inflammation and an improvement of symptoms [70], the regular administration seems challenging for families with young children [71], a scenario reflected in studies showing an average adherence of ≤50% [72, 73]. To address this problem, smartphone applications with a focus on adherence reminders have been developed. The AsthmaCare™ app (Nationwide Children's Hospital, USA) features several functions, such as medication reminders, information on triggers of exacerbations, and the individual treatment plan [74]. After 6 months, no significant decrease in emergency department utilization, urgent care visits, and hospitalizations between both groups could be detected. However, participants using the AsthmaCare app had a higher probability of improved asthma management (79% vs 64%; $p = 0.06$).

Multifunctional apps - When the question arises about which app feature is more important for extensive asthma management, several reviews in the field conclude that multifunctional smartphone applications have good potential in increasing asthma control [75–77].

An app combining a multitude of functions has been tested in a multicenter RCT with 152 children (aged 6–11ys), resulting in a higher adherence and asthma control (children (Δ(intervention-control) =1.9 points; $p < 0.05$), as well as a reduction of respiratory tract infections when compared to conventional treatment [78]. Other apps combining a multitude of functions are still in the making [79], or feasibility tests are ongoing.

Among these, a multifunctional app still in an early test stage has been evaluated by Iio et al., in 60 children aged 2–12 ys and their caregivers [80]. Aiming to provide asthma education to children in a fun way, participants were encouraged to continue taking and recording their medication via digital animals hatching from eggs if they continued to enter the medication applied. Caregivers could also improve their asthma knowledge with quizzes, and the app allowed feedback messages regarding the use of medications to be displayed for the children and their parents. After the 3-to-6-month study period, the high feasibility of the app could be shown, even though the number of access logs to the app decreased over time, identifying possible app utilization difficulties.

In terms of eHealth solutions, smartphone applications offer a variety of opportunities, such as recording symptoms, sending medication reminders, and enabling an overall support system for managing pediatric asthma and wheezing. Though many applications have yet to be further improved and tested, they may potentially become a widely adopted digital health intervention for children with asthma and wheezing in the future.

10.6 Gamification of Asthma Education

In the era of smartphones, laptops, and a multitude of gaming devices, children and teenagers are increasingly engaging in video game behaviors, with 90% using a gaming application irrespective of the device type [81]. Game-based asthma education may further motivate children with asthma to gain knowledge, acquire specific skills to manage their asthma symptoms, and improve adherence to therapy [82]. The concept of "serious games" combining an attractively designed digital platform with a scoring system motivating the player and providing them feedback may improve acceptance of therapy and promote positive attitudes in children regarding asthma therapy [83, 84].

An example for a gamified mobile application aimed at young children and adolescents is ASTHMAXcel Adventures™ (Montefiore Applications, USA), which combines short informative video sessions with corresponding interactive games, testing the acquired asthma knowledge regarding medication usage, asthma exacerbation triggers, and more. The mini-games are imbedded by a 5- level system, displayed on an animated game map with touch-screen functionality [85]. Throughout the game, the children are able to complete a total of 11 chapters, training and testing specific asthma management-related topics such as "How to use an inhaler and spacer" and "How asthma affects your airways." At the follow-up visits, the AsthmaXcel Adventures App has shown to improve asthma control (increase in controlled asthma in patients from 30.8% to 59.0%; $p = 0.02$), asthma-related knowledge, as well as reduce emergency departments visits (0.46 vs 0.02; $p = 0.02$), and medication use (0.49 vs 0.03; $p = 0.003$). It also resulted in high patient satisfaction [85].

The CHANGE™ Asthma App (Cincinnati Children's Hospital Medical Center, USA) also uses gamified features for asthma education [86]. In an RCT with children aged 4 to 11ys with poorly controlled asthma, there was no significant increase in overall asthma control scores when compared to the control group, but a dose-dependent increase in the c-ACT score, depending on the total app usage time score could be detected (children-asthma control test; bivariate regression beta = 0.004; $p = 0.03$) [86].

A computer-based serious game is MIRACLE™ (Taipei Medical University, Taiwan), which is aiming to increase asthma self-management and train correct inhaler usage more in children aged 6–12 years old [87]. The game is tailored specifically to the cultural preferences of Indonesian children, including story lines such as Indonesian children visiting their grandparents in a village during religious holidays. It consists of "sessions" covering different aspects of asthma education, each session made appealing by colorful visualization and corresponding sounds for different gaming formats such as adventures, quizzes, and puzzles [87].

All in all gamification of asthma education has widely received positive feedback and likability by children, and may therefore be a promising approach to motivate children in the self-management of their respiratory symptoms.

10.7   Multi-component Digital Asthma Interventions

Among the multitude of digital health interventions featuring smart devices, adherence reminders, gaming applications, and telehealth options for children with wheeze and/or asthma [15], several solutions aim at combining different electronical features in multi-component applications [6].

InSpire™ is a mobile smartphone app (Duke University School of Medicine Durham, USA) which motivates children to assess their forced expiratory volume via a handheld portable spirometer and integrates it in an interactive game setting [88]. The concept of the game relies on role playing based on the world, where the young player must join hands with their health care specialist in order to manage their asthma symptoms. The data is sent to the physician, who is in turn able to give feedback and recommendations to the patients in real time via a messaging system. The children testing the app have given positive feedback on the app, and it has received a high likability of almost 100% in the children surveyed (aged 7–14 ys) [88].

Another multi-component digital intervention is the AirBuddy™ App [89] (The State University of New Jersey, USA). The mobile app is able to monitor indoor air quality, measured by an off-the-shelf air quality sensor and could therefore help children to reduce symptom severity and frequency triggered by a substandard indoor quality. All children testing the app have given positive feedback regarding to the usefulness and usability of Airbuddy [89].

A combination of different interventions to improve asthma self-management among children and their caretakers has been evaluated in an RCT in 305 children being diagnosed with poorly controlled asthma [90]. The system supports the affected child by offering asthma education in a gamified format and establishing contact with other children with asthma via a peer discussion platform. In combination with this, a case manager can make an overall assessment of the child's adherence to therapy through monthly phone calls. The summarized data collected by the case manager is available to the parents, who are in turn able to receive support through helpful links and can directly contact the case manager via phone call. After a 12-month study period, the authors concluded that the intervention did not increase medication adherence significantly but led to an improved asthma control in the children suffering from poorly controlled asthma (Asthma Control Questionnaire: $d = -0.31$, 95% CL-0.88, 1.60; $p = 0.01$) [90].

A multi-component platform combining a smartwatch application with a commercially available wireless dust-sensor and a smart spirometer was developed to evaluate real-time asthma exacerbation risk [91]. The system is able to assess asthma risk with $80.10 \pm 14.13\%$ accuracy and it has also received positive results on its usability according to pre-testing [91].

10.8 Discussion

In the recent past, diverse digital health interventions have been developed to improve the management of preschool wheeze and childhood asthma. While wheeze and cough detectors may support parents in recognizing and monitoring wheezing and cough in preschool children at home [19, 34, 35], there are also various devices tailored for older children with asthma, targeting different aspects of disease management: smart devices are able to monitor and improve medication adherence, correct inhaler technique, measure lung function parameters, and promote a healthy disease-related lifestyle [43, 47, 92, 93]. Telemedicine options improve access to doctor's evaluation and asthma education [60, 62]. Apps are easily available monitoring devices to record symptoms and send adherence reminders [68, 94], and gamification is a highly attractive option for children to increase motivation for self-management, adherence and gain disease-related knowledge. [85, 87]

Although several studies have reported positive trends for asthma symptom control, therapy adherence, as well as reduced visits to the emergency department and hospitalization among children, broad evidence of clinical efficacy is still lacking for many technologies, specifically considering their use in preschool children [6,

95, 96]. Most identified publications focus on user-centered development, feasibility studies, and small-scale clinical trials, often sharing limitations, such as low participant numbers, missing control groups and heterogeneous, non-standardized patient outcomes. However, these may be the next steps to come once the developmental stages and exploratory studies have been completed successfully.

Overall, even though digital health interventions show substantial potential in various settings of pediatric asthma and wheeze management, future research focused on standardized disease outcomes, larger patient populations, and randomization is vital to enable a widespread integration into routine clinical care for young patients suffering from preschool wheeze or childhood asthma.

Disclosure of Potential Conflict of Interest Yen Hoang Do has nothing to disclose. Paolo M. Matricardi received grants and personal fees from OMRON Healthcare Co. Ltd. Stephanie Dramburg received personal fees from OMRON Healthcare Co. Ltd.

References

1. Rajapakse Mudiyanselage SIR, Amarasiri W, Yasaratne B, Warnasekara J, Agampodi S. Epidemiology of wheeze among preschool children: a population-based cross-sectional study from rural Sri Lanka. BMJ Open. 2021;11(7):e046688.
2. Ducharme FM, Tse SM, Chauhan B. Diagnosis, management, and prognosis of preschool wheeze. Lancet. 2014;383(9928):1593–604.
3. Doss AMA, Stokes JR. Viral Infections and Wheezing in Preschool Children. Immunol Allergy Clin N Am. 2022;42(4):727–41.
4. Brand PL, Baraldi E, Bisgaard H, et al. Definition, assessment and treatment of wheezing disorders in preschool children: an evidence-based approach. Eur Respir J. 2008;32(4):1096–110.
5. Morrison D. Digital asthma self-management interventions: a systematic review. J Med Internet Res. 2014;16(2):e51.
6. Ferrante G, Licari A, Marseglia GL, La Grutta S. Digital health interventions in children with asthma. Clin Exp Allergy. 2021;51(2):212–20.
7. Stokes JR, Bacharier L. Prevention and treatment of recurrent viral-induced wheezing in the preschool child. Ann Allergy Asthma Immunol. 2020;125(2):156–62.
8. Tenero L, Tezza G, Cattazzo E, Piacentini G. Wheezing in preschool children. Early Hum Dev. 2013;89(Suppl. 3):S13–7.
9. https://www.asthmafoundation.org.nz/stories/what-is-preschool-wheeze.
10. Duncan CL, Hogan MB, Tien KJ, Graves MM, Chorney JM, Zettler MD, Koven L, Wilson NW, Dinakar C, Portnoy J. Efficacy of a parent-youth teamwork intervention to promote adherence in pediatric asthma. J Pediatr Psychol. 2013;38(6):617–28.
11. Mosnaim GS, Pappalardo AA, Resnick SE, et al. Behavioral interventions to improve asthma outcomes for adolescents: a systematic review. J Allergy Clin Immunol Pract. 2016;4(1):130–41.
12. Eccles MP, Armstrong D, Baker R, et al. An implementation research agenda. Implement Sci Engl. 2009;4:18.
13. Normansell R, Kew KM, Stovold E. Interventions to improve adherence to inhaled steroids for asthma. Cochrane Database Syst Rev. 2017;4(4):Cd012226.
14. Shah AC, Badawy SM. Telemedicine in pediatrics: systematic review of randomized controlled trials. JMIR Pediatr Parent. 2021;4(1):e22696.

15. Alvarez-Perea A, Dimov V, Popescu FD, Zubeldia JM. The applications of eHealth technologies in the management of asthma and allergic diseases. Clin Transl Allergy. 2021;11(7):e12061.
16. Brand PL, Caudri D, Eber E, et al. Classification and pharmacological treatment of preschool wheezing: changes since 2008. Eur Respir J. 2014;43(4):1172–7.
17. Lozano P, Finkelstein JA, Hecht J, Shulruff R, Weiss KB. Asthma medication use and disease burden in children in a primary care population. Arch Pediatr Adolesc Med. 2003;157(1):81–8.
18. Vasilopoulou I. Underdiagnosis and undertreatment of asthma in children: a tertiary hospital's experience. Clin Transl Allergy. 2015;5:1.
19. Dramburg S, Dellbrügger E, van Aalderen W, Matricardi PM. The impact of a digital wheeze detector on parental disease management of pre-school children suffering from wheezing-a pilot study. Pilot Feasibility Stud. 2021;7(1):185.
20. Birring SS, Fleming T, Matos S, Raj AA, Evans DH, Pavord ID. The Leicester Cough Monitor: preliminary validation of an automated cough detection system in chronic cough. Eur Respir J. 2008;31(5):1013–8.
21. Eising JB, Uiterwaal CS, van der Ent CK. Nocturnal wheeze measurement in preschool children. Pediatr Pulmonol. 2014;49(3):257–62.
22. Urban C, Kiefer A, Conradt R, et al. Validation of the LEOSound® monitor for standardized detection of wheezing and cough in children. Pediatr Pulmonol. 2022;57(2):551–9.
23. Theodore AC, Tseng CH, Li N, Elashoff RM, Tashkin DP. Correlation of cough with disease activity and treatment with cyclophosphamide in scleroderma interstitial lung disease: findings from the Scleroderma Lung Study. Chest. 2012;142(3):614–21.
24. Li AM, Tsang TW, Chan DF, et al. Cough frequency in children with mild asthma correlates with sputum neutrophil count. Thorax. 2006;61(9):747–50.
25. Kevat AC, Kalirajah A, Roseby R. Digital stethoscopes compared to standard auscultation for detecting abnormal paediatric breath sounds. Eur J Pediatr. 2017;176(7):989–92.
26. Lee SH, Kim YS, Yeo MK, et al. Fully portable continuous real-time auscultation with a soft wearable stethoscope designed for automated disease diagnosis. Sci Adv. 2022;8(21):eabo5867.
27. Lee SH, Kim YS, Yeo WH. Advances in microsensors and wearable bioelectronics for digital stethoscopes in health monitoring and disease diagnosis. Adv Healthc Mater. 2021;10(22):e2101400.
28. Rennoll V, McLane I, Emmanouilidou D, West J, Elhilali M. Electronic stethoscope filtering mimics the perceived sound characteristics of acoustic stethoscope. IEEE J Biomed Health Inform. 2021;25(5):1542–9.
29. Kevat A, Kalirajah A, Roseby R. Artificial intelligence accuracy in detecting pathological breath sounds in children using digital stethoscopes. Respir Res. 2020;21(1):253.
30. Kim Y, Hyon Y, Lee S, Woo S-D, Ha T, Chung C. The coming era of a new auscultation system for analyzing respiratory sounds. BMC Pulm Med. 2022;22(1):119.
31. Habukawa C, Ohgami N, Matsumoto N, et al. A wheeze recognition algorithm for practical implementation in children. PLoS One. 2020;15(10):e0240048.
32. Kantar A. Phenotypic presentation of chronic cough in children. J Thorac Dis. 2017;9:907–13.
33. Goldsobel AB, Chipps BE. Cough in the pediatric population. J Pediatr. 2010;156(3):352–8.
34. Kruizinga MD, Zhuparris A, Dessing E, et al. Development and technical validation of a smartphone-based pediatric cough detection algorithm. Pediatr Pulmonol. 2022;57(3):761–7.
35. Koehler U, Brandenburg U, Weissflog A, Sohrabi K, Groß V. LEOSound, an innovative procedure for acoustic long-term monitoring of asthma symptoms (wheezing and coughing) in children and adults. Pneumologie. 2014;68(4):277–81.
36. Global Initiative for Asthma (2020) GINA report, global strategy for asthma management and prevention.
37. Cerveri I, Locatelli F, Zoia MC, Corsico A, Accordini S, De Marco R. International variations in asthma treatment compliance: the results of the European Community. Eur Respir J. 1999;14(2):288–94.
38. Zhou Y, Lu Y, Zhu H, Zhang Y, Li Y, Yu Q. Short-term effect of a smart nebulizing device on adherence to inhaled corticosteroid therapy in Asthma Predictive Index-positive wheezing children. Patient Prefer Adher. 2018;12:861–8.

39. Chan AH, Stewart AW, Harrison J, Camargo CA Jr, Black PN, Mitchell EA. The effect of an electronic monitoring device with audiovisual reminder function on adherence to inhaled corticosteroids and school attendance in children with asthma: a randomised controlled trial. Lancet Respir Med. 2015;3(3):210–9.
40. Vasbinder EC, Goossens LM, Rutten-van Mölken MP, et al. e-Monitoring of Asthma Therapy to Improve Compliance in children (e-MATIC): a randomised controlled trial. Eur Respir J. 2016;48(3):758–67.
41. Gupta RS, Fierstein JL, Boon KL, et al. Sensor-based electronic monitoring for asthma: a randomized controlled trial. Pediatrics. 2021;147(1)
42. Merchant RK, Inamdar R, Quade RC. Effectiveness of population health management using the propeller health asthma platform: a randomized clinical trial. J Allergy Clin Immunol Pract. 2016;4(3):455–63.
43. Chrystyn H, Saralaya D, Shenoy A, et al. Investigating the accuracy of the digihaler, a new electronic multidose dry-powder inhaler, in measuring inhalation parameters. J Aerosol Med Pulm Drug Deliv. 2022;35(3):166–77.
44. Eichenberger PA, Diener SN, Kofmehl R, Spengler CM. Effects of exercise training on airway hyperreactivity in asthma: a systematic review and meta-analysis. Sports Med. 2013;43(11):1157–70.
45. Wanrooij VH, Willeboordse M, Dompeling E, van de Kant KD. Exercise training in children with asthma: a systematic review. Br J Sports Med. 2014;48(13):1024–31.
46. Zhang W, Wang Q, Liu L, Yang W, Liu H. Effects of physical therapy on lung function in children with asthma: a systematic review and meta-analysis. Pediatr Res. 2021;89(6):1343–51.
47. Brons A, Braam K, Broekema A, et al. Translating promoting factors and behavior change principles into a blended and technology-supported intervention to stimulate physical activity in children with asthma (foxfit): design study. JMIR Form Res. 2022;6(7):e34121.
48. Siering L, Ludden GDS, Mader A, van Rees H. A theoretical framework and conceptual design for engaging children in therapy at home-the design of a wearable breathing trainer. J Pers Med. 2019;9(2)
49. Brown W, Odenthal D. The uses of telemedicine to improve asthma control. J Allergy Clin Immunol Pract. 2015;3(2):300–1.
50. Kew KM, Cates CJ. Remote versus face-to-face check-ups for asthma. Cochrane Database Syst Rev. 2016;4(4):Cd011715.
51. McDaniel NL, Novicoff W, Gunnell B, Cattell GD. Comparison of a novel handheld telehealth device with stand-alone examination tools in a clinic setting. Telemed J E Health. 2019;25(12):1225–30.
52. Leng S, Tan RS, Chai KT, Wang C, Ghista D, Zhong L. The electronic stethoscope. Biomed Eng Online. 2015;14:66.
53. Bender BG, Cvietusa PJ, Goodrich GK, et al. Pragmatic trial of health care technologies to improve adherence to pediatric asthma treatment: a randomized clinical trial. JAMA Pediatr. 2015;169(4):317–23.
54. Buescher PA, Jones-Vessey K. Using Medicaid data to estimate state- and county-level prevalence of asthma among low-income children. Matern Child Health J. 1999;3(4):211–6.
55. Chrischilles E, Ahrens R, Kuehl A, et al. Asthma prevalence and morbidity among rural Iowa schoolchildren. J Allergy Clin Immunol. 2004;113(1):66–71.
56. Pesek RD, Vargas PA, Halterman JS, Jones SM, McCracken A, Perry TT. A comparison of asthma prevalence and morbidity between rural and urban schoolchildren in Arkansas. Ann Allergy Asthma Immunol. 2010;104(2):125–31.
57. Van Houten L, Deegan K, Siemer M, Walsh S. A telehealth initiative to decrease no-show rates in a pediatric asthma mobile clinic. J Pediatr Nurs. 2021;59:143–50.
58. Creary SE, Gladwin MT, Byrne M, Hildesheim M, Krishnamurti L. A pilot study of electronic directly observed therapy to improve hydroxyurea adherence in pediatric patients with sickle-cell disease. Pediatr Blood Cancer. 2014;61(6):1068–73.

59. Munoz F, Collins K, Moser K, Cerecer-Callu P, et al. Video-directly observed therapy: a promising solution for monitoring TB and HIV treatment adherence for binational Mobile direct observation therapy of inhaler use. 2012.
60. Shields MD, F AL, Rivey MP, McElnay JC. Mobile direct observation of therapy (MDOT)—a rapid systematic review and pilot study in children with asthma. PLoS One. 2018;13(2):e0190031.
61. Halterman JS, Fagnano M, Tajon RS, et al. Effect of the school-based telemedicine enhanced asthma management (SB-TEAM) program on asthma morbidity: a randomized clinical trial. JAMA Pediatr. 2018;172(3):e174938.
62. Perry TT, Halterman JS, Brown RH, et al. Results of an asthma education program delivered via telemedicine in rural schools. Ann Allergy Asthma Immunol. 2018;120(4):401–8.
63. Ofcom. 2016. Communications Market Report 2018. Retrieved from http://www.ofcom.org.uk/research/cm/cmr08/.
64. Research2Guidance—mHealth Economics 2017—Current Status and Future Trends in Mobile Health. (n.d.). Retrieved October 29, 2019, from https://research2guidance.com/product/mhealth-economics-2017-current-status-and-future-trends-in-mobile-health/.
65. Marcano Belisario JS, Huckvale K, Greenfield G, Car J, Gunn LH. Smartphone and tablet self management apps for asthma. Cochrane Database Syst Rev. 2013;2013(11):Cd010013.
66. Burbank AJ, Lewis SD, Hewes M, et al. Mobile-based asthma action plans for adolescents. J Asthma. 2015;52(6):583–6.
67. Meirte J, Hellemans N, Anthonissen M, et al. Benefits and disadvantages of electronic patient-reported outcome measures: systematic review. JMIR Perioper Med. 2020;3(1):e15588.
68. Clark M, Romano C, Olayinka-Amao O, et al. Development and content validation of a self-completed, electronic pediatric asthma symptom diary. J Patient Rep Outcomes. 2022;6(1):25.
69. Mayoral K, Garin O, Caballero-Rabasco MA, et al. Smartphone App for monitoring Asthma in children and adolescents. Qual Life Res. 2021;30(11):3127–44.
70. Baraldi E, Rossi GA, Boner AL. Beclomethasone and salbutamol treatment for children study G. Budesonide in preschool-age children with recurrent wheezing. N Engl J Med. 2012;366:570–1. author reply 571
71. Bårnes CB, Ulrik CS. Asthma and adherence to inhaled corticosteroids: current status and future perspectives. Respir Care. 2015;60(3):455–68.
72. Jentzsch NS, Camargos P, Sarinho ES, Bousquet J. Adherence rate to beclomethasone dipropionate and the level of asthma control. Respir Med. 2012;106(3):338–43.
73. Rachelefsky G. Inhaled corticosteroids and asthma control in children: assessing impairment and risk. Pediatrics. 2009;123(1):353–66.
74. Stukus DR, Farooqui N, Strothman K, et al. Real-world evaluation of a mobile health application in children with asthma. Ann Allergy Asthma Immunol. 2018;120(4):395–400.e391.
75. Hui CY, Walton R, McKinstry B, Jackson T, Parker R, Pinnock H. The use of mobile applications to support self-management for people with asthma: a systematic review of controlled studies to identify features associated with clinical effectiveness and adherence. J Am Med Inform Assoc. 2017;24(3):619–32.
76. Unni E, Gabriel S, Ariely R. A review of the use and effectiveness of digital health technologies in patients with asthma. Ann Allergy Asthma Immunol. 2018;121(6):680–691.e681.
77. Farzandipour M, Nabovati E, Sharif R, Arani MH, Anvari S. Patient self-management of asthma using mobile applications to support self-management of asthma using mobile applications: a systematic review of the functionalitities and effects. Appl Clin Inform. 2017;8(4):1068–81.
78. Lv S, Ye X, Wang Z, et al. A randomized controlled trial of a mobile application-assisted nurse-led model used to improve treatment outcomes in children with asthma. J Adv Nurs. 2019;75(11):3058–67.
79. Sonney J, Cho EE, Zheng Q, Kientz JA. Refinement of a parent-child shared asthma management mobile health app: human-centered design study. JMIR Pediatr Parent. 2022;5(1):e34117.
80. Iio M, Sato M, Narita M, et al. Development and feasibility of a mobile asthma app for children and their caregivers: mixed methods study. JMIR Form Res. 2022;6(5):e34509.

81. Anderson M, Jiang J. Teens, social media & technology. https//www.pewresearch.org/internet/2018/05/31/teens-social-media-technology-2018/. 2018.
82. Whiteley L, Mena L, Craker LK, Healy MG, Brown LK. Creating a theoretically grounded gaming app to increase adherence to pre-exposure prophylaxis: lessons from the development of the viral combat mobile phone game. JMIR Serious Games. 2019;7(1):e11861.
83. Kato PM, Cole SW, Bradlyn AS, Pollock BH. A video game improves behavioral outcomes in adolescents and young adults with cancer: a randomized trial. Pediatrics. 2008;122(2):e305–17.
84. Howell K. "Quest for the code": a study of a computer-based education program for children with asthma. Thesis and Dissertations—Syracuse University; 2005.
85. Hsia BC, Singh AK, Njeze O, et al. Developing and evaluating ASTHMAXcel adventures: a novel gamified mobile application for pediatric patients with asthma. Ann Allergy Asthma Immunol. 2020;125(5):581–8.
86. Real FJ, Beck AF, DeBlasio D, et al. Dose matters: a smartphone application to improve asthma control among patients at an urban pediatric primary care clinic. Games Health J. 2019;8(5):357–65.
87. Sarasmita MA, Larasanty LPF, Kuo LN, Cheng KJ, Chen HY. A computer-based interactive narrative and a serious game for children with asthma: development and content validity analysis. J Med Internet Res. 2021;23(9):e28796.
88. Elias P, Rajan NO, McArthur K, Dacso CC. InSpire to promote lung assessment in youth: evolving the self-management paradigms of young people with asthma. Medicine 20. 2013;2(1):e1.
89. Kim S, Stanton K, Park Y, Thomas S. A mobile app for children with asthma to monitor indoor air quality (AirBuddy): development and usability study. JMIR Form Res. 2022;6(5):e37118.
90. Gustafson D, Wise M, Bhattacharya A, et al. The effects of combining web-based eHealth with telephone nurse case management for pediatric asthma control: a randomized controlled trial. J Med Internet Res. 2012;14(4):e101.
91. Hosseini A, Buonocore CM, Hashemzadeh S, et al. Feasibility of a secure wireless sensing smartwatch application for the self-management of pediatric asthma. Sensors (Basel). 2017;17(8)
92. Vasbinder EC, Janssens HM, Rutten-van Mölken MP, et al. e-Monitoring of asthma therapy to improve compliance in children using a real-time medication monitoring system (RTMM): the e-MATIC study protocol. BMC Med Inform Decis Mak. 2013;13:38.
93. Ljungberg H, Carleborg A, Gerber H, et al. Clinical effect on uncontrolled asthma using a novel digital automated self-management solution: a physician-blinded randomised controlled crossover trial. Eur Respir J. 2019;54(5)
94. Coker TR, Mitchell SJ, Lowry SJ, et al. Text2Breathe: text-message intervention for parent communication and pediatric asthma. Acad Pediatr. 2023;23(1):123–9.
95. Ramsey RR, Plevinsky JM, Kollin SR, Gibler RC, Guilbert TW, Hommel KA. Systematic review of digital interventions for pediatric asthma management. J Allergy Clin Immunol Pract. 2020;8(4):1284–93.
96. Doshi H, Hsia B, Shahani J, Mowrey W, Jariwala SP. Impact of technology-based interventions on patient-reported outcomes in asthma: a systematic review. J Allergy Clin Immunol Pract. 2021;9(6):2336–41.

Chapter 11
Digital Health and Chronic Urticaria

Marcus Maurer, Pavel Kolkhir, Aiste Ramanauskaite, and Ivan Cherrez-Ojeda

Contents

Marcus Maurer, Pavel Kolkhir, Aiste Ramanauskaite, and Ivan Cherrez-Ojeda contributed equally to this work.

Marcus Maurer died before publication of this work was completed.

M. Maurer (Deceased) · P. Kolkhir (✉) · A. Ramanauskaite
Urticaria Center of Reference and Excellence, Institute of Allergology, Charité—
Universitätsmedizin Berlin, Corporate Member of Freie Universität Berlin and Humboldt-
Universität zu Berlin, Berlin, Germany

Fraunhofer Institute for Translational Medicine and Pharmacology ITMP, Immunology and
Allergology, Berlin, Germany
e-mail: marcus.maurer@charite.de; pavel.kolkhir@charite.de;
aiste.ramanauskaite@charite.de

I. Cherrez-Ojeda
Urticaria Center of Reference and Excellence, Espiritu Santo University,
Samborondón, Ecuador

P. M. Matricardi, S. Dramburg, *Digital Allergology*, Health Informatics,
https://doi.org/10.1007/978-3-031-71021-6_11

Abstract Chronic urticaria (CU) is a common chronic inflammatory skin disease characterized by recurrent itchy wheals and angioedema for longer than 6 weeks. CU significantly impacts patients' quality of life and needs effective long-term treatment aimed at complete control. To achieve this aim, digital resources can help in multiple ways. Here, we review digital health measures currently used in urticaria management and urticariology. Several digital tools and platforms aim to improve patient and physician education on urticaria as well as monitoring of CU activity, impact, control, and response to treatment. CRUSE, the chronic urticaria self-evaluation app and an example of the latter, can also enhance digital patient–physician communication, another important aim of digital tools used in CU. Leveraging digital technologies such as online platforms like UCARE 4 U and LevelUp and telemedicine can play a positive role in advancing comprehensive patient care. Furthermore, data obtained with digital health measures such as registries, e.g., Chronic Urticaria Registry (CURE), can improve CU understanding and aid the development of novel treatment approaches and personalized therapy. In the following, we summarize the latest knowledge on the use and potential of digital health technologies in CU.

11.1   Unmet Needs in Chronic Urticaria

Chronic urticaria (CU) is a chronic inflammatory skin disease of more than 6 weeks duration. The signs and symptoms of CU, i.e., itchy wheals (hives) and angioedema, can appear spontaneously (chronic spontaneous urticaria, CSU) or be induced by a specific and definite trigger such as cold or pressure (chronic inducible urticaria, CIndU). About one-third of CU patients have both, CSU and CIndU [1, 2]. CU is a common and debilitating disease with a point prevalence ranging from ≤1.5% to 3–4% globally. CU lasts for more than 1 year in most patients, longer in CIndU than CSU (2–12 years vs. ~1–4 years), and considerably impairs quality of life. Second-generation antihistamines, the first-line treatment, are not effective in up to half of the patients [1].

Many CU patients are seen by primary care physicians [3], but <20% of general practitioners (GPs) are familiar with urticaria guideline recommendations [4, 5]. About two-thirds of GPs have inadequate knowledge of urticaria, and up to 75% of GPs have an urgent learning need regarding urticaria. As demonstrated by a French study, many GPs have difficulties with CU diagnosis (19%), differential diagnosis (33%), choice of treatment (45%), and access to specialist physicians (55%) [6]. Furthermore, many physicians do not use patient-reported outcome measures (PROMs), the best available means to assess urticaria activity, impact, and control [7]. The consequences are diagnostic and treatment delay (mean time to diagnosis is 2 years), considerable decrease in patients' QoL, and high healthcare as well as societal costs [8]. Patients are frustrated with the time it takes to reach a diagnosis and with cycling through different therapies until treatment success is achieved [9]. CU requires new and more effective treatments that target its underlying mechanisms.

This highlights many unmet needs, including shortcomings in patient/physician communication, patient and physician information and education, and means of monitoring disease activity, impact, control, and response to treatment. Moreover, we need to understand how and why CU can present differently in different patients, to develop individualized treatment approaches that consider the patient's particular symptoms, triggers, and comorbidities. All of that will permit to develop a targeted treatment strategy and algorithm as well as global improvements in decision-making around initiating, maintaining, modifying, switching, and stopping the treatment of CU [10]. Addressing these unmet needs would also facilitate earlier diagnosis, minimizing unnecessary investigations, and early identification of patients who may benefit from a specialist care.

11.2   How Can Digital Health Measures Help Address the Unmet Needs in CU

Person-centered care (PCC) is an approach that acknowledges patients as experts on their own lives and the lived experience with their disease. PCC increases the involvement of patients in their own health care across nine themes: empathy, respect, engagement, relationship, communication, joint decision-making, holistic focus, individualized focus, and coordinated care [11]. Increasingly, politicians and policymakers are interested in adopting and implementing PCC.

Patient activation (PA) and engagement in shared decision-making (SDM) are important components of PCC and may benefit the patient–physician relationship, ease frustration, as well as encourage a more collaborative approach to long-term disease management [9]. PA and SDM are linked bidirectionally, and this relationship is driven by baseline PA, i.e., higher PA is associated with greater benefit in SDM. Low PA is an important barrier to SDM. Interventions that promote PA such as Digital Care Pathways (DCP) should be prioritized, and patients with high activation should be engaged in SDM interventions [12, 13].

DCPs use digital technologies to support patients through their healthcare journey and to improve our ability to enhance the delivery of healthcare, empowering patients to have more control over their disease and to make better informed decisions about their health [14]. These digital technologies include online platforms, programs, and activities for patient information and physician education, telemedicine, and apps.

DCP instruments are in and of use in the management of CU (Fig. 11.1). Examples include online listings of urticaria specialists such as Urticaria Centers of Reference and Excellence (UCAREs, https://ga2len-ucare.com). The UCARE network is a global GA²LEN consortium of urticaria expert centers dedicated to improving the diagnosis, treatment, and management of chronic urticaria with the

Fig. 11.1 Digital health initiatives for chronic urticariaAbbreviations: *PROMs* patient-reported outcome measures, *UCT* urticaria control test, *CRUSE* chronic urticaria self-evaluation app, *CURE* the chronic urticaria registry

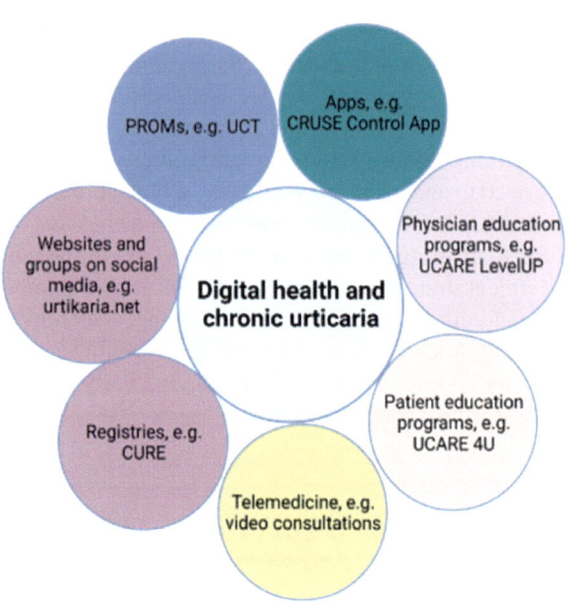

Fig. 11.1 Digital health initiatives for chronic urticariaAbbreviations: *PROMs* patient-reported outcome measures, *UCT* urticaria control test, *CRUSE* chronic urticaria self-evaluation app, *CURE* the chronic urticaria registry

ultimate aim of improving patient outcomes and quality of life [15]. Many UCAREs offer tele-consultation with a urticaria specialist and provide patients, via email, with a screening questionnaire and PROMs triggered by the patient's responses. Other urticaria DCP instruments support effective communication and patient education outside of the office, e.g., the UCARE 4 U program, mobile applications to monitor patients' disease activity and control, e.g., the CRUSE App, urticaria-related websites and groups on social media, webinars, and urticaria seminars. Similarly, physician education on urticaria can be improved by means of digital initiatives including UCARE LevelUp webinars and publications as an outcome of the analysis of data from the Chronic Urticaria Registry (CURE) [16] (Fig. 11.2).

11.3 Digital Patient and Physician Education

The use of digital technology for patient and physician education, particularly through mobile platforms, can help to improve the quality of care for patients with chronic diseases including urticaria and can be adapted quickly on a large scale at low cost. Recently, digital healthcare technologies have undergone a significant leap in development, accompanied by an additional increase in implementation due to the COVID pandemic [17].

In a recent study, one-to-many information and communication technology (ICT), e.g., web browsers, YouTube, Facebook, was used by three of four CU patients to obtain information about their disease [18]. Furthermore, more than half of the patients who were asked about the quality of information obtained from

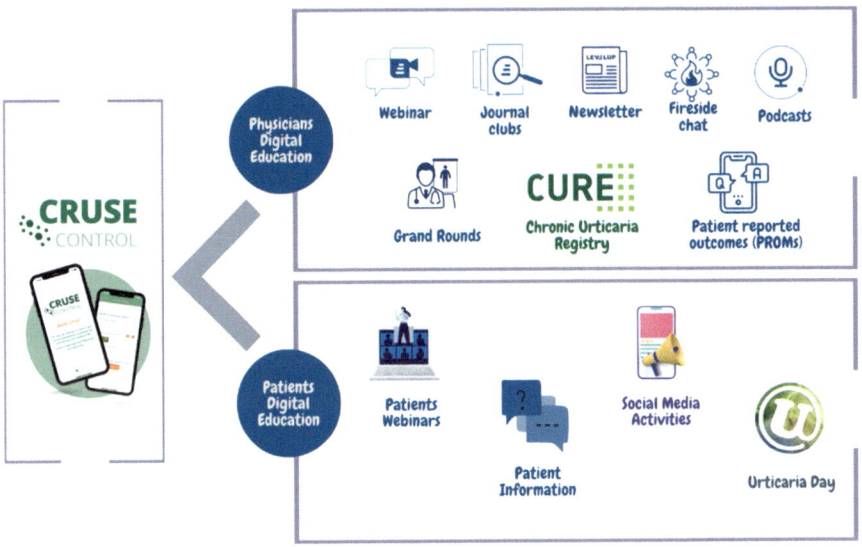

Fig. 11.2 Digital education for patients and physicians: information and communication technologies tools

one-to-many ICT reported that the information was of good or very good quality. This suggests that future efforts to improve patient education and information regarding CU should prioritize one-to-many platforms, particularly websites and YouTube videos provided by accredited urticaria experts and centers such as UCAREs [19].

Digital physician education is an equally important strategy for improving CU management. Recent studies have identified major knowledge gaps in physicians who treat urticaria [20], and online CME online education has been shown to yield significant gains in physicians' knowledge of diagnosis and management of CU. One study reported that 50% of physicians who completed an online education activity improved their knowledge related to guideline recommendations for the management of CU, with a 62% relative increase in correct responses from pre- to post-CME [21] Importantly, incorporating the patient voice into online education for physicians can increase competence and confidence in optimizing CU treatment and improve physicians' ability to accurately diagnose and effectively manage CU [22].

11.3.1 Digital Patient Education

Comprehensive disease education and information empower CU patients to make well-informed decisions and adhere to their treatment plan. The GA²LEN UCARE network recognized this need and launched, in 2021, the UCARE 4 U initiative

[23]. It includes four digital formats and activities: patient webinars (https://ucare-4u.com/en/webinars/), online information on the 4 U website (https://ucare-4u.com/en/learn-about-urticaria/), social media postings (https://ucare-4u.com/en/social-media/), and urticaria day activities. With these formats, patients are provided with a comprehensive overview of all things urticaria, developed by urticaria specialists. The main goal of the UCARE 4 U initiative is to keep patients engaged in learning about CU triggers, comorbidities, and treatments and to increase and improve communication with their treating physicians. To this end, the information and education provided by UCARE 4 U are continuously updated and developed further, free of charge, and made available in various languages. UCARE 4 U also informs CU patients how to connect with patient organizations, as well as how to start new ones if none exist in their area. Furthermore, patients can keep up to date on ongoing research as well as opportunities to engage in research projects and clinical studies.

A new approach to providing digital CU patient information is the use of an app such as UCARE's CRUSE app (Chronic Urticaria Self Evaluation; https://cruse-control.com). CRUSE is a state-of-the-art digital platform developed specifically for patients with CSU. CRUSE allows CSU patients to monitor their disease activity and control and also provides them with information on their condition (Fig. 11.3).

11.3.2 Digital Physician Education

Physician education on CU is in high demand and much needed, as shown by recent studies, for example, on the knowledge and use of patient-reported outcomes measures (PROMs). The use of CU PROMs is generally recommended and aims to

Fig. 11.3 CRUSE control app

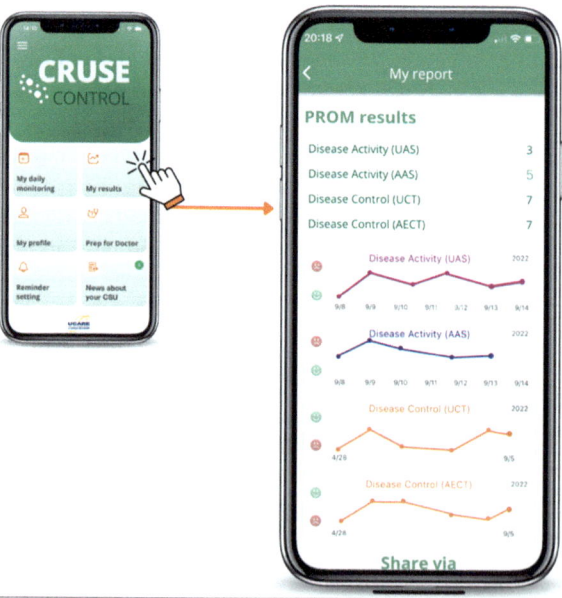

gather information regarding CU disease activity, impact, and control. A recent study showed that only 20% of physicians who treat CU patients are aware of these PROMs. These [24] results indicate that more physician information and education are urgently needed.

Currently, several digital physician education and information platforms for CU are operated by medical societies, pharmaceutical industry, digital medical publishing and communication companies, and UCARE. The most comprehensive of these platforms is UCARE LevelUp, which was launched with the purpose of developing an ongoing teaching program for physicians [25]. The goal of UCARE LevelUp is to create an interactive, virtual, and all-encompassing environment in which healthcare professionals from around the world may learn, strengthen their network, and share best clinical practices in CU to keep physicians updated on the latest advances in the field of urticaria, to optimize treatment of their patients.

The UCARE LevelUp program uses different formats to keep clinicians engaged and updated on CU, i.e., webinars, podcasts, websites, journal clubs, grand rounds, and newsletters. Across these formats, physicians are educated on a wide range of topics, including guideline recommendations, new publications, studies, clinical trials, and UCARE project outcomes; new webinars come online every 8, episode of the UCARE podcast "All Things Urticaria" are aired every 2 weeks, with more than 60 episodes so far [26]. The UCARE LevelUp digital journal club hosts rotating presenters of recent urticaria publications, and the grand round format allows physicians to present exceptional cases and receive input from top urticariologists, via live online sessions. All activities are announced and summarized in the UCARE LevelUp newsletter.

Digital education of physicians who treat CU patients, in family practice, specialist settings, or at UCAREs plays a crucial role in improving patient outcomes and quality of life as well as can improve physician knowledge. Future efforts to improve physician education and information on CU should aim to use formats that align with the learning profiles and expectations of physicians and to prioritize information of high relevance for different health care settings and geographical regions.

11.4 Digital Monitoring of CU Activity, Impact, Control, and Response to Treatment

The use of PROMs for assessing CU activity, impact, and control is of key importance to achieving treatment goals. This includes the use of the urticaria and angioedema activity scores, UAS and AAS [27–31] and of the urticaria and angioedema control tests, UCT and AECT [29–33]. At present, these tools are not used enough, despite their broad and free of charge availability as paper and digital versions (MOXIE, Berlin; https://moxie-gmbh.de). Because of this, UCARE developed CRUSE, an app that allows CSU patients to monitor their disease with the help of PROMs such as the UAS, AAS, UCT, and AECT. The development of CRUSE was supported by the finding of the UCARE CURICT project that more than half of CU patients have a significant interest in the use of an app to monitor their condition [34] and a subsequent study that showed the lack of suitable apps for CSU [35]. The CRUSE app was launched in 2022 and has since served over 4000 patients from around the world. CRUSE is available in 13 countries (Germany, Austria, Switzerland, Italy, Spain, Portugal, Turkey, France, UK, Ecuador, Argentina, Brazil, and Peru) adapted to the local language and medication, and globally, in English and Ukrainian.

CRUSE provides patients and their healthcare providers with real-time, data-driven insights, thus facilitating the implementation of personalized treatment plans. CRUSE also strengthens patient–physician communication and active patient engagement in their disease management. Furthermore, CRUSE data enable novel insights into CSU progression and treatment response, which may be enhanced by integrating AI and machine learning algorithms that analyze patient data and may help with the identification and characterization of CSU phenotypes, similar to allergic respiratory diseases [36].

11.5   Digital Patient–Physician Communication

High quality and patient-centered healthcare is based on efficient patient–physician communication [37]. Digital health is all about bringing a positive and significant transformation in the practice and organization of healthcare. This transformation is made possible by monitoring patient health and enhancing quality of life through digital tools beyond the traditional healthcare environment [38].

As digital patient–physician communication becomes increasingly prevalent in healthcare, concerns have arisen regarding its safety and effectiveness. Some experts caution that the integration of digital health technologies could fundamentally alter the patient–physician relationship. They argue that replacing face-to-face consultations with virtual interactions could be hazardous and undesirable, as digital technologies may miss crucial information that doctors would ordinarily observe. Additionally, critics warn of the risk of imposing an unseen burden of work on patients, who may be required to invest substantial time and effort in actively participating in the treatment process. Another concern pertains to the roles and responsibilities of patients, as some fear that patients could be held accountable for tasks that traditionally fall under the purview of physicians [38, 39].

The experience with digital tools in urticariology suggests that these concerns are unfounded in the case of treating patients with CU. Through digital patient–physician communication, education, and disease monitoring, CU patients and their treating physicians share a common sense of empowerment. Specifically, CU patients at our UCAREs report to have gained a more comprehensive grasp of their disease and its impact on their quality of life as well as a better understanding of treatment responses and how to improve them. At the same time, physicians who treat CU patients have developed a new and more positive outlook on the management of this disease. The use of digital tools, from their point of view, saves time, streamlines communication, and allows for more efficient CU management. As a result, both patients and their physicians have achieved a newfound sense of equality, with the exchange of information facilitating their alignment as equal partners in making informed decisions regarding the treatment of CU.

Across the various digital tools and platforms used in CU, the CRUSE app is seen as a gamechanger in patient–physician communication. With the help of CRUSE, PROMs are used by patients and shared with their physicians before visits, allowing physicians to review current UAS and AAS values and UCT and AECT scores and prepare for the consultation. This is facilitated by the comprehensive report generated by the app generates, which includes patient pictures, medication, and a detailed documentation of symptoms and triggering factors. This report accurately reflects the current disease status and its changes over time, forming the foundation for continued and qualified patient–physician collaboration in optimizing outcomes.

Online consultations are another digital cornerstone of improved CU management. Previous studies have demonstrated that video visits can reduce stress levels among physicians, improve their usage and attention to body language, and amplify overall satisfaction [40, 41]. Furthermore, when combined with objectively provided data, such as that obtained through the CRUSE control app, video consultations have the potential to enhance healthcare sector efficiency and provide mutual benefits for both patients and doctors [42].

11.6 Improving CU Understanding by Data Obtained with Digital Health Measures

Data obtained with digital tools and platforms can help to improve the understanding of CU and its treatment and the factors that influence them. Here, digital registries are of key importance as they capture data from routine care settings [43]. CU registries can be national, e.g., the Danish National Patient Registry [44], multinational, e.g., Latin American CU registry [45], and international, e.g., Chronic Urticaria Registry (CURE; https://www.urticaria-registry.com) [16].

CURE is an ongoing, prospective, international, multicenter, observational, and voluntary registry of patients with CU [16]. The main advantage of CURE over national registries is its very large sample size collected from many centers and physicians around the world. Its results can thus teach us about similarities and differences in different regions of the world. Any physician dealing with CU patients can participate in CURE and enter the data of their patients. CURE collects baseline and follow-up data on all CU patients including the patient's demographics, history, symptoms, trigger and risk factors, therapies as well as healthcare utilization. As of May 2023, 59 centers from 27 countries worldwide have joined the registry and have entered baseline data on more than 5000 CU patients.

The first analyses of CURE data resulted in two publications [7, 16], and there are at least three more under development. The first publication shed light on the rationale, methods, and initial implementation of CURE [16]. The following study analyzed baseline and follow-up data of 2078 CSU patients to assess factors associated with complete response to CSU treatment [7]. Urticaria Control Test (UCT), weekly Urticaria Activity Score (UAS7), and Physician Global Assessment (PhyGA) of treatment response were used to evaluate complete response/control to treatment. Complete response/control was seen at baseline in 9.8%, 17.9%, and 42.3% of patients as assessed by UCT = 16, UAS7 = 0, and PhyGA = CR, respectively, which increased at 6 and 12 months. Patients with higher UCT scores or UAS7 had better sleep and quality of life. Factors associated with complete control of CSU included presence of angioedema without wheals, episodic disease, omalizumab treatment, and male sex. Agreement between UCT = 16 and UAS7 = 0 measurements was moderate, but poor between UCT = 16 and PhyGA = CR. The results of this study support the urticaria guideline recommendation to aim for complete control/response in CSU treatment [2]. This analysis also revealed that CSU complete control/response is more accurately measured by using PROMs, i.e., UCT and UAS7, than physician global assessment [7], in line with the international urticaria guideline [2].

Further CURE-based publications will include comparisons in terms of symptom patterns, risk factors, treatment responses, costs to the health system, and deeper analysis of some of the rarer subtypes of CU.

Patient data including the results from the use of PROMs, collected by using CRUSE, can be included in the Chronic Urticaria Registry (CURE) using a common identifier (ID). This allows improving current CU management of a specific patient as well as keeping the data for scientific analyses within CURE.

11.7   Open Questions and Future Developments

The advancement and widespread adoption of digital health measures are poised to greatly enhance the management of CU and drive future research in this field. Active self-management programs are increasingly recognized as integral to the comprehensive management of chronic disease, including CU [46].

Digital health measures for CU, today, encompass various technological platforms and tools, including mobile applications, telemedicine services, and online platforms. One class of digital tools that remains largely unexplored in CU are wearable devices. Wearables are defined as sensory devices that can be attached to clothing or worn as an accessory, which allow the tracking of health information through a multitude of onboard sensors of disease-related outcomes [47]. Furthermore, wearables enable continuous, real-time monitoring of health status [48]. As research and development in wearable technology progress, we expect that these devices will play an increasing role in supporting the monitoring of CU, for example, heart rate, sleep quality, energy expenditure, and scratching.

Further research in the field of digital CU tools has the potential to expand the range of healthcare-related services available online and lead to increased accessibility, accuracy, trust, and engagement in remote consultations for both patients and physicians. At the same time, to assure security and privacy in digital healthcare, it will be crucial to develop robust encryption methods, secure data storage, and authentication protocols to protect patient information and maintain confidentiality. By addressing these challenges, research can contribute to building a trustworthy and secure digital health ecosystem, further fostering CU patient–physician collaboration.

The expanding digital health landscape holds immense potential for future CU research. With the integration of data analytics and machine learning algorithms, large-scale datasets generated by digital health measures can be analyzed to uncover patterns, identify risk factors, and develop predictive models for CU outcomes [49]. Here, artificial intelligence represents a new exciting tool in urticariology. For example, it might help in the differential diagnosis of CU and as and educational resource for training physicians who treat patients with CU [50].

Additionally, digital platforms can facilitate the recruitment of diverse and geographically dispersed participants for clinical trials and scientific projects, accelerating the pace of research and enabling more comprehensive investigations into the underlying mechanisms, treatment options, and long-term outcomes of CU and its comorbidities. Further development of CURE, for example, will contribute to improving knowledge of urticaria and angioedema. The latter will be also be aided by the Chronic Angioedema Registry (CARE), a CURE twin registry under development by the network of angioedema centers of reference and excellence (ACARE; https://acare-network.com) [51]. We firmly hold the integration, development, and expansion of digital health tools as essential for improving the understanding and management of CU.

References

1. Kolkhir P, Giménez-Arnau AM, Kulthanan K, Peter J, Metz M, Maurer M. Urticaria. Nat Rev Dis Primers. 2022;8(1):61.
2. Zuberbier T, Abdul Latiff AH, Abuzakouk M, Aquilina S, Asero R, Baker D, et al. The international EAACI/GA²LEN/EuroGuiDerm/APAAACI guideline for the definition, classification, diagnosis, and management of urticaria. Allergy. 2022;77(3):734–66.
3. Wagner N, Zink A, Hell K, Reinhardt M, Romer K, Hillmann E, et al. Patients with chronic urticaria remain largely undertreated: results from the DERMLINE Online Survey. Dermatol Ther (Heidelb). 2021;11(3):1027–39.
4. Ryan D, Angier E, Gomez M, Church D, Batsiou M, Nekam K, et al. Results of an allergy educational needs questionnaire for primary care. Allergy. 2017;72(7):1123–8.
5. Weller K, Maurer M, Bauer A, Wedi B, Wagner N, Schliemann S, et al. Epidemiology, comorbidities, and healthcare utilization of patients with chronic urticaria in Germany. J Eur Acad Dermatol Venereol. 2022;36(1):91–9.
6. Dezoteux F, Adam B, Pape E, Azib-Meftah S, Calafiore M, Staumont-Sallé D. A real-life assessment of the management of chronic urticaria in primary care by general practitioners in the North of France. Ann Dermatol Venereol. 2021;148(4):266–8.

7. Kolkhir P, Laires PA, Salameh P, Asero R, Bizjak M, Košnik M, et al. The benefit of complete response to treatment in patients with chronic spontaneous Urticaria-CURE Results. J Allergy Clin Immunol Pract. 2023;11(2):610–20.e5.
8. Maurer M, Abuzakouk M, Bérard F, Canonica W, Oude Elberink H, Giménez-Arnau A, et al. The burden of chronic spontaneous urticaria is substantial: real-world evidence from ASSURE-CSU. Allergy. 2017;72(12):2005–16.
9. Goldstein S, Eftekhari S, Mitchell L, Winders TA, Kaufman L, Dudas D, et al. Perspectives on living with chronic spontaneous Urticaria: from onset through diagnosis and disease management in the US. Acta Derm Venereol. 2019;99(12):1091–8.
10. De Bruin-Weller M, Biedermann T, Bissonnette R, Deleuran M, Foley P, Girolomoni G, et al. Treat-to-target in atopic dermatitis: an international consensus on a set of core decision points for systemic therapies. Acta Derm Venereol. 2021;101(2):adv00402.
11. Hakansson Eklund J, Holmstrom IK, Kumlin T, Kaminsky E, Skoglund K, Hoglander J, et al. "Same same or different?" A review of reviews of person-centered and patient-centered care. Patient Educ Couns. 2019;102(1):3–11.
12. Poon BY, Shortell SM, Rodriguez HP. Patient activation as a pathway to shared decision-making for adults with diabetes or cardiovascular disease. J Gen Intern Med. 2020;35(3):732–42.
13. Smith SG, Pandit A, Rush SR, Wolf MS, Simon CJ. The role of patient activation in preferences for shared decision making: results from a National Survey of U.S. Adults J Health Commun. 2016;21(1):67–75.
14. Awad A, Trenfield SJ, Pollard TD, Ong JJ, Elbadawi M, McCoubrey LE, et al. Connected healthcare: Improving patient care using digital health technologies. Adv Drug Deliv Rev. 2021;178:113958.
15. Thøgersen M. UCARE. https://ga2len-ucare.com/; 2023.
16. Weller K, Giménez-Arnau A, Grattan C, Asero R, Mathelier-Fusade P, Bizjak M, et al. The chronic Urticaria registry: rationale, methods and initial implementation. J Eur Acad Dermatol Venereol. 2021;35(3):721–9.
17. Marcolino MS, Oliveira JAQ, D'Agostino M, Ribeiro AL, Alkmim MBM, Novillo-Ortiz D. The impact of mHealth interventions: systematic review of systematic reviews. JMIR Mhealth Uhealth. 2018;6(1):e23.
18. Cherrez-Ojeda I, Vanegas E, Cherrez A, Felix M, Weller K, Magerl M, et al. How are patients with chronic urticaria interested in using information and communication technologies to guide their healthcare? A UCARE study. World Allergy Organ J. 2021;14(6):100542.
19. Maurer M, Weller K, Magerl M, Maurer RR, Vanegas E, Felix M, et al. The usage, quality and relevance of information and communications technologies in patients with chronic urticaria: a UCARE study. World Allergy Organ J. 2020;13(11):100475.
20. Pozo-Beltran CF, Larenas-Linnemann D, Arteche JDC. CME suggestions for pediatricians, allergists, and dermatologists, directed by an online survey on urticaria knowledge. Allergol Immunopathol (Madr). 2021;49(1):87–94.
21. Calle M, Stan A, Schoonheim P, Lebwohl M, Kaplan A. Online education yields significant gains in physicians' knowledge of diagnosis and management of chronic spontaneous Urticaria. J Allergy Clin Immunol. 2022;149(2):AB177.
22. Drexel C, Bixler E, Lee J, Lang D, Eftekhari S. Online education with the patient voice highlights continuous gaps in care and needs for therapeutic options for chronic spontaneous urticaria (CSU). Manage J Allergy Clin Immunol. 2023;151(2):AB138.
23. Activities—UCARE 4U. https://ucare-4u.com/en/activities/; 2023.
24. Maurer M, Bousquet J, Zuberbier T, Robles-Velasco K, Ramon G, Krasowska D, et al. Barriers of use of proms among allergists who treat atopic dermatitis and chronic urticaria. Ann Allergy Asthma Immunol. 2022;129(5):S33–S4.
25. Soltész R. Levelup—Educational program. UCARE https://ga2len-ucare.com/levelup-educational-program/; 2023.
26. Föll J. All things urticaria podcast. UCARE. https://ga2len-ucare.com/all-things-urticaria-podcast/; 2023.

27. Hawro T, Ohanyan T, Schoepke N, Metz M, Peveling-Oberhag A, Staubach P, et al. The urticaria activity score—validity, reliability, and responsiveness. J Allergy Clin Immunol Pract. 2018;6(4):1185–90. e1
28. Hawro T, Ohanyan T, Schoepke N, Metz M, Peveling-Oberhag A, Staubach P, et al. Comparison and interpretability of the available urticaria activity scores. Allergy. 2018;73(1):251–5.
29. Ohanyan T, Schoepke N, Bolukbasi B, Metz M, Hawro T, Zuberbier T, et al. Responsiveness and minimal important difference of the urticaria control test. J Allergy Clin Immunol. 2017;140(6):1710–3. e11
30. Weller K, Groffik A, Church MK, Hawro T, Krause K, Metz M, et al. Development and validation of the urticaria control test: a patient-reported outcome instrument for assessing urticaria control. J Allergy Clin Immunol. 2014;133(5):1365–72. e6
31. Weller K, Groffik A, Magerl M, Tohme N, Martus P, Krause K, et al. Development, validation, and initial results of the angioedema activity score. Allergy. 2013;68(9):1185–92.
32. Buttgereit T, Salameh P, Sydorenko O, Zuberbier T, Metz M, Weller K, et al. The 7-day recall period version of the Urticaria Control Test–UCT7. J Allergy Clin Immunol. 2023;152(5):1210–7.
33. Weller K, Donoso T, Magerl M, Aygören-Pürsün E, Staubach P, Martinez-Saguer I, et al. Validation of the Angioedema Control Test (AECT)—a patient-reported outcome instrument for assessing angioedema control. J Allergy Clin Immunol Pract. 2020;8(6):2050–7. e4
34. Cherrez-Ojeda I, Vanegas E, Cherrez A, Felix M, Weller K, Magerl M, et al. Chronic urticaria patients are interested in apps to monitor their disease activity and control: a UCARE CURICT analysis. Clin Transl Allergy. 2021;11(10):e12089.
35. Anto A, Maurer R, Gimenez-Arnau A, Cherrez-Ojeda I, Hawro T, Magerl M, et al. Automatic screening of self-evaluation apps for urticaria and angioedema shows a high unmet need. Allergy. 2021;76(12):3810–3.
36. Bousquet J, Melen E, Haahtela T, Koppelman GH, Togias A, Valenta R, et al. Rhinitis associated with asthma is distinct from rhinitis alone: the ARIA-MeDALL hypothesis. Allergy. 2023;78(5):1169–203.
37. Rathert C, Mittler JN, Banerjee S, McDaniel J. Patient-centered communication in the era of electronic health records: what does the evidence say? Patient Educ Couns. 2017;100(1):50–64.
38. Jongsma KR, Bekker MN, Haitjema S, Bredenoord AL. How digital health affects the patient-physician relationship: an empirical-ethics study into the perspectives and experiences in obstetric care. Pregn Hypertens. 2021;25:81–6.
39. Mesko B, Drobni Z, Benyei E, Gergely B, Gyorffy Z. Digital health is a cultural transformation of traditional healthcare. Mhealth. 2017;3:38.
40. Byrne MHV, Ashcroft J, Alexander L, Wan JCM, Harvey A. Systematic review of medical student willingness to volunteer and preparedness for pandemics and disasters. Emerg Med J. 2021;39(10):e6.
41. Primholdt Christensen N, Skou KE, Boe DD. Health care professionals' experiences with the use of video consultation: qualitative study. JMIR Form Res. 2021;5(7):e27094.
42. Birnbaum F, Lewis D, Rosen RK, Ranney ML. Patient engagement and the design of digital health. Acad Emerg Med. 2015;22(6):754–6.
43. Gómez RM, Jares E, Canonica GW, Baiardini I, Passalacqua G, Sánchez Borges M, et al. Why a registry of Chronic Urticaria (CUR) is needed. World Allergy Organ J. 2017;10(1):16.
44. Ghazanfar MN, Kibsgaard L, Thomsen SF, Vestergaard C. Risk of comorbidities in patients diagnosed with chronic urticaria: a nationwide registry-study. World Allergy Organ J. 2020;13(1):100097.
45. Gómez RM, Jares E, Borges MS, Baiardini I, Canonica GW, Passalacqua G, et al. Latin American chronic urticaria registry (CUR) contribution to the understanding and knowledge of the disease in the region. World Allergy Organ J. 2019;12(6):100042.
46. Chodosh J, Morton SC, Mojica W, Maglione M, Suttorp MJ, Hilton L, et al. Meta-analysis: chronic disease self-management programs for older adults. Ann Intern Med. 2005;143(6):427–38.

47. Kamei T, Kanamori T, Yamamoto Y, Edirippulige S. The use of wearable devices in chronic disease management to enhance adherence and improve telehealth outcomes: a systematic review and meta-analysis. J Telemed Telecare. 2022;28(5):342–59.
48. Sharma A, Badea M, Tiwari S, Marty JL. Wearable biosensors: an alternative and practical approach in healthcare and disease monitoring. Molecules. 2021;26(3):748.
49. Pathania Y. Artificial intelligence in chronic urticaria: unsupervised versus supervised machine learning. Actas Dermo-Sifiliogr. 2023;114(7):659.
50. Liopyris K, Gregoriou S, Dias J, Stratigos AJ. Artificial intelligence in dermatology: challenges and perspectives. Dermatol Ther. 2022:1–15.
51. Maurer M, Aberer W, Agondi R, Al-Ahmad M, Al-Nesf MA, Ansotegui I, et al. Definition, aims, and implementation of GA2LEN/HAEi Angioedema Centers of Reference and Excellence. Allergy. 2020;75(8):2115–23.

Chapter 12
Digital Health and Atopic Dermatitis

Sebastian Sitaru and Alexander Zink

Contents

Abstract Atopic dermatitis is a chronic inflammatory skin disease associated with allergic diseases and can lead to significant disease burden and loss of quality of life despite modern treatments. Digital tools for AD patients include online resources such as web searches and social media platforms, wearable biosensors (*wearables*), mobile apps, and new diagnostic tools such as 3D full body scanners and optical coherence tomography. While the analysis of online data can provide insights into the needs and wants of AD patients, the general quality of AD-related online information seems to be low and laced with misinformation. There is still insufficient clinical data validating the clinical use of apps in AD. Digital data, especially from new diagnostic methods, lends itself to machine learning and artificial intelligence analysis. New data is constantly being generated, and algorithms are being created and improved, so there are exciting future perspectives especially for this field in digital tools in AD.

S. Sitaru (✉) · A. Zink
Department of Dermatology and Allergy, School of Medicine, Technical University of Munich, Munich, Germany
e-mail: sebastian.sitaru@tum.de; alexander.zink@tum.de

© The Author(s), under exclusive license to Springer Nature Switzerland AG 2025
P. M. Matricardi, S. Dramburg, *Digital Allergology*, Health Informatics, https://doi.org/10.1007/978-3-031-71021-6_12

Atopic dermatitis (AD) is a prevalent chronic inflammatory skin disease associated with allergies [1]. AD leads to the formation of itchy, recurrent rashes which are characterized by vesicles and erythematous papules and plaques, as well as fine scaling. Although the disease can affect the whole body and all age groups, it is predominantly present in children and young adults. Pathophysiologically, genetic and environmental factors lead to an inflammation driven by type 2 T helper cells [2]. It is still not completely understood what happens upstream of this inflammation and therefore, AD is currently mostly seen as a heterogeneous inflammatory response to a plethora of potential exacerbating factors, including genetic predisposition, microbiome, stress, dryness of the skin (xerosis), and environmental factors including exposure to allergens [1]. Even though novel therapies with small molecules and biologics have greatly improved therapeutic outcomes, there are still many patients who do not adequately respond to these therapies, so that overall, AD still directly and indirectly leads to a severely impaired quality of life [3–6]. One major factor contributing to the decrease in quality of life is the intense itch and associated sleeplessness [7]. Recently, discussions have opened up regarding different endotypes of atopic dermatitis based on the spectrum of observed response to systemic treatments and serum biomarkers [8, 9].

In AD, more and more digital data are being generated; this includes biochemical data related to the microbiome, clinical parameters such as scores and device measurements, but also patient questionnaire responses and clinical 2D and 3D images [10, 11]. For AD, recommendations regarding high-quality biomarkers have been established by expert interviews [12]. Together with the fact that AD affects predominantly younger patients, digital tools are increasingly impacting AD research and patient care.

12.1 Crowd-Sourced Data and Social Media

Many dermatological patients including AD patients use "Dr. Google" and social media to inform themselves about their disease and discuss it with others [13]. Therefore, crowd-sourced data such as Google web search data and social media analyses can provide insights into population level needs and estimates of disease burden in correlation to different environmental factors [14–16]. Especially in AD, patients are predominantly younger and therefore more likely to use web and social media platforms.

An analysis of publicly available AD-related web information in 2020 revealed a mixed landscape with a presence of patient support groups, but also businesses, disseminating mostly general information about AD [17]. AD-related online forum posts in France revealed that discussions were mostly about tips to manage AD, therapy failure, AD in infants, and quality of life [18]. In general, the quality of AD-related online information seems to be mixed to low: 17–48% of AD-related videos on YouTube were categorized as misleading and around one-third as potentially harmful [19, 20]. Also on TikTok, in 2020, the quality of information presented by health care professionals and non-health care professionals alike was deemed low [21]. Noted deficiencies, especially in content from health care professionals, included failure to discuss risks of treatments and to cite sources, which could be in part due to the overall short length of the videos being on TikTok.

Indeed, one challenge in chronic inflammatory skin conditions like AD is to maintain long-term treatment adherence. Misinformation, such as the scientifically largely unfounded topical corticosteroid withdrawal ("steroid addition") syndrome, are discussed on social media and can impact disease control [22–24]. In extreme cases, exposure to social media misinformation can trigger complete cessation of all AD therapy, resulting in predictable and avoidable flares [25].

Beyond providing passive data for analysis, social media was also used successfully to recruit AD participants for a clinical study [26].

Taken together, crowd-sourced data is a powerful tool providing a direct window into the publicly (social media) and privately (Google web search data) addressed concerns and stories of AD patients and is therefore important to both research and direct patient care. Special attention should be paid to AD-related information found online since it is mostly of low quality, therefore patients should be educated accordingly.

12.2 Mobile Apps

Mobile apps can help patients by providing educational material and monitoring disease severity by patient-reported outcomes [27, 28]. For AD specifically, there is clinical data suggesting that mobile apps can boost AD treatment adherence and improve quality of life [29–31]. The major challenges and needs of adult patients, as well as caregivers of younger patients, regarding mobile apps for AD have been identified as a possibility to uncover triggers leading to flare-ups, pipelines to physicians, empowerment to improve disease condition by education, and helping with the correct treatment, among others [32, 33]. Even though a plethora of AD-related apps can be found in app stores, many of them still lack clinical validation data for their efficacy [34, 35]. A recent example of a validated app is the "Atopic App," which addresses many of the needs mentioned above and showed a significant reduction of AD severity scores among its users [35]. When combining future apps with novel algorithms (see below) to, e.g., automatically determine scores from images or to predict flares, even more benefit could be generated for AD patients.

12.3 Wearables

A topic which is gaining traction in dermatological research is digital wearable sensors or *wearables* [36]. Recent advances in material science lay the groundwork for ever smaller and more capable wearables which can provide a plethora of measurements from minimally invasive or non-invasive sensors [37, 38]. For AD, scratch measurement by wrist-worn non-invasive sensors was recently established in research [39]. Currently, wearables are being researched which track the level of skin dryness (xerosis) (Fig. 12.1). Data from transepithelial water loss (TEWL) sensors and electrodermal activity (EDA) sensors, which are patterns of skin conductance changes, is being collected in a wearable context in the real world. It is hypothesized that this data cannot be used only for reactive disease monitoring, but also to proactively predict flares. However, even more biosensors already exist, e.g., measuring skin resistance, pH, or even cytokines in body fluids [40–42]. Many of these sensors have promising validation data, e.g., correct measurements of cytokines compared to traditional methods in healthy volunteers [40]; however, data from larger clinical trials in patients with AD or other skin diseases are currently still lacking. In the future, we can expect more and more such trials, and ultimately wearables providing significant benefit to patients with AD.

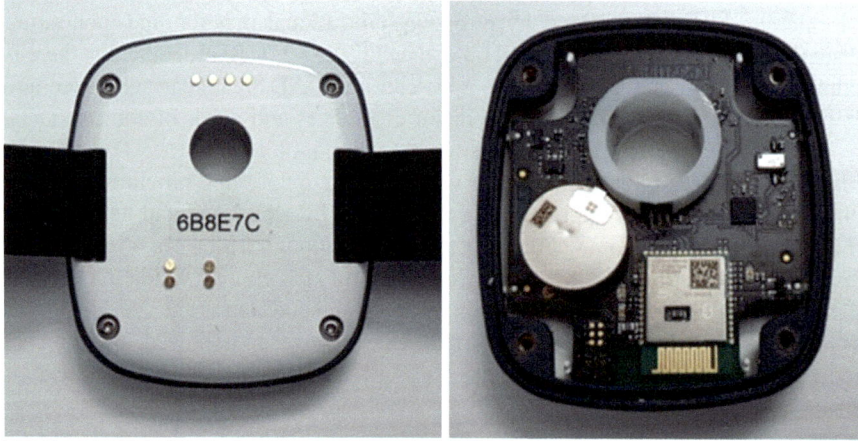

Fig. 12.1 Development version of a wearable device for measuring the skin parameters transepithelial water loss (TEWL) and electrodermal activity (EDA). Reproduced with permission by Eltroplan GmbH, Endingen, Germany © 2024. All Rights Reserved

12.4   Machine Learning and Artificial Intelligence

Once digitalized, data can be processed and analyzed in many ways, including artificial intelligence (AI) and machine learning (ML) algorithms [43, 44]. ML is a subset of artificial intelligence and has recently seen a rise in popularity and research output due to the advancement of underlying key technologies such as artificial neural networks [44]. Especially in the field of dermatology and for AD, the expansion of possible data sources including new digital biomarkers, 2D and 3D image data, and data from novel techniques such as line-field confocal optical coherence tomography (LC-OCT) and of course, wearables, opens new possibilities for ML and AI analysis.

Already, 2D clinical images can be analyzed for outliers, as well as affected body parts with good accuracy using AI algorithms [45].

3D body scanners have been recently introduced to dermatology [11]. They can capture almost the whole skin surface using off-the-shelf camera chips in an instant and reconstruct the images to a 3D model (Fig. 12.2). By simplifying and standardizing image capture, these devices can provide a plethora of benefits for many skin diseases including AD. For example, they enable easy store-and-forward models for diagnosis or follow-ups and can generate standardized data needed for ML and AI analysis [11].

Similarly, data from new non-invasive microscopic imaging tools like LC-OCT could be used for ML and AI analysis, e.g., to diagnose or follow-up skin diseases including AD [46]. In fact, there is data that LC-OCT can have a similar value to conventional histology in the diagnosis of AD [47].

One strength of ML algorithms is their inference abilities on never-before-seen data: for example, predicting persistence of AD diagnosed in infancy with good accuracy based on clinical variables and serum cytokine levels becomes possible

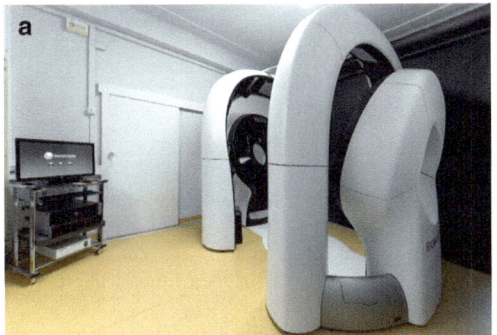
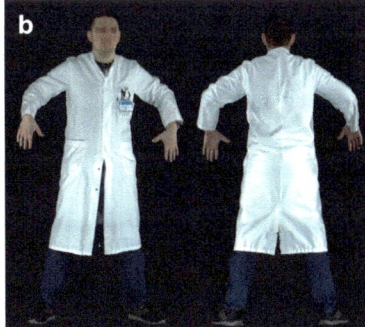

Fig. 12.2 3D whole body scanner (**a**) and its output (**b**). The 3D whole body scanner simultaneously captures almost the whole skin surface using multiple cameras and reconstructs a 3D model from the images (**b**). (Source: [11])

[48]. Furthermore, biomarkers which can predict quality of life impairment in AD are being systematically analyzed [49].

More and more digital data are being generated using traditional and novel techniques, so it can be predicted that the field of ML and AI will offer exciting perspectives in the research and treatment of AD.

12.5   Summary

In summary, atopic dermatitis is a chronic inflammatory skin disease associated with allergic diseases. It affects mostly younger patients and can lead to significant disease burden and loss of quality of life despite modern treatments. Digital tools are increasingly being researched and used in AD. Patients suffering from AD can use online resources including web searches and social media platforms to inform themselves about their disease and to discuss relevant topics with others. The analysis of these data can provide insights into the needs and wants of AD patients and could be used in future to estimate disease burden. Importantly however, the general quality of AD-related information online seems to be low and laced with misinformation, which can negatively affect treatment adherence. Wearable biosensors (*wearables*) are becoming increasingly smaller and more powerful and might soon be clinically used for AD diagnosis and follow-up. A plethora of mobile apps have been published in the app stores, and initial studies confirm beneficial effects in AD; however, there is still insufficient clinical data validating their widespread use in AD. Digital data lends itself to machine learning and artificial intelligence analysis. Already today, it is possible to estimate persistence of AD beyond childhood based on biomarkers and predict quality of life impairment. Since more and more digital data are generated, and new digital diagnostic tools like optical coherence tomography and 3D full body scanners are being established in dermatology, we can expect many more exciting applications of machine learning algorithms in skin diseases and AD.

References

1. Weidinger S, Beck LA, Bieber T, Kabashima K, Irvine AD. Atopic dermatitis. Nat Rev Dis Primer. 2018;4(1):1.
2. Schäbitz A, Eyerich K, Garzorz-Stark N. So close, and yet so far away: the dichotomy of the specific immune response and inflammation in psoriasis and atopic dermatitis. J Intern Med. 2021;290(1):27–39.
3. Birdi G, Cooke R, Knibb RC. Impact of atopic dermatitis on quality of life in adults: a systematic review and meta-analysis. Int J Dermatol. 2020;59(4):e75–91.
4. Rogner D, Biedermann T, Lauffer F. Treatment of atopic dermatitis with Baricitinib: first real-life experience. Acta Derm Venereol. 2022;102:adv00677.
5. Lauffer F, Ring J. Target-oriented therapy: emerging drugs for atopic dermatitis. Expert Opin Emerg Drugs. 2016;21(1):81–9.

6. Augustin M, Bauer A, Ertner K, von Kiedrowski R, Schenck F, Ramaker-Brunke J, et al. Dupilumab demonstrates rapid onset of action in improving signs, symptoms and quality of life in adults with atopic dermatitis. Dermatol Ther. 2023;13(3):803–16.
7. Podder I, Mondal H, Kroumpouzos G. Nocturnal pruritus and sleep disturbance associated with dermatologic disorders in adult patients. Int J Womens Dermatol. 2021;7(4):403–10.
8. Kim J, Ahn K. Atopic dermatitis endotypes: knowledge for personalized medicine. Curr Opin Allergy Clin Immunol. 2022;22(3):153–9.
9. Wu Y, Gu C, Wang S, Yin H, Qiu Z, Luo Y, et al. Serum biomarker-based endotypes of atopic dermatitis in China and prediction for efficacy of dupilumab. Br J Dermatol. 2023;188(5):649–60.
10. Preis S, Schmidt L, Tizek L, Schielein M, Lang V, Bleuel R, et al. Munich atopy prediction study (MAPS): protocol for a prospective birth cohort addressing clinical and molecular risk factors for atopic dermatitis in early childhood. BMJ Open. 2022;12(9):e059256.
11. Sitaru S, Kaczmarczyk R, Erdmann M, Biedermann T, Zink A. [3D whole body scans in dermatology-a new era in clinical practice and research?]. Dermatol Heidelb Ger. 2022;73(7):575–9.
12. Ziehfreund S, Tizek L, Hangel N, Fritzsche MC, Weidinger S, Smith C, et al. Requirements and expectations of high-quality biomarkers for atopic dermatitis and psoriasis in 2021-a two-round Delphi survey among international experts. J Eur Acad Dermatol Venereol JEADV. 2022;36(9):1467–76.
13. Hongler VNS, Navarini A, Brandt O, Goldust M, Mueller SM. Global trends in YouTube and Google search activity for psoriasis and atopic eczema: detecting geographic hot spots, blind spots and treatment strategies. Dermatol Ther. 2020;33(4):e13510.
14. Schober A, Tizek L, Johansson EK, Ekebom A, Wallin JE, Buters J, et al. Monitoring disease activity of pollen allergies: what crowdsourced data are telling us. World Allergy Organ J. 2022;15(12):100718.
15. Sitaru S, Tizek L, Buters J, Ekebom A, Wallin JE, Zink A. Assessing the national burden of allergic asthma by web-search data, pollen counts, and drug prescriptions in Germany and Sweden. World Allergy Organ J. 2023;16(2):100752. https://www.worldallergyorganization-journal.org/article/S1939-4551(23)00012-1/fulltext.
16. Gesualdo F, Stilo G, D'Ambrosio A, Carloni E, Pandolfi E, Velardi P, et al. Can twitter be a source of information on allergy? Correlation of pollen counts with tweets reporting symptoms of allergic rhinoconjunctivitis and names of antihistamine drugs. PLoS One. 2015;10(7):e0133706.
17. Iglesias-Puzas Á, Conde-Taboada A, Campos-Muñoz L, Belinchón-Romero I, López-Bran E. Social networks and atopic dermatitis: cross-sectional descriptive study. Actas Dermosifiliogr. 2020;111(8):665–70.
18. Voillot P, Riche B, Portafax M, Foulquié P, Gedik A, Barbarot S, et al. Social media platforms listening study on atopic dermatitis: quantitative and qualitative findings. J Med Internet Res. 2022;24(1):e31140.
19. Freemyer B, Drozd B, Suarez A. A cross-sectional study of YouTube videos about atopic dermatitis. J Am Acad Dermatol. 2018;78(3):612–3.
20. Mueller SM, Hongler VNS, Jungo P, Cajacob L, Schwegler S, Steveling EH, et al. Fiction, falsehoods, and few facts: cross-sectional study on the content-related quality of atopic eczema-related videos on YouTube. J Med Internet Res. 2020;22(4):e15599.
21. Khan S, Yee D, Khan S, Mehta M, Zagona-Prizio C, Maynard N, et al. Biologics to breast milk: a cross-sectional study of popular eczema treatment content on TikTok. Pediatr Dermatol. 2022;39(6):920–2.
22. Hajar T, Leshem YA, Hanifin JM, Nedorost ST, Lio PA, Paller AS, et al. A systematic review of topical corticosteroid withdrawal ("steroid addiction") in patients with atopic dermatitis and other dermatoses. J Am Acad Dermatol. 2015;72(3):541–549.e2.
23. Finnegan P, Murphy M, O'Connor C. #corticophobia: a review on online misinformation related to topical steroids. Clin Exp Dermatol. 2023;48(2):112–5.
24. Nickles MA, Coale AT, Henderson WJA, Brown KE, Morrell DS, Nieman EL. Steroid phobia on social media platforms. Pediatr Dermatol. 2023;40:479.

25. Wilson A, Cowan TL, Rivero ADL, Murrell DF. The dangers of social media: patients with atopic dermatitis ceasing their basic treatment. Clin Exp Dermatol. 2023;48(2):142–3.
26. Baker A, Mitchell EJ, Thomas KS. A practical guide to implementing a successful social media recruitment strategy: lessons from the eczema monitoring online trial. Trials. 2022;23(1):905.
27. Richter JG, Nannen C, Chehab G, Acar H, Becker A, Willers R, et al. Mobile app-based documentation of patient-reported outcomes—3-months results from a proof-of-concept study on modern rheumatology patient management. Arthritis Res Ther. 2021;23(1):121.
28. Benze G, Nauck F, Alt-Epping B, Gianni G, Bauknecht T, Ettl J, et al. PROutine: a feasibility study assessing surveillance of electronic patient reported outcomes and adherence via smartphone app in advanced cancer. Ann Palliat Med. 2019;8(2):104–11.
29. Gudmundsdóttir SL, Ballarini T, Ámundadóttir ML, Mészáros J, Eysteinsdóttir JH, Thorleifsdóttir RH, et al. Clinical efficacy of a digital intervention for patients with atopic dermatitis: a prospective single-center study. Dermatol Ther. 2022;12(11):2601–11.
30. Gudmundsdóttir SL, Ballarini T, Ámundadóttir ML, Mészáros J, Eysteinsdottir JH, Thorleifsdottir RH, et al. Engagement, retention and acceptability in a digital health program for atopic dermatitis: prospective interventional study. JMIR Form Res. 2023.
31. Shah S, Kemp JM, Kvedar JC, Gracey LE. A feasibility study of the burden of disease of atopic dermatitis using a smartphone research application, myEczema. Int J Womens Dermatol. 2020;6(5):424–8.
32. Gracey LE, Zan S, Gracz J, Miner JJ, Moreau JF, Sperber J, et al. Use of user-centered design to create a smartphone application for patient-reported outcomes in atopic dermatitis. NPJ Digit Med. 2018;1:33.
33. Xu X, Griva K, Koh M, Lum E, Tan WS, Thng S, et al. Creating a smartphone app for caregivers of children with atopic dermatitis with caregivers, health care professionals, and digital health experts: participatory co-design. JMIR Mhealth Uhealth. 2020;8(10):e16898.
34. Schuster B, Dugas M, Zink A. Medizinische Apps—Möglichkeiten bei Pruritus. Hautarzt Z Dermatol Venerol Verwandte Geb. 2020;71(7):528–34.
35. Zvulunov A, Lenevich S, Migacheva N. A Mobile health app for facilitating disease Management in Children with Atopic Dermatitis: feasibility and impact study. JMIR Dermatol. 2023;6:e49278.
36. Kiani C, Kain A, Zink A. Wearables and smart skin as new tools for clinical practice and research in dermatology. JEADV Clin Pract. 2022;1:66.
37. Guk K, Han G, Lim J, Jeong K, Kang T, Lim EK, et al. Evolution of wearable devices with real-time disease monitoring for personalized healthcare. Nano. 2019;9(6):813.
38. Todorov A, Torah R, Ardern-Jones MR, Beeby SP. Electromagnetic sensing techniques for monitoring atopic dermatitis-current practices and possible advancements: a review. Sensors. 2023;23(8):3935.
39. Ji J, Venderley J, Zhang H, Lei M, Ruan G, Patel N, et al. Assessing nocturnal scratch with actigraphy in atopic dermatitis patients. NPJ Digit Med. 2023;6(1):72.
40. Chu H, Hu X, Lee CY, Zhang A, Ye Y, Wang Y, et al. A wearable electrochemical fabric for cytokine monitoring. Biosens Bioelectron. 2023;232:115301.
41. De Silva T, Fawzy M, Hasani A, Ghanbari H, Abnavi A, Askar A, et al. Ultrasensitive rapid cytokine sensors based on asymmetric geometry two-dimensional MoS2 diodes. Nat Commun. 2022;13(1):7593.
42. Zhu L, Spachos P, Ng PC, Yu Y, Wang Y, Plataniotis K, et al. Stress detection through wrist-based Electrodermal activity monitoring and machine learning. IEEE J Biomed Health Inform. 2023;27:2155.
43. Mintz Y, Brodie R. Introduction to artificial intelligence in medicine. Minim Invasive Ther Allied Technol. 2019;28(2):73–81.
44. Young AT, Xiong M, Pfau J, Keiser MJ, Wei ML. Artificial intelligence in dermatology: a primer. J Invest Dermatol. 2020;140(8):1504–12.
45. Schielein MC, Christl J, Sitaru S, Pilz AC, Kaczmarczyk R, Biedermann T, et al. Outlier detection in dermatology: performance of different convolutional neural networks for binary classification of inflammatory skin diseases. J Eur Acad Dermatol Venereol JEADV. 2023;37(5):1071–9.

46. Ruini C, Schuh S, Sattler E, Welzel J. Line-field confocal optical coherence tomography—practical applications in dermatology and comparison with established imaging methods. Skin Res Technol. 2021;27(3):340–52.

47. Verzì AE, Broggi G, Micali G, Sorci F, Caltabiano R, Lacarrubba F. Line-field confocal optical coherence tomography of psoriasis, eczema and lichen planus: a case series with histopathological correlation. J Eur Acad Dermatol Venereol JEADV. 2022;36(10):1884–9.

48. Lauffer F, Baghin V, Standl M, Stark SP, Jargosch M, Wehrle J, et al. Predicting persistence of atopic dermatitis in children using clinical attributes and serum proteins. Allergy. 2021;76(4):1158–72.

49. Balato A, Zink A, Babino G, Buononato D, Kiani C, Eyerich K, et al. The impact of psoriasis and atopic dermatitis on quality of life: a literature research on biomarkers. Life Basel Switz. 2022;12(12):2026.

Chapter 13
Machine Learning for the Management of Allergies and Asthma in Childhood

Adnan Custovic, Darije Custovic, and Sara Fontanella

Contents

Abstract Atopic diseases (asthma, eczema, rhinitis) are heterogeneous, both in their course (curricular heterogeneity, i.e., differences in the time-course of their development) and their cause (aetiological heterogeneity, i.e., differences in the underpinning pathological mechanisms). Despite this diversity of mechanisms and

This chapter is a major update and adaptation of: Custovic D, Fontanella S, Custovic A. Understanding progression from pre-school wheezing to school-age asthma: Can modern data approaches help? *Pediatr Allergy Immunol* 2023; **34**(12): e14062.

A. Custovic (✉) · D. Custovic · S. Fontanella
National Heart and Lung Institute, Imperial College London, London, UK
e-mail: a.custovic@imperial.ac.uk; darije.custovic@imperial.ac.uk;
s.fontanella@imperial.ac.uk

P. M. Matricardi, S. Dramburg, *Digital Allergology*, Health Informatics,
https://doi.org/10.1007/978-3-031-71021-6_13

later outcomes, at symptom onset, clinical presentation in different subgroups of patients (such as transient or persistent wheezers) may be similar. Consequently, it is difficult to predict the course of allergies in individual patients, and the mechanisms associated with the persistence and remission of symptoms are poorly understood. Collection of vast amounts of longitudinal clinical data and high-throughput technologies may help us to understand the complexity of the development of childhood allergies. However, it is challenging to process, analyze, and interpret the large volumes of clinical and biological data. Machine Learning (ML) is a fundamental technology which may meaningfully process data that exceed the capacity of the human brain to comprehend, and ML models can digest large amounts of data quickly and identify underlying patterns within large data sets. However, it is important to emphasize that these patterns do not necessarily correspond to underlying biologic pathways. This chapter provides examples on how different ML approaches and methodologies (predictive and explanatory) have been used in pediatric allergy research, focussing on two specific exemplars: (1) understanding heterogeneity of childhood wheezing illness, including prediction models for childhood asthma and (2) understanding heterogeneity of childhood allergic sensitization and its relationship with asthma.

13.1   Introduction

Atopic diseases (including asthma, eczema, rhinitis) are heterogeneous, both in the time-course of the development and progression of symptoms (curricular heterogeneity) and in their underpinning pathological mechanisms (aetiological heterogeneity) [1]. The current diagnostic labels are mostly based on "typical" symptoms and/ or medication use (e.g., wheezing is considered a key symptom of asthma) and do not map precisely onto underlying disease mechanisms [2]. The burden of allergic diseases is considerable for patients, their families, and the society; for example, despite considerable improvements in the quality of care, asthma remains a cause of death among children and young people [3, 4]. Over recent decades, numerous epidemiological studies have demonstrated a close relationship between specific immunoglobulin E (sIgE) antibody responses and asthma, rhinitis, and eczema [5–7] (thereby justifying the label atopic diseases). However, the data about the strength of this association are inconsistent across studies [8–11], and there are no reliable and reproducible sensitisation parameters on which clinicians can base accurate diagnosis and risk prediction [9, 12, 13].

13.2   Curricular Heterogeneity of Preschool Wheezing and School-Age Asthma

Approximately half of children in the developed countries experience at least one episode of wheezing by school-age, and the majority of hospital admissions for acute wheeze attacks occur among preschool children [14]. In many patients, wheezing remits by mid-school age, but other children develop persisting symptoms, which are often diagnosed as asthma [15–17]. However, despite heterogeneity in long-term outcomes, clinically, at the onset of symptoms, patients whose wheeze will remit ("transient wheezers") and those in whom wheeze will persist ("persistent wheezers") clinically appear very similar, and differentiating those preschool wheezers who will stop wheezing from those whose wheezing will persist is difficult [18]. In addition, mechanisms associated with persistence or remission of wheezing are poorly understood [16, 19]. The persistence likely involves numerous factors, including immunological [20], genetic [21], environmental [22] and their interplay [23] (reviewed in [24]). Some of the key areas of unmet need for both patients/families and healthcare professionals are accurate diagnosis and long-term prognosis. In addition, identification of factors associated with persistence of wheeze may also help identify novel therapeutic and intervention targets.

Over the last decades, substantial effort has been devoted to understanding the heterogeneity of childhood wheezing [15, 25–27]. In 1989, Nicola Wilson provided an exceptional account of the complexities of wheezing illness in preschool children, including the suggestion for the introduction of the term virus-associated wheeze, and another clinical observation that shaped our thinking that of the differences in temporal patterns of wheezing between different patients, including remission, relapse, and persistence [28]. Martinez et al probed the natural history of wheezing using data collected at ages 3 and 6 years in the Tucson birth cohort and described three wheezing phenotypes in preschool age (transient early, late-onset, and persistent); different phenotypes were associated with different risk factors [29]. These findings were confirmed in several cohorts [30–32].

13.3   The Big Data Era: Meeting Unmet Needs Using Modern Data Approaches (MDAs)

After these early observational studies, the long-term follow-up of birth cohorts and recent rapid technological advances resulted in collections of vast amounts of longitudinal clinical information spanning decades, with associated data from high-throughput technologies. However, such large volumes of data are challenging to process, analyze, and interpret, and underlying patterns within such data sets are often impossible for human eye to observe, i.e., they are hidden (latent) [33, 34]. The detailed analysis of this sort of "big data" [35] holds the promise for better understanding of asthma and atopic diseases. Machine learning (ML) is a technology that allows to meaningfully process data that exceed the capacity of the human brain to comprehend, and ML models can digest large amounts of data and identify patterns/clusters that humans cannot find. It is important to emphasize that although these different clusters are sometimes referred to as "endotypes," such patterns may [36] or may not [37] correspond to different underlying mechanisms. In other words, the scientific discoveries made using ML should be both interpretable and verified [37], and clusters identified using data-driven methodologies remain hypothetical constructs until their underlying mechanisms confirmed in carefully conducted studies [34, 37].

Modern data approaches (MDAs) grounded in artificial intelligence (AI) and ML are fundamentally dependent on having large-scale high-quality data sets and the computational power and algorithms to analyze that data. The emergence of these methods has led to a new approach to doing science, often called the data-driven approach, and over the last 15 years, substantial effort has been devoted to understanding the heterogeneity of childhood allergic diseases using these modern data analysis techniques (reviewed in [1, 15, 25–27]).

13.4 ML, AI, and Data Science

ML, AI, and data science have had a profound influence on medical research in the last few decades. The annual rate of scientific papers on AI increased tenfold from 2012 to 2021 [38], with a similar pattern in AI/ML for allergic diseases [39, 40]. However, in their rapid uptake, the meaning of the various terms that fall under the MDA umbrella (multivariable statistics, AI, ML, data science, etc.) have often been confused [1, 39].

In general, statistics is concerned with the collection, organization, and interpretation of data. Statistical analysis can be divided into descriptive and inferential, with inferential analysis being particularly important to the topic of this chapter. Inferential statistics deals with drawing conclusions from data when the observations are subject to chance variation, i.e., evaluating hypotheses when there is a considerable element of uncertainty. To address this, statisticians adopted the mathematical tools of probability theory; however, in contrast to mathematics which in general answered the question "what data result from this chance process?" the statisticians sought to answer "what chance process do the data result from?" [1].

The development of the digital computer marked the beginning of computer science, with AI at its heart. Computer science is concerned with the automation of calculation, which had historically been a *mental* work; the takeover of this unique human function by mechanical-electrical systems opened the question of whether other aspects of natural intelligence could also be emulated in artificial systems (e.g., whether we can build a computer system capable of performing a mental task better than a human). This is relevant for the application of AI in medicine as an aid to clinical diagnosis, treatment selection, and decision-making, which are tasks traditionally performed by doctors. A prime example of such application is the use of AI in radiology [41].

Machine learning is a branch of AI generally concerned with the development and study of algorithms that can learn from data and generalize to unseen data and make predictions.

13.5   Machine Learning: Supervised and Unsupervised Approaches

The main objective of supervised ML is to predict output variables from input variables. The success of the trained model is validated by its ability to correctly predict the output variable when given unlabelled inputs [1]. Classical regression models, support vector machines, and deep learning (using artificial neural networks) are all methods of supervised ML.

The task of unsupervised ML is to find patterns in large data sets. Clustering is one example, and statistical models at the heart of unsupervised ML proceed from two mathematical definitions, one of the abstract patterns (e.g., clusters) being recognized in the data set, and the other of what a "close fit" of data to a pattern means [1]. The success of a model is measured by its ability to re-establish the same patterns when asked to look at the data multiple times, as well as to reproduce the same/similar patterns in similar data sets.

Some AI/ML researchers draw distinction between two classes of objectives when using ML in medical research, predictive, and explanatory [42]. Predictive ML seeks to make accurate and useful predictions, without requiring an explanation of the predictions (for example, when we don't care what features of the radiological image a software is "using" to come to its conclusion, as long as the pathological feature is correctly identified). Explanatory ML is done to describe, explain, or understand patterns in the data; it is conducted when the processes that give rise to the data are of primary interest. Such work is usually model-based; the assumptions about the medical problem domain are made explicit and re-expressed in a precise mathematical form, from which a bespoke algorithm to answer specific question about the problem at hand is determined [42].

In this chapter, we will give examples on how these different approaches and methodologies (predictive and explanatory) have been used in pediatric allergy research, using two specific exemplars: (1) understanding heterogeneity of childhood wheezing illness, including prediction models for childhood asthma and (2) Understanding heterogeneity of childhood allergic sensitisation and its relationship with asthma.

13.6   Prediction Models for Childhood Asthma: Are We Trying to Predict the Unpredictable?

ML approaches for the prediction of childhood asthma have been reported to have better performance and generalizability over regression-based models (such as the Asthma Prediction Index) [43]. For example, ML has been used to develop and externally validate a "Childhood Asthma Preschool Prediction" model (CAPP) [43], but although promising, this approach is not sufficiently useful for a roll-out to clinical practice (with the AUC of 0.82). Subsequent extension of this work aimed to establish whether inclusion of large-scale genetic and epigenetic information improves the prediction ability [44]. The genomic risk scores per se had modest discriminative performance (e.g., AUC, for polygenic risk score was only 0.64), and their integration only marginally improved the performance of the ML prediction CAPP model (from AUC of 0.82 to AUC of 0.84) [44]. The limited predictive performance of genomic risk scores and their inability to improve upon the performance of ML asthma prediction models may suggest that predictors of the highly heterogeneous phenotype of "asthma diagnosis" are unlikely to be clinically useful, and that studies predicting specific, more homogenous phenotypes (clusters) of wheezing are required.

13.7   Data-Driven Methods to Understand Wheezing Phenotypes

Most data-driven analyses to date to understand childhood wheezing phenotypes used the latent class analysis (LCA) [45–50], in which repeated information on wheeze presence is used to uncover temporal patterns over a specified time interval (reviewed in [51]). These analyses revealed structure within the datasets which may be viewed as similar, but more granular to the original description of the three phenotypes (transient, persistent, and late-onset [29]), suggesting the existence of one [52, 53], or two further intermediate phenotypes [48–50]. Of note, although "wheeze phenotypes" derived from different analyses often share the same nomenclature, they often differ in the age of onset, resolution, prevalence, and associated risk factors [15, 26]. Some of these inconsistencies are partly due to the sample size, frequency, and timing of data collection, which all influence the number and type of phenotypes [54].

Ultimately, the key question is whether different wheeze phenotypes are different disease, i.e., whether they are underpinned by different mechanisms [55]. In relation to this point, if the genetic associates of these different latent classes/phenotypes are different, it would suggest that different mechanisms may be at work. However, one study suggested that the associations between multiple 17q12–21 variants were similar for all wheeze phenotypes, indicating a shared genetic origin [56]. In contrast, a large study which derived wheeze phenotypes from birth to adolescence in >15,000 individuals recently suggested that genetic associates are phenotype-unique [57]. A multivariate genome-wide association study (GWAS) of wheezing phenotypes derived using LCA reported subsets of independent single nucleotide polymorphisms (SNPs) which were exclusively associated with persistent wheeze, preschool remitting mid-childhood remitting, or late-onset wheeze [57], with little evidence of shared genetic architecture between different phenotypes. The analysis also identified two GWAS-significant loci associated exclusively with persistent wheeze (but not any other wheeze phenotype): 17q12–21, $p < 5.5 \times 10^{-9}$, and a novel locus on chr9q21.13 close to *annexin 1* (*ANXA1*), $p < 6.7 \times 10^{-9}$. Functional studies in a mouse model demonstrated that both ANXA1 protein and mRNA expression were significantly increased in lung tissue following exposure to dust mite allergen, and experiments in ANXA1-/- deficient mice indicated that loss of ANXA1 resulted in increased airway hyperreactivity and T2 inflammation upon allergen challenge [57]. A further study provided mechanistic explanation for how ANXA1 may be associated with persistent wheezing [58]. This series of studies suggest that annexin 1 may be important in wheezing persistence, and the potential power of data-driven methodologies in deep phenotyping to better understand mechanisms underpinning complex traits.

13.8 Homogeneity and Stability of Wheeze Phenotypes Discovered Using MDAs

When using some of the data-driven methods such as LCA, a proportion of children may be classified imprecisely [56], and there may be a transition of individual children between different phenotypes in different runs of the model (e.g., one study has shown that as many as 23% of participants may move into a different phenotype when using complete and incomplete data set) [59]. The impact of this on the assessment of mechanisms underpinning different phenotypes is unclear. Recently, we developed a novel data-driven method which improves the assignment to wheeze phenotypes, at least in terms of internal homogeneity and stability [60]. Through clustering of multi-dimensional variables of wheezing spells (including duration, temporal sequencing, and extent of persistence/recurrence), we derived wheeze clusters which were more homogenous and stable compared to previous methods [60]. However, it is not certain that greater internal homogeneity will necessarily result in a better classification that maps more closely to underlying pathologic mechanisms.

Irrespective of some uncertainties outlined above, one important point needs to be emphasized: all phenotypes of preschool wheezing (even the transient ones) are associated with impaired lung function in early adulthood [59–62]. Given that diminished lung function at the physiological peak in the third decade is associated with adverse health outcomes through life course (from COPD to premature death of all causes) [63–67], we need to pursue research to understand mechanisms of all childhood wheeze phenotypes. End-organ pathology may be crucial for ascertaining such mechanisms. Recent unsupervised ML analysis of data on lower airway inflammation and infection from bronchoalveolar lavage in preschool children with severe wheeze who underwent clinically indicated bronchoscopy revealed four pathophysiological clusters, which had distinct allergic sensitisation profiles and blood eosinophils, and also differed in BAL microbial profiles [68], demonstrating the power of MDAs in helping us to move from diagnostic labels to underlying mechanisms.

13.9   Allergic Sensitization and Atopic Diseases

Another important question which needs to be answered is whether different clusters of wheeze/asthma described above, and other allergic diseases (rhinitis [69], eczema [70, 71], and allergic multimorbidity [17]) differ in their association with allergic sensitization. It is interesting that despite different genetic architecture [57], highly concordant longitudinal sensitization patterns were associated with different wheeze phenotypes, with sensitization trajectories from infancy to adolescence being almost identical in persistent and late-onset wheezing [59, 60]. However, wheeze preceded sensitization in persistent cluster, while sensitization preceded wheeze in late-onset wheezing [60]. In contrast to these findings, similar unsupervised analysis in South African birth cohort study has shown no association between persistent wheeze and sensitisation [72]. Overlapping sensitisation trajectories were recently reported also in relation to different lung function trajectories [73].

Consistent with the above data on wheeze phenotypes and sensitization, recent study reported very similar association between allergic sensitization and different eczema clusters which were derived using data-driven methodologies [70]. All eczema clusters were associated with allergic sensitization in early-school age; however, eczema preceded sensitization in the persisting clusters, while children with late-onset eczema tended to develop sensitization before the onset of symptoms [70].

Finally, recent study reported interesting data on the relationship between allergic multimorbidity and sensitization [17]. Children with multimorbidity of eczema, wheeze, and rhinitis were more likely to be sensitized, but more than half of subjects with persistent multimorbidity of all three "atopic" diseases were not sensitized at age 5, and ~30% were not sensitized in adolescence [17].

This relative lack of clarity and consistency on the role of sensitization in childhood atopic disease, both among individual patients and at population level, may indicate that the term "allergic sensitisation" as used currently in clinical practice may compose of several distinct types of sensitization that differ in their association with asthma and other atopic diseases [45, 74]. Some of these subtypes of sensitization may be "benign" (i.e., not associated with clinical symptoms), and some are "pathologic" [75], but we lack tools at the point of care in primary practice to determine in sensitized individual patients whether sensitization is important, or a chance finding. In a finding consistent with this idea, a pioneering ML analysis which took into account the type of allergen, and the timing of onset and remission of IgE responses from infancy to school-age, suggested existence of several distinct clusters of sensitization, and identified one of these (described as "Multiple early") as a strong associate of asthma diagnosis, and among patients with asthma, a marker of disease severity [45, 74]. However, currently, individuals can be assigned to these different sensitization clusters only through modeling of longitudinal data on allergy tests collected over many years. What we need for diagnostic and prognostic purposes are biomarkers to differentiate in individual sensitized patients, preferably at a single clinical consultation, whether sensitization is important for current or future symptoms, or whether it is a chance finding of little or no relevance to the disease. Ultimately, knowing which sensitization subtype an individual patient has, and how this will develop throughout life course, may help predict whether a sensitized individual will have specific clinical symptoms, their severity, and allergic comorbidity.

13.10 Disaggregating Allergic Sensitization

Traditionally, whole allergen extracts (either in skin prick tests and/or measurement of sIgE) are used to diagnose allergic sensitization. However, confirmation of sensitization using these standard diagnostic tests does not confirm that patient's symptoms are caused by an IgE-mediated reaction [5, 76]. Quantification of allergic sensitization through IgE titre or size of skin test wheal rather than commonly used binary cut-offs can increase the specificity (both in terms of diagnostic accuracy [77, 78] and the ability to predict the persistence of symptoms [79]). However, the problem of a significant number of false-positive test results remains [5, 6]. Consequently, although asthma is closely associated with allergic sensitization, most current guidelines do not recommend assessment of sensitization in asthma diagnosis or monitoring [22]; in contrast, most individual physicians caring for children with asthma considered monitoring of allergy to be of a high priority for monitoring childhood asthma [80].

We can now describe sensitization in much greater detail using component-resolved diagnostics (CRD, also known as molecular allergy tests) that measures sIgE to a large number of allergenic molecules or allergen components (component-specific IgE, c-sIgE). For example, in allergy to peanut [81–83] and other foods [84, 85], sensitization-specific allergenic proteins in allergen extracts are important for making a distinction between true allergy and asymptomatic sensitisation. Consequently, CRD is established in clinical practice in food allergy [86, 87], but the data to support similar approach in allergic airway diseases is lacking.

The field of molecular allergology is fast-moving, and European Academy of Allergy and Clinical Immunology (EAACI) established a Taskforce to summarize state-of-the-art information on allergen molecules, their clinical relevance, and their application in diagnostic algorithms for clinical practice, which recently published The Molecular Allergology User's Guide 2.0 to provide a comprehensive guidance on CRD [88]. Technological developments have led to products in which c-sIgE to hundreds of allergen components can be measured using the multiplex-based assays (reviewed in [89, 90]). This has created conditions to test the notion that measuring sensitization using CRD multiplex array data may be more informative than standard tests in respiratory allergy, to allow us to identify clinically relevant sensitization more accurately. As an example, several specific c-sIgEs in early life may be risk molecules for predicting asthma in school-age and adolescence [91, 92], and c-sIgE polysensitization to house dust mite (HDM) components predicts allergic disease [93].

13.11 CRD and Asthma: Application of ML Techniques

CRD arrays produce complex data sets which are ideal for the application of ML techniques to interrogate the data [94]. In previous studies, to shed light on the relationship between allergic sensitization and respiratory diseases, we applied ML techniques to the CRD microarrays data [95–98]. Our initial analysis identified three patterns of c-sIgE responses measured by a commercial CRD array, with a strong association between asthma and sensitisation to a group of 27 components of plant, animal, and fungal origin [96]. In further studies, we demonstrated a clear association of different longitudinal trajectories of c-sIgE responses with clinical outcomes; for example, an early-onset grass trajectory increased the risk of asthma substantially [97]; in contrast, a similar pattern starting 2–3 years later (late-onset trajectory) was not associated with asthma, but was strongly predictive of rhinitis. In a follow-up study that looked at the whole panel of >100 allergenic molecules longitudinally, specific component clusters at age 5 years were strong predictors of asthma at age 16 years [98], suggesting that it may be possible to develop ML interpretation algorithms for CRD multiplex arrays which practising physicians may use to predict the future risk of asthma [98].

It is reassuring that unsupervised ML approaches identified component clusters which are biologically plausible, reflecting the sources of allergenic proteins (e.g., grass and HDM clusters) [96] or their structural homogeneity within protein families (e.g., pathogenesis-related [PR]-10 and profilin clusters [98]). Also of note is the finding that almost identical component clusters were uncovered using different ML methodologies in studies of children and adults with asthma [99]. These studies suggest a remarkable similarity in the structure of the CRD component sensitization patterns in the general population [98, 100] and among patients with asthma [99].

Taking into account the findings of previous studies which reduced dimensionality of the multiplex array data using different ML techniques to cluster components or patients [95–98], and recently published observation that the number of c-sIgE responses within each cluster and their specific within-cluster patterns add further information improving the diagnosis and prediction of asthma and rhinitis [101], we developed a different ML approach to analysis of the complex CRD data by applying network analysis to investigate interactions and connectivity patterns between c-sIgE on a CRD array and related these to asthma diagnosis [100]. This study has shown that in contrast to peanut allergy, in which sensitization to a specific peanut protein predicts clinical reactivity, what predicted asthma was not c-sIgE to any individual molecule, but the pattern of interaction between c-sIgEs [100]. Importantly, underlying structure was very similar to that described in other analyses using different unsupervised techniques [96–98]. Further analyses revealed a differential network of pairwise interactions between a limited number of c-sIgEs from different component clusters, which predicted asthma with an excellent balance between sensitivity and specificity [100].

We then applied a similar approach to investigate whether, among sensitized patients with asthma, we can differentiate those with severe disease from patients with mild/moderate asthma [99]. These studies in the U-BIOPRED severe asthma cohort demonstrated that the pattern of connectivity and interactions between c-sIgE and multiple allergenic proteins is a potentially important biomarker of asthma severity in sensitized asthmatics, both among school-age children and adult patients [99]. We have shown that there is higher connectivity among c-sIgEs in severe asthma, although these connections were weaker than those in mild asthma. The mild asthma c-sIgE network had less co-sensitizations, but these were stronger [99]. Of note, although patients were recruited from seven different European countries with considerable differences in the pattern of allergen exposure and sensitization, we found remarkable consistencies in the connectivity structure among c-sIgEs compared to our previous studies at the UK general population level [99]. These data suggest that it may be possible to develop algorithms to differentiate clinically important sensitization patterns associated with asthma severity.

13.12 Prospects for Future Work

The acknowledgment that asthma and other atopic diseases, as well as allergic sensitization, are principally diagnostic label, rather than diagnoses pointing to well-understood pathophysiological mechanisms, raises several prospects for research which can be handled by combining different data approaches.

In relation to current clinical diagnoses, ML models are taught to predict the diagnostic label from examples; if that label does not map onto any underlying disease processes and mechanisms, our ability to accurately predict development of "disease" within individuals will be limited. To address this, one potential avenue of research is to disaggregate childhood atopic diseases using MDAs to better represent their mechanistic heterogeneity, and to use different disease phenotypes/classes/clusters as the inputs in supervised ML models. By integrating longitudinal clinical data with rich biomarker, biological and -omics data, this could help us answer questions about the biological associates of the various disease clusters.

In parallel, we could aim for clinical application by seeking to find a small set of features which could be easily obtained in early childhood, and which would strongly predict various clusters to aid prognosis, thus enabling clinicians to better manage patients, and help parents with the uncertainty surrounding the disease. However, to achieve this will require large international collaborations to guarantee validation and generalizability of any findings. Once this is completed, we should aim to reform the taxonomy of childhood atopic diseases from traditional symptom/medication-based criteria toward a mechanism-based framework.

References

1. Custovic D, Fontanella S, Custovic A. Understanding progression from pre-school wheezing to school-age asthma: can modern data approaches help? Pediatr Allergy Immunol. 2023;34(12):e14062.
2. Custovic A, Siddiqui S, Saglani S. Considering biomarkers in asthma disease severity. J Allergy Clin Immunol. 2022;149(2):480–7.
3. Wolfe I. Why children die: death in infants, children and young people in the UK. Royal College of Paediatrics and Child Health and National Children's Bureau; 2014.
4. Physicians RCo. Why asthma still kills: the National Review of asthma deaths (NRAD) Confidential Enquiry report. 2014.
5. Custovic A, Custovic D, Kljaic Bukvic B, Fontanella S, Haider S. Atopic phenotypes and their implication in the atopic march. Expert Rev Clin Immunol. 2020;16(9):873–81.
6. Custovic A, Lazic N, Simpson A. Pediatric asthma and development of atopy. Curr Opin Allergy Clin Immunol. 2013;13(2):173–80.
7. Oksel C, Custovic A. Development of allergic sensitization and its relevance to paediatric asthma. Curr Opin Allergy Clin Immunol. 2018;18(2):109–16.
8. Arshad SH, Kurukulaaratchy RJ, Fenn M, Matthews S. Early life risk factors for current wheeze, asthma, and bronchial hyperresponsiveness at 10 years of age. Chest. 2005;127(2):502–8.
9. Brockow I, Zutavern A, Hoffmann U, et al. Early allergic sensitizations and their relevance to atopic diseases in children aged 6 years: results of the GINI study. J Investig Allergol Clin Immunol. 2009;19(3):180–7.
10. Carroll WD, Lenney W, Child F, et al. Asthma severity and atopy: how clear is the relationship? Arch Dis Child. 2006;91(5):405–9.
11. Weinmayr G, Weiland SK, Bjorksten B, et al. Atopic sensitization and the international variation of asthma symptom prevalence in children. Am J Respir Crit Care Med. 2007;176(6):565–74.
12. Illi S, von Mutius E, Lau S, et al. The natural course of atopic dermatitis from birth to age 7 years and the association with asthma. J Allergy Clin Immunol. 2004;113(5):925–31.
13. Illi S, von Mutius E, Lau S, et al. The pattern of atopic sensitization is associated with the development of asthma in childhood. J Allergy Clin Immunol. 2001;108(5):709–14.
14. Keeble E, Kossarova L. Focus on: emergency hospital care for children and young people, what has changed in the part 10 years? The Health Foundation and Nuffield Trust; 2017.
15. Belgrave D, Simpson A, Custovic A. Challenges in interpreting wheeze phenotypes: the clinical implications of statistical learning techniques. Am J Respir Crit Care Med. 2014;189(2):121–3.
16. Belgrave DC, Custovic A, Simpson A. Characterizing wheeze phenotypes to identify endotypes of childhood asthma, and the implications for future management. Expert Rev Clin Immunol. 2013;9(10):921–36.
17. Haider S, Fontanella S, Ullah A, et al. Evolution of eczema, wheeze, and rhinitis from infancy to early adulthood: four birth cohort studies. Am J Respir Crit Care Med. 2022;206(8):950–60.
18. Koefoed HJL, Vonk JM, Koppelman GH. Predicting the course of asthma from childhood until early adulthood. Curr Opin Allergy Clin Immunol. 2022;22(2):115–22.

19. Saglani S, Custovic A. Childhood asthma: advances using machine learning and mechanistic studies. Am J Respir Crit Care Med. 2019;199(4):414–22.
20. Tang HH, Teo SM, Belgrave DC, et al. Trajectories of childhood immune development and respiratory health relevant to asthma and allergy. elife. 2018;7:7.
21. Slob EMA, Longo C, Vijverberg SJH, et al. Persistence of parental-reported asthma at early ages: a longitudinal twin study. Pediatr Allergy Immunol. 2022;33(3):e13762.
22. Custovic A, de Moira AP, Murray CS, Simpson A. Environmental influences on childhood asthma: allergens. Pediatr Allergy Immunol. 2023;34(2):e13915.
23. Tutino M, Granell R, Curtin JA, et al. Dog ownership in infancy is protective for persistent wheeze in 17q21 asthma-risk carriers. J Allergy Clin Immunol. 2023;151(2):423–30.
24. Laubhahn K, Schaub B. From preschool wheezing to asthma: immunological determinants. Pediatr Allergy Immunol. 2023;34(10):e14038.
25. Deliu M, Belgrave D, Sperrin M, Buchan I, Custovic A. Asthma phenotypes in childhood. Expert Rev Clin Immunol. 2017;13(7):705–13.
26. Howard R, Rattray M, Prosperi M, Custovic A. Distinguishing asthma phenotypes using machine learning approaches. Curr Allergy Asthma Rep. 2015;15(7):38.
27. Just J, Bourgoin-Heck M, Amat F. Clinical phenotypes in asthma during childhood. Clin Exp Allergy. 2017;47(7):848–55.
28. Wilson NM. Wheezy bronchitis revisited. Arch Dis Child. 1989;64(8):1194–9.
29. Martinez FD, Wright AL, Taussig LM, Holberg CJ, Halonen M, Morgan WJ. Asthma and wheezing in the first six years of life. N Engl J Med. 1995;332(3):133–8.
30. Cano-Garcinuño A, Mora-Gandarillas I. Wheezing phenotypes in young children: an historical cohort study. Prim Care Respir J. 2014;23:60–6.
31. Kurukulaaratchy R, Fenn M, Waterhouse L, Matthews S, Holgate S, Arshad S. Characterization of wheezing phenotypes in the first 10 years of life. Clin Exp Allergy. 2003;33(5):573–8.
32. Lowe LA, Simpson A, Woodcock A, et al. Wheeze phenotypes and lung function in preschool children. Am J Respir Crit Care Med. 2005;171(3):231–7.
33. Tang HHF, Sly PD, Holt PG, Holt KE, Inouye M. Systems biology and big data in asthma and allergy: recent discoveries and emerging challenges. Eur Respir J. 2020;55(1):1900844.
34. Belgrave D, Henderson J, Simpson A, Buchan I, Bishop C, Custovic A. Disaggregating asthma: big investigation versus big data. J Allergy Clin Immunol. 2017;139(2):400–7.
35. Leonelli S. Scientific research and big data. In: Zalta EN, editor. The stanford encyclopedia of philosophy. Summer 2020 ed; 2020.
36. Saria S, Goldenberg A. Subtyping: what it is and its role in precision medicine. IEEE Intell Syst. 2015;30(4):70–5.
37. Rajkomar A, Dean J, Kohane I. Machine learning in medicine. N Engl J Med. 2019;380(14):1347–58.
38. Zhu S, Gilbert M, Chetty I, Siddiqui F. The 2021 landscape of FDA-approved artificial intelligence/machine learning-enabled medical devices: an analysis of the characteristics and intended use. Int J Med Inform. 2022;165:104828.
39. Fontanella S, Cucco A, Custovic A. Machine learning in asthma research: moving toward a more integrated approach. Expert Rev Respir Med. 2021;15(5):609–21.
40. Duverdier A, Custovic A, Tanaka RJ. Data-driven research on eczema: systematic characterization of the field and recommendations for the future. Clin Transl Allergy. 2022;12(6):e12170.
41. Hosny A, Parmar C, Quackenbush J, Schwartz LH, Aerts H. Artificial intelligence in radiology. Nat Rev Cancer. 2018;18(8):500–10.
42. Winn JM. Model-based machine learning. CRC Press; 2023.
43. Kothalawala DM, Murray CS, Simpson A, et al. Development of childhood asthma prediction models using machine learning approaches. Clin Transl Allergy. 2021;11(9):e12076.
44. Kothalawala DM, Kadalayil L, Curtin JA, et al. Integration of genomic risk scores to improve the prediction of childhood asthma diagnosis. J Pers Med. 2022; 12(1).
45. Lazic N, Roberts G, Custovic A, et al. Multiple atopy phenotypes and their associations with asthma: similar findings from two birth cohorts. Allergy. 2013;68(6):764–70.

46. Spycher BD, Silverman M, Brooke AM, Minder CE, Kuehni CE. Distinguishing phenotypes of childhood wheeze and cough using latent class analysis. Eur Respir J. 2008;31(5):974–81.

47. Lodge CJ, Zaloumis S, Lowe AJ, et al. Early-life risk factors for childhood wheeze phenotypes in a high-risk birth cohort. J Pediatr. 2014;164(2):289–94. e2

48. Henderson J, Granell R, Heron J, et al. Associations of wheezing phenotypes in the first six years of life with atopy, lung function and airway responsiveness in mid childhood. Thorax. 2008;63(11):974–80.

49. Granell R, Henderson AJ, Sterne JA. Associations of wheezing phenotypes with late asthma outcomes in the Avon longitudinal study of parents and children: a population-based birth cohort. J Allergy Clin Immunol. 2016;138(4):1060–70. e11

50. Savenije OE, Granell R, Caudri D, et al. Comparison of childhood wheezing phenotypes in 2 birth cohorts: ALSPAC and PIAMA. J Allergy Clin Immunol. 2011;127(6):1505–12. e14.

51. Oksel C, Haider S, Fontanella S, Frainay C, Custovic A. Classification of pediatric asthma: from phenotype discovery to clinical practice. Front Pediatr. 2018;6:258.

52. Belgrave DC, Simpson A, Semic-Jusufagic A, et al. Joint modeling of parentally reported and physician-confirmed wheeze identifies children with persistent troublesome wheezing. J Allergy Clin Immunol. 2013;132(3):575–83. e12

53. Valk R, Caudri D, Savenije O, et al. Childhood wheezing phenotypes and FeNO in atopic children at age 8. Clin Exp Allergy. 2012;42(9):1329–36.

54. Oksel C, Granell R, Mahmoud O, et al. Causes of variability in latent phenotypes of childhood wheeze. J Allergy Clin Immunol. 2019;143(5):1783–90 e11.

55. Koppelman GH, Kersten ETG. Understanding how asthma starts: longitudinal patterns of wheeze and the chromosome 17q locus. Am J Respir Crit Care Med. 2021;203(7):793–5.

56. Hallmark B, Wegienka G, Havstad S, et al. Chromosome 17q12-21 variants are associated with multiple wheezing phenotypes in childhood. Am J Respir Crit Care Med. 2021;203(7):864–70.

57. Granell R, Curtin JA, Haider S, et al. A meta-analysis of genome-wide association studies of childhood wheezing phenotypes identifies ANXA1 as a susceptibility locus for persistent wheezing. elife. 2023;12:12.

58. Irie M, Kabata H, Sasahara K, et al. Annexin A1 is a cell-intrinsic metalloregulator of zinc in human ILC2s. Cell Rep. 2023;42(6):112610.

59. Oksel C, Granell R, Haider S, et al. Distinguishing wheezing phenotypes from infancy to adolescence. A pooled analysis of five birth cohorts. Ann Am Thorac Soc. 2019;16(7):868–76.

60. Haider S, Granell R, Curtin J, et al. Modeling wheezing spells identifies phenotypes with different outcomes and genetic associates. Am J Respir Crit Care Med. 2022;205(8):883–93.

61. Custovic A, Fontanella S. Evolution of lung function within individuals: clinical insights and data-driven methods. Am J Respir Crit Care Med. 2023;207(4):379–81.

62. Belgrave DCM, Granell R, Turner SW, et al. Lung function trajectories from pre-school age to adulthood and their associations with early life factors: a retrospective analysis of three population-based birth cohort studies. Lancet Respir Med. 2018;6(7):526–34.

63. Agusti A, Noell G, Brugada J, Faner R. Lung function in early adulthood and health in later life: a transgenerational cohort analysis. Lancet Respir Med. 2017;5(12):935–45.

64. Lange P, Celli B, Agusti A, et al. Lung-function trajectories leading to chronic obstructive pulmonary disease. N Engl J Med. 2015;373(2):111–22.

65. Cuttica MJ, Colangelo LA, Dransfield MT, et al. Lung function in young adults and risk of cardiovascular events over 29 years: the CARDIA study. J Am Heart Assoc. 2018;7(24):e010672.

66. Cheng YJ, Chen ZG, Yao FJ, Liu LJ, Zhang M, Wu SH. Airflow obstruction, impaired lung function and risk of sudden cardiac death: a prospective cohort study. Thorax. 2022;77(7):652–62.

67. Guerra S, Sherrill DL, Venker C, Ceccato CM, Halonen M, Martinez FD. Morbidity and mortality associated with the restrictive spirometric pattern: a longitudinal study. Thorax. 2010;65(6):499–504.

68. Robinson PFM, Fontanella S, Ananth S, et al. Recurrent severe preschool wheeze: from Prespecified diagnostic labels to underlying Endotypes. Am J Respir Crit Care Med. 2021;204(5):523–35.
69. Yavuz ST, Oksel Karakus C, Custovic A, Kalayci O. Four subtypes of childhood allergic rhinitis identified by latent class analysis. Pediatr Allergy Immunol. 2021;32(8):1691–9.
70. Haider S, Granell R, Curtin JA, et al. Identification of eczema clusters and their association with filaggrin and atopic comorbidities: analysis of five birth cohorts. Br J Dermatol. 2023;190(1):45–54.
71. Nakamura T, Haider S, Fontanella S, Murray CS, Simpson A, Custovic A. Modelling trajectories of parentally reported and physician-confirmed atopic dermatitis in a birth cohort study. Br J Dermatol. 2022;186(2):274–84.
72. McCready C, Haider S, Little F, et al. Early childhood wheezing phenotypes and determinants in a south African birth cohort: longitudinal analysis of the Drakenstein child health study. Lancet Child Adolesc Health. 2023;7(2):127–35.
73. Ullah A, Granell R, Haider S, et al. Obstructive and restrictive spirometry from school age to adulthood: three birth cohort studies. eClinicalMedicine. 2024;67:102355.
74. Simpson A, Tan VY, Winn J, et al. Beyond atopy: multiple patterns of sensitization in relation to asthma in a birth cohort study. Am J Respir Crit Care Med. 2010;181(11):1200–6.
75. Holt PG, Strickland D, Bosco A, et al. Distinguishing benign from pathologic TH2 immunity in atopic children. J Allergy Clin Immunol. 2016;137(2):379–87.
76. Wise SK, Damask C, Roland LT, et al. International consensus statement on allergy and rhinology: allergic rhinitis—2023. Int Forum Allergy Rhinol. 2023;13(4):293–859.
77. Marinho S, Simpson A, Soderstrom L, Woodcock A, Ahlstedt S, Custovic A. Quantification of atopy and the probability of rhinitis in preschool children: a population-based birth cohort study. Allergy. 2007;62(12):1379–86.
78. Marinho S, Simpson A, Marsden P, Smith JA, Custovic A. Quantification of atopy, lung function and airway hypersensitivity in adults. Clin Transl Allergy. 2011;1(1):16.
79. Simpson A, Soderstrom L, Ahlstedt S, Murray CS, Woodcock A, Custovic A. IgE antibody quantification and the probability of wheeze in preschool children. J Allergy Clin Immunol. 2005;116(4):744–9.
80. Papadopoulos NG, Mathioudakis AG, Custovic A, et al. Current and optimal practices in childhood asthma monitoring among multiple international stakeholders. JAMA Netw Open. 2023;6(5):e2313120.
81. Nicolaou N, Poorafshar M, Murray C, et al. Allergy or tolerance in children sensitized to peanut: prevalence and differentiation using component-resolved diagnostics. J Allergy Clin Immunol. 2010;125(1):191–7. e1–13.
82. Nicolaou N, Murray C, Belgrave D, Poorafshar M, Simpson A, Custovic A. Quantification of specific IgE to whole peanut extract and peanut components in prediction of peanut allergy. J Allergy Clin Immunol. 2011;127(3):684–5.
83. Kotsapas C, Nicolaou N, Haider S, et al. Early-life predictors and risk factors of peanut allergy, and its association with asthma in later-life: population-based birth cohort study. Clin Exp Allergy. 2022;52(5):646–57.
84. Saf S, Borres MP, Sodergren E. Sesame allergy in children: new insights into diagnosis and management. Pediatr Allergy Immunol. 2023;34(8):e14001.
85. Labrosse R, Graham F, Caubet JC. Recent advances in the diagnosis and management of tree nut and seed allergy. Curr Opin Allergy Clin Immunol. 2022;22(3):194–201.
86. Riggioni C, Ricci C, Moya B, et al. Systematic review and meta-analyses on the accuracy of diagnostic tests for IgE-mediated food allergy. Allergy 2023.
87. Patel N, Shreffler WG, Custovic A, Santos AF. Will oral food challenges still be part of allergy care in 10 years' time? J Allergy Clin Immunol Pract. 2023;11(4):988–96.
88. Dramburg S, Hilger C, Santos AF, et al. EAACI molecular Allergology user's guide 2.0. Pediatr Allergy Immunol. 2023;34(Suppl 28):e13854.

89. Hamilton RG, Croote D, Lupinek C, Matsson P. Evolution toward chip-based arrays in the laboratory diagnosis of human allergic disease. J Allergy Clin Immunol Pract. 2023;11(10):2991–9.
90. Sampson HA, Hamilton RG. Advances in the assessment and Management of Allergic Sensitization. J Allergy Clin Immunol Pract. 2023;11(10):3008–9.
91. Wickman M, Lupinek C, Andersson N, et al. Detection of IgE reactivity to a handful of allergen molecules in early childhood predicts respiratory allergy in adolescence. EBioMedicine. 2017;26:91–9.
92. Farraia M, Mendes FC, Sokhatska O, et al. Component-resolved diagnosis in childhood and prediction of asthma in early adolescence: a birth cohort study. Pediatr Allergy Immunol. 2023;34(12):e14056.
93. Posa D, Perna S, Resch Y, et al. Evolution and predictive value of IgE responses toward a comprehensive panel of house dust mite allergens during the first 2 decades of life. J Allergy Clin Immunol. 2017;139(2):541–9 e8.
94. van Breugel M, Fehrmann RSN, Bugel M, et al. Current state and prospects of artificial intelligence in allergy. Allergy. 2023;78(10):2623–43.
95. Prosperi MC, Belgrave D, Buchan I, Simpson A, Custovic A. Challenges in interpreting allergen microarrays in relation to clinical symptoms: a machine learning approach. Pediatr Allergy Immunol. 2014;25(1):71–9.
96. Simpson A, Lazic N, Belgrave DC, et al. Patterns of IgE responses to multiple allergen components and clinical symptoms at age 11 years. J Allergy Clin Immunol. 2015;136(5):1224–31.
97. Custovic A, Sonntag H-J, Buchan IE, Belgrave D, Simpson A, Prosperi MCF. Evolution pathways of IgE responses to grass and mite allergens throughout childhood. J Allergy Clin Immunol. 2015;136(6):1645–52.e8.
98. Howard R, Belgrave D, Papastamoulis P, Simpson A, Rattray M, Custovic A. Evolution of IgE responses to multiple allergen components throughout childhood. J Allergy Clin Immunol. 2018;142(4):1322–30.
99. Roberts G, Fontanella S, Selby A, et al. Connectivity patterns between multiple allergen specific IgE antibodies and their association with severe asthma. J Allergy Clin Immunol. 2020;146(4):821–30.
100. Fontanella S, Frainay C, Murray CS, Simpson A, Custovic A. Machine learning to identify pairwise interactions between specific IgE antibodies and their association with asthma: a cross-sectional analysis within a population-based birth cohort. PLoS Med. 2018;15(11):e1002691.
101. Howard R, Fontanella S, Simpson A, Murray CS, Custovic A, Rattray M. Component-specific clusters for diagnosis and prediction of allergic airway diseases. Clin Exp Allergy. 2024;54:339.

Chapter 14
Digital Health and Drug Allergies

Shuayb Elkhalifa, Haggar Elbashir, Inmaculada Cerecedo, and Fulvio Salvo

Contents

S. Elkhalifa (✉)
Allergy and Clinical Immunology Department, Respiratory Institute, Cleveland Clinic Abu Dhabi, Abu Dhabi, United Arab Emirates

Centre for Musculoskeletal Research, Faculty of Biology, Medicine and Health, The University of Manchester, Manchester, UK
e-mail: shuayb@doctors.net.uk

H. Elbashir
Department of Allergy and Clinical Immunology, Lancashire Teaching Hospitals NHS Foundation Trust, Preston, UK
e-mail: Haggar@doctors.net.uk

I. Cerecedo · F. Salvo
Allergy and Clinical Immunology Department, Respiratory Institute, Cleveland Clinic Abu Dhabi, Abu Dhabi, United Arab Emirates
e-mail: cerecei@clevelandclinicabudhabi.ae; SalvoF@clevelandclinicabudhabi.ae

© The Author(s), under exclusive license to Springer Nature Switzerland AG 2025
P. M. Matricardi, S. Dramburg, *Digital Allergology*, Health Informatics, https://doi.org/10.1007/978-3-031-71021-6_14

Abstract As the healthcare landscape undergoes a digital revolution, new avenues are emerging for ensuring patient safety, fostering real-time clinical decision support, and enhancing personalized medical care. One area of significant impact is in the management of drug allergies. Drug allergies, potentially life-threatening responses to medications, present a ubiquitous challenge to clinicians and patients alike. Accurate diagnosis, documentation, and communication of these reactions are vital for preventing adverse events. Digital health, encompassing electronic health records (EHRs), mobile health (mHealth) applications, wearable technologies, and data analytics, is reshaping the way drug allergies are identified, documented, and managed. This chapter delves into the interplay between digital health solutions and drug allergy management, highlighting the advancements, current challenges, and the future trajectory of integrating technology to enhance patient safety and care quality. The intersection of digital health and drug allergies promises not only improved patient outcomes but also a paradigm shift in proactive and personalized allergy management.

14.1 Introduction

The management of drug allergies has traditionally relied on manual record-keeping and communication among healthcare providers. This approach, however, has proven to be error-prone, time-consuming, and sometimes ineffective in preventing allergic and adverse reactions. Digitalization offers a solution to these challenges by leveraging electronic health records (EHRs), health information exchange (HIE) systems, and other technological tools.

In recent years, the integration of digital health technologies has revolutionized the healthcare landscape, offering innovative solutions for various medical challenges. One area where digital health has shown promise is in managing drug allergies.

Before delving into the impact of digital health on managing drug allergies, it is important to understand what drug allergies are. A drug allergy is an adverse reaction of the immune system to a medication. Unlike side effects, which are often predictable and dose-dependent, allergies are unpredictable and can range from mild skin rashes to severe anaphylaxis or multi-organ failure in severe delayed cutaneous reactions (SCARS). These severe allergic reactions can be fatal if not treated promptly. The challenge with drug allergies lies not only in their diverse manifestations but also in the difficulty of predicting who will experience an allergic reaction to a particular medication.

Digital health technologies, including electronic health records (EHRs), wearable devices, and mobile apps, are playing a crucial role in transforming how we understand drug allergies.

This chapter explores the intersection of digital health and drug allergies, highlighting various applications that enhance drug allergy management, patient education, and healthcare provider communication.

14.2   The Role of Digital Health

Digital health encompasses a wide range of technologies designed to improve healthcare delivery and patient outcomes using digital, electronic, and mobile tools. When it comes to managing drug allergies, digital health solutions offer several crucial benefits:

1. Improved Patient Safety
   Digitalizing drug allergies significantly improves patient safety by reducing the risk of medication errors. With readily accessible allergy information, healthcare providers can make more informed decisions about prescribing medications, reducing the likelihood of adverse reactions. This is especially critical in emergency situations where quick decisions must be made.
2. Enhanced Healthcare Efficiency
   Efficiency in healthcare delivery is another notable benefit of digitalizing drug allergies. Rapid access to patient allergy information streamlines the medication reconciliation process, enabling healthcare providers to prescribe appropriate drugs more efficiently. This can lead to shorter hospital stays, reduced administrative burdens, and improved patient satisfaction.
3. Accurate Data Management
   Digitalization allows for standardized and consistent recording of drug allergy information. This contributes to more accurate data management and analysis, facilitating research on drug allergies, their prevalence, and patterns. Such insights can inform clinical practices and improve patient care strategies.
4. Interoperability and Continuity of Care
   Interoperability is a key advantage of digitalizing drug allergies. When integrated with EHRs and HIE systems, allergy information can seamlessly travel across different healthcare facilities, ensuring continuity of care even when patients visit different providers. This is particularly valuable for individuals with complex medical histories.

14.3   Digital Health Solutions for Drug Allergies

14.3.1   Data Collection and Aggregation: Electronic Health Records (EHRs)

Electronic Health Records (EHRs) [1] have revolutionized the way patient information is stored and shared across healthcare settings. In recent years, EHR systems have evolved to include comprehensive drug allergy profiles for patients. These profiles are not only accessible to healthcare providers within a particular institution but also facilitate information exchange across different healthcare facilities. This interoperability ensures that vital allergy information is available to emergency responders and specialists, thereby reducing the risk of adverse reactions due to lack of data. Also, this data can be aggregated and analyzed to identify trends and risk factors associated with drug allergies. Machine learning algorithms can sift through large datasets to find patterns that might not be obvious to human researchers.

While potentially being the perfect solution for recording drug allergy information, it also raises several issues. Drug allergies are documented in the allergy section in most EHR systems, often together with non-allergic adverse reactions, contraindications, environmental allergies, and patient's preferences, but while these are usually clearly described and differentiated inside the subsection, the information is often displayed as "allergy" in the shortcut layout, contributing to confusion in the users. Most of the EHRs allows recording of both coded and non-coded information: this can bring in turn to oversimplification or to an excess of details. The same category "rash" can be used for a severe cutaneous adverse reaction or for a benign delayed maculopapular rash. On the contrary, the use of "other" plus a detailed description of the reaction entered as free text, while being potentially useful for future users, may also cause several issues, like the need to access a subsection to get to the actual information or the problematic exportation of data while migrating to a different EHR or during data analysis.

Information under the allergy section may be entered by several different healthcare professionals, including physicians, physician assistants, nurses, and pharmacists. Interestingly, allergists are responsible only for a small minority of the allergy records [1]. Most of non-allergist professionals have a very limited knowledge of immune-mediated drug reactions and how to distinguish them from non-immune adverse drug reaction reactions or from pharmacological side effects.

Several retrospective studies [1, 2] have shown that the quality of allergy documentation in EHRs is overall poor or requires active efforts for reconciliation [2]. For example, a retrospective study analyzing the quality of documentation of contrast media allergy in EHR in the greater Boston area showed that more than two thirds of the entries were of low quality, i.e., did not even specify if the contrast was iodinated or gadolinium-based [3]. Interestingly, the vast majority of the low-quality entries were coded data in which the generic term "contrast medium" was selected without any additional information. This again highlights the need of standard definitions for drug adverse reactions and of providing specific training on adverse drug reaction nomenclature and definition to all the healthcare workers in charge of editing the allergy section in the EHR.

Drug allergy information recorded in EHR should ideally be able to facilitate decision-making by triggering clinical decision support (CDS). CDS is potentially a very powerful tool: it prevents ordering medications responsible for previous reactions, it alerts the clinician or pharmacist of possible cross-reactions when prescribing a new medication by providing an alert message [4]. However, there are few potential flaws in the system: over recording of mild and non-immune mediated reactions can produce a high number of alerts, causing the well-described phenomenon of the "alert fatigue" in the healthcare providers [5]. On the other hand, incorrectly entered allergy information (e.g., using free text or generic categories) may fail to activate the CDS system.

Considering all these challenges, specific workforces have been created by scientific societies in the allergy filed with the aim of producing agreed definitions, promoting good clinical practices, providing education to the healthcare staff responsible for drug allergy documentation, and liaising with EHR software companies to reshape the allergy module in order to improve its effectiveness [6, 7].

14.3.2   Mobile Applications for Patient Empowerment

Mobile applications [8] have empowered patients to take charge of their health, and this trend extends to managing drug allergies. Patients can now utilize smartphone apps to input and update their allergy information in real time. These apps often come with features like barcode scanning, allowing patients to quickly check whether a specific medication contains allergens. Additionally, some apps provide personalized alerts and reminders to help users avoid potential allergens in over-the-counter drugs and supplements.

Apps like "AllergyAlert" and "Medisafe" enable users to input their allergies, including drug sensitivities, and receive personalized alerts and reminders. These apps often integrate with electronic health records (EHRs) and can notify users about potential drug interactions, helping patients and caregivers manage their medications safely.

14.3.3   Wearable Medical Devices

Wearable devices [9] equipped with sensors and biometric tracking capabilities can provide real-time monitoring of physiological parameters, helping to detect early signs of allergic reactions. For instance, smartwatches with heart rate monitors and skin conductivity sensors can alert users to abnormal changes that might indicate an allergic response.

14.3.4   Telemedicine and Virtual Consultations

Telemedicine platforms [10] have gained prominence, especially in remote or underserved areas, allowing patients to consult allergists and healthcare professionals virtually. There are many studies supporting virtual consultation for various medical practices. However, the management of penicillin allergy through virtual consultation during the COVID-19 pandemic was a unique example, Ghassemian et al. [11] addressed the challenges of traditional in-person oral provocation tests, which are essential but were disrupted by social distancing measures, the researchers implemented a virtually supported platform for penicillin allergy delabeling. The process involved initial virtual assessments and subsequent virtual oral amoxicillin challenges under remote supervision by allergists, proving not only feasible but also safe, with all 23 participants successfully completing the challenge without adverse reactions.

The outcomes of this study highlight the broader applicability of virtual health services in allergy management, suggesting that such models could be extended beyond the pandemic to offer a cost-effective, accessible, and efficient alternative for allergy delabeling. This shift could significantly reduce the strain on healthcare facilities while ensuring patient safety and improving access to necessary care, particularly in remote or underserved areas. This virtual approach aligns with other literature that has demonstrated the efficacy of telemedicine in improving patient outcomes across various medical fields, thereby supporting the integration of digital health strategies into more permanent healthcare practices.

14.3.5   AI-Powered Decision Support Systems

The integration of artificial intelligence (AI) and machine learning (ML) algorithms has given rise to Allergy Decision Support Systems. These systems analyze patient data, medical histories, and medication regimens to predict potential drug allergies and recommend safer alternatives. By assessing large datasets, these systems can identify hidden patterns and correlations that might not be apparent through traditional methods. Such predictive capabilities empower healthcare professionals to make informed decisions and prescribe medications that align with a patient's allergy profile.

Drug allergies documented in the electronic health record (EHR), including penicillin allergies, are common and often inaccuarte [12] with up to 15% of hospitalized patients [13, 14] and 10% of the general population [15, 16] reporting a penicillin allergy. Of these individuals, more than 90% can tolerate penicillin after formal allergy testing, and many of the intolerances during testing are not representative of serious allergic responses. Incorrect penicillin allergy labels are recognized as both a public health concern and a medication safety issue because of the many associated harms which include increased multidrug-resistant infections and increased mortality [17–19].

The burden and impact of penicillin and antibiotic allergies have been established by many studies (Table 14.1). However, the main challenge is how to implement a safe clinical decision support tool to delabel patients with inaccurate Penicillin allergy label; moreover, given the limited numbers of allergy and immunology services [19]. This huge task cannot be undertaken by immunologists and allergists alone; hence, the way forward is to empower non-immunologists and non-allergists to champion this process.

14.4 Clinical Decision Support Tool in Practice Across the Globe

There have been many successful attempts by non-immunologists and non-allergists to delabel penicillin allergy across the globe to establish a risk stratification pathways (Table 14.1); approximately 25–30% of patients with penicillin allergy label could have been delabeled [20] on the basis of clinical history alone, without the need for allergy tests; several studies [21, 22] have explored models of non-specialist PenA delabeling. Studies have taken place in emergency department, inpatient (pharmacy led), preoperative, and in the outpatient settings. The risk stratification processes, inclusion and exclusion criteria have varied [21, 23]. Delabeling has been based on history alone in some cases, and others have included skin testing and/or direct oral challenge testing. The outcomes have overall been positive with very few adverse reactions, all of which would be classified as mild without any cases of anaphylaxis or delayed severe hypersensitivity occurring. A recent systematic review confirms the safety of direct oral provocation, after risk assessment, in low-risk non-specialist cohorts. The global experience is strongly supportive of non-specialist delabeling using risk assessment and/or decision support tools such as our proposed Drug Allergy App. The British Society for Allergy and Clinical Immunology (BSACI) is encouraging such practice, and there are current plans of setting up a national working group to address this issue of inaccurate PenA by empowering non-immunologists and non-allergists to champion these initiatives [21].

14.5 Practical Example: The Drug Allergy App

An example of a validated digital tool to support drug allergy delabeling is the drug allergy app (Fig. 14.1) [19]. the details of the development and retrospective validation of the mobile clinical decision support tool for the diagnosis of drug allergy can be found in the original publication [19]; it is one of the first of its kind which may

Table 14.1 A summary of few published studies and reports that have established the impact of penicillin allergy label vs. de-labelling upon patients, clinicians, hospitals and communities

Reference	Description	Summary and recommendations
(a) The impact of drug allergy label/de-labelling upon healthcare:		
Powell et al. 2020, UK	Multi-variable log-linear modelling was used to determine associations between patients labelled as penicillin allergic and total antibiotic costs and length of stay in 750-bed NHS Hospital	Patients with a penicillin allergy record accounted for an excess antibiotic spend of £10,637 (2.61% of annual antibiotic drug spend) and 3522 excess bed-days (3.87% of annual bed-days). Delabelling 50% of patients with a self-reported penicillin allergy record would save an estimated £5501 in antibiotic costs and £503,932 through reduced excess bed-days
Sousa-Pinto et al. 2020, Portugal	An economic evaluation study. Models were built to project the economic impact of (1) diagnostic testing (drug challenges, with or without skin tests) vs. (2) no diagnostic testing	Penicillin allergy testing was found to be cost-saving in all decision models built. Allergy testing resulted in average savings of $657 for inpatients (United States of America: $1444, Europe: $489) and $2746 for outpatients (United States of America: $256, Europe: $6045). 75% of simulations obtained through probabilistic sensitivity analysis identified testing as the less costly option. Hence, supporting the adoption of policies promoting widespread testing of patients with a penicillin allergy label
Blumenthal et al. 2020, USA	The prevalence and impact of a reported penicillin allergy in high-cost, high-need (HCHN) patients using multivariable logistic regression models	20% (383) of 1870 patients have reported penicillin allergy which resulted in fourfold increased odds of beta-lactam alternative antibiotic use with all the potential associated complications. A detailed drug allergy evaluation to optimize antibiotic use in these high risk patients is recommended to reduce cost and improve quality of life
Blumenthal et al. 2020, USA	a multisite prospective study of patients seen for drug allergy at the first sites of the United States Drug Allergy Registry (USDAR)	Patients with a label of drug or antibiotic allergy were concerned about their options for receiving medical treatment, new medications, developing an allergic reaction; addressing these concerns may have great impact on patient journey and engagement with drug allergy testing
Chan et al. 2020, Hong Kong	A total of 6081 rheumatology patients were recruited. Prevalence and clinical outcomes of reported drug allergies were calculated and compared to control cohort	The prevalence of reported drug allergies was found to be significantly higher in rheumatology patients, which was found to be associated with increased rate of infection-related admissions

(continued)

Table 14.1 (continued)

Reference	Description	Summary and recommendations
Vyles et al., 2020, USA	The public health impact and safety of de-labelling children with reported penicillin allergy	Prescription costs are 30 to 40% higher in children with suspected penicillin allergy. Estimated savings of prescribing amoxicillin instead of cefdinir for 50% of children with otitis media would result in annual savings exceeding $34 million
Shenoy ES et al., 2019, USA	Literature review of the current practice of evaluation and management of penicillin allergy	Consequences of penicillin allergy label were concluded as: less effective agent chosen e.g. vancomycin for MSSA, more surgical site infections when non-Penicillins used for peri-operative prophylaxis, more susceptibility to develop multi-resistant organisms and increased healthcare costs
Moran R et, 2019, Australia	A literature review of the current impacts of inaccurate antibiotic allergy labelling in hospitalised and critically ill adults	15–25% of the reported inpatients had an antibiotic allergy label (evenmore among immunocompromised patients); 30–40% did not receive first line antibiotics and had a significant delay in time to first administration of antimicrobial treatment (50 min). For critically ill patients this disbalance worsened; often time-critical decisions were delayed whilst detailed allergy history was not available
Blumenthal et al. 2018, USA	Estimated cost of penicillin allergy evaluation using time-driven activity-based costing	Lower cost estimates were achieved when only a graded drug challenge was performed in comparison to the detailed penicillin evaluation. For drug test with direct challenge only by nurse the cost was $40. For consultant led challenge with skin testing beforehand cost was $220. Estimated cost of penicillin allergy label during acute admission with inaccurate antibiotics allergy label and subsequent adverse events, treatment failure, health care associated infection $3023–$14,269 per patient
(b) The impact of digital health upon drug allergy delabelling:		
Elkhalifa et al. 2021 [19]	Development and validation of a mobile clinical decision support tool for the diagnosis of drug allergy in adults: the Drug Allergy App	A clinical algorithm based on the NICE classification of drug allergy to make the delabeling easier and safer for non-immunologists and non-allergists through the Drug Allergy App. The algorithm has the lowest risk for misclassification of outcomes compared with reference standard drug allergy investigations in allergy and dermatology clinics. The Drug Allergy App may represent a useful clinical decision support tool for clinicians to diagnose drug allergy correctly and support appropriate antibiotic prescribing

(continued)

Table 14.1 (continued)

Reference	Description	Summary and recommendations
Ghassemian et al. 2023 [11]	Virtually supported penicillin allergy de-labelling during COVID-19	Addressed the challenges of traditional in-person oral provocation tests, which are essential but were disrupted by social distancing measures, the researchers implemented a virtually supported platform for penicillin allergy de-labeling. The process involved initial virtual assessments and subsequent virtual oral amoxicillin challenges under remote supervision by allergists, proving not only feasible but also safe, with all 23 participants successfully completing the challenge without adverse reactions
Guyer et al. [6]	Allergy electronic health record documentation: a 2022 work group report of the AAAAI adverse reactions to drugs, biologicals, and latex committee	This document includes a proposal for the creation, education, and implementation of a drug allergy labeling system that may allow for more accurate EHR documentation for improved patient safety the main recommendation is that, allergy and immunology specialists with training and understanding of complex drug reactions can lead allergy reconciliation, which includes new documentation, edits to existing documentation, and removal of inaccurate, erroneous, or inconsequential entries. However, a multidisciplinary approach with training and improved tech-nologies from EHR vendors is needed for optimal use of EHR allergy modules

MSSA methicillin sensitive *Staphylococcus aureus*; *C diff* clostridium difficile; *MRSA* methicillin resistant *Staphylococcus aureus*; *VRE* vancomycin-resistant enterococcus

represent a useful clinical decision support tool for non-allergists to diagnose drug allergy correctly and support appropriate antibiotic prescribing as an attempt to address antimicrobial stewardship. Correct identification of drug allergy may reduce costs by preventing further reactions, some of which could be severe or fatal. In addition, fewer people would be prescribed inappropriate treatments that are some-times at higher cost due to a false recording of drug allergy (see Table 14.1).

For example, in a patient with inaccurate Penicillin Allergy Label and frequent requirement for antibiotic therapy (e.g., due to diabetic foot infection), the cost of a specialist allergy outpatient appointment to undertake the gold-standard testing (skin and/or intradermal drug allergy testing followed by drug challenges) might be lower than the cost of alternative more expensive and less effective antimicrobial options that can result in increased toxicity and prolonged hospitalization.

We are proposing a clinical flow chart incorporating the Drug Allergy App as a useful clinical decision support tool for non-allergists to diagnose drug allergy cor-rectly and encourage referrals to drug allergy services as appropriate in order to support appropriate antibiotic prescribing as an attempt to address antimicrobial stewardship [19].

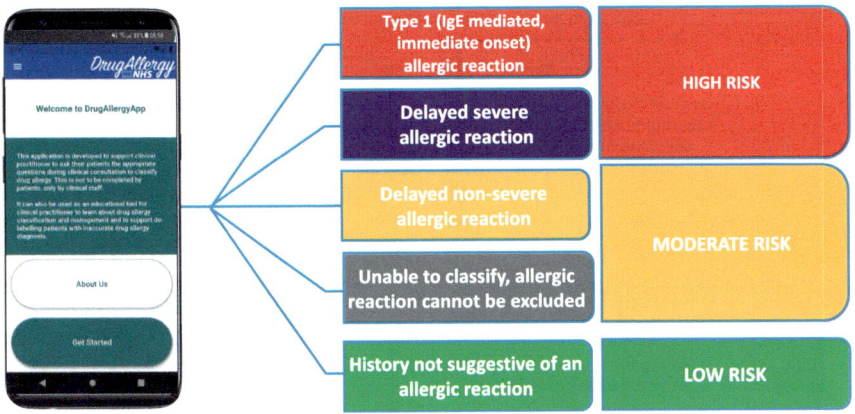

Fig. 14.1 The Drug Allergy App: developed by Dr. Elkhalifa et al. [19]

Moreover, this drug Allergy App can be a platform that enhances visual presentation and user interaction which could be further improved by including VR/AR technology (Virtual reality/Augmented reality). This would not only facilitate learning through 3D representations of potential allergy symptoms, but also improve accuracy for intuitively recognizing allergies and various skin manifestations in such patients. Recent work in innovative research is using machine learning algorithms to automate and improve medical investigation and diagnosis such as histological images of human colorectal cancer, digital mammograms, and COVID19 chest X-ray images.

14.6   Challenges and Considerations

While digital health presents numerous opportunities, it also comes with challenges:

1. Data Privacy and Security
   One of the foremost challenges is ensuring the privacy and security of sensitive patient information. Digitalizing drug allergies requires robust cybersecurity measures to protect against data breaches and unauthorized access. Striking a balance between data accessibility and protection is essential to maintain patient trust. Compliance with regulations such as the Health Insurance Portability and Accountability Act (HIPAA) is paramount.
2. Accessibility
   Not all patients have access to the necessary technology, such as smartphones or wearable devices. Ensuring equitable access to digital health tools is crucial to avoid exacerbating healthcare disparities.
3. Data Accuracy and Updating

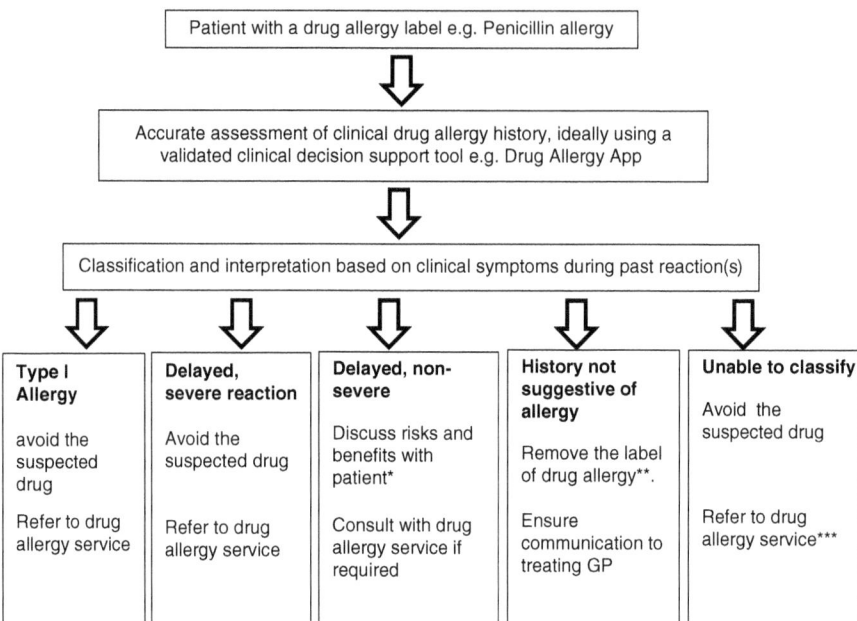

Patient with a drug allergy label e.g. Penicillin allergy

⇩

Accurate assessment of clinical drug allergy history, ideally using a
validated clinical decision support tool e.g. Drug Allergy App

⇩

Classification and interpretation based on clinical symptoms during past reaction(s)

⇩   ⇩   ⇩   ⇩   ⇩

Type I Allergy	**Delayed, severe reaction**	**Delayed, non-severe**	**History not suggestive of allergy**	**Unable to classify**
avoid the suspected drug	Avoid the suspected drug	Discuss risks and benefits with patient*	Remove the label of drug allergy**.	Avoid the suspected drug
Refer to drug allergy service	Refer to drug allergy service	Consult with drug allergy service if required	Ensure communication to treating GP	Refer to drug allergy service***

* In case of penicillin allergy, use of 2nd or 3rd generation cephalosporins with low risk of cross reactivity (e.g. cefuroxime & ceftriaxone) or carbapenems is unlikely to result in serious allergic reactions.

** For example gastrointestinal intolerance, such as diarrhoea or nausea. If the suspected drug is indicated the same medication can be given following discussion with patient. Delabelling of drug allergy can take place at this stage of clinical consultation.

*** In case of penicillin allergy, use of alternative β-lactam antibiotics should be discussed with drug allergy or infection specialists on a case by case basis. Discussing the risks and benefits with patient is recommended.

Fig. 14.2 A proposed clinical flow chart incorporating the Drug Allergy App as a clinical decision support tool for non-allergists to accurately diagnose drug allergy and encourage referrals as appropriate; Concrete examples for penicillin allergy are indicated by *,**,***; *GP* general practitioner

The accuracy and reliability of digital health tools must be rigorously validated to ensure they provide trustworthy information and recommendations. Regulatory bodies need to adapt to the evolving landscape of digital health to ensure patient safety. Maintaining accurate and up-to-date allergy information is crucial. Patients, healthcare providers, and EHR systems must collaborate to ensure that changes in allergy status are promptly recorded and reflected in the digital records. Inaccurate or outdated information could lead to adverse events.

4. Technological Infrastructure

Widespread digitalization requires a robust technological infrastructure across healthcare facilities. This includes adopting compatible EHR systems, training healthcare professionals, and addressing potential technical glitches that might arise during implementation.

5. Patient Education
   Using digital health tools effectively requires a certain level of digital literacy. Patients need to be educated about how to use these tools, interpret the information they provide, and collaborate effectively with healthcare professionals.

14.6.1   Online Resources and Educational Platforms

Numerous websites, forums, and educational platforms provide information about drug allergies, including common allergens, symptoms, and management strategies. These resources can potentially be confusing or misleading for patients and healthcare professionals who are not specialized in drug allergy.

14.6.2   Social Media Support Groups

Social media platforms host support groups where individuals with drug allergies share their experiences, exchange advice, and offer emotional support. These groups foster a sense of community and enable members to learn from others' journeys. However, social media can play both positive and negative roles, for example:

– *Misinformation*: Social media platforms are filled with information, but not all of it is accurate or reliable. Individuals with drug allergies might come across misleading advice or incorrect information regarding their allergies, which can lead to potentially harmful decisions. It's crucial for users to verify information from credible sources.

– *Self-Diagnosis*: Social media can sometimes encourage self-diagnosis, where individuals rely on information from others to determine if they have a drug allergy. This can lead to misinterpretation of symptoms and unnecessary avoidance of medications, affecting their health management.

– *Anecdotal Experiences*: While personal anecdotes shared on social media can provide insights into others' experiences with drug allergies, they might not be applicable to everyone. Allergies can manifest differently in each individual, and what works for one person might not work for another.

– *Sharing Medical Information*: Some individuals might share their detailed medical histories and allergic reactions on social media platforms. While this can create a sense of community and support, it also poses privacy concerns as sensitive health information becomes publicly accessible.

– *Promotion of Alternative Treatments*: Social media can promote unverified alternative treatments for drug allergies, which might lack scientific evidence or even be dangerous. Individuals should be cautious when considering alternative therapies and consult medical professionals.

- *Fear and Anxiety*: Overexposure to negative or sensationalized information about drug allergies on social media can amplify fear and anxiety among individuals. It's important to strike a balance between staying informed and avoiding undue stress.
- *Lack of Professional Guidance*: While social media can provide general information and emotional support, it cannot replace advice from healthcare professionals. Seeking proper medical guidance is crucial for accurate diagnosis, treatment, and management of drug allergies.
- *Reporting Adverse Reactions*: Social media can be a platform for reporting adverse reactions to medications, potentially leading to more comprehensive data collection for regulatory agencies. However, such reports should also be validated and reported through official channels for accurate documentation.

14.7 What Is an Ideal Platform for Digitalizing Drug Allergy?

The gold-standard of drug allergy information in electronic medical records requires the creation, networking, and management of newer forms of individual patient data programs such as mobile applications and multi-location software programs. Currently, in many hospitals around the world, patient records are only immediately accessible at the patient's main medical center or local network. Although this helps to ensure the privacy of patient data behind strong electronic data protection software programs, this more isolated system produces difficulties for which a singularly networked system would not have. Should a patient need to transfer to another location or see a specialist elsewhere for any multitude of reasons, these records need to move from one confidential software enclave to another. This creates additional administration burdens and costs on both the sending and receiving structures. In a wider, more uniform patient record system, this process would be redundant. Furthermore, utilizing this type of record management produces both a safer and more beneficial medical environment for patients because it ensures higher levels of data accuracy. For instance, if a patient is first demonstrated to be allergic to penicillin at the emergency room of one hospital, both their general practitioner in another center and local pharmacist would immediately be able to access this information. Inverse information pathways would also be true and medically significant details and terminology would be handled by qualified medical professionals removing the need for patients or unqualified personnel to potentially introduce misinformation.

To maximize the benefit of a wider networked patient record system, individual hospitals should strengthen their local data management protocols. Explicitly, hospitals should review current electronic data records to ensure now-tolerated medicines from the allergy list have been removed or inactivated. Along the same lines, patients who have demonstrated through allergy challenges to not have suspected allergies must have their electronic health records reconcile accurately to reflect test results. Also critically important to maintaining accurate records is the appropriate training of the many possible healthcare professionals who have access to these software systems and possess various levels of allergy-specific knowledge. Most pertinently, staff should be trained in the correct terminology including definitions and types of adverse reactions, as well as the standardization of recording expectations to ensure uniform practices.

Patient education and empowerment is the ultimate aim in digitalizing drug allergy [24, 25]. The power and security of current mobile devices allow patients the opportunity to create and maintain their own electronic records. For instance, in a patient's daily life they may take an ibuprofen tablet to relieve a headache and then develop a skin rash. In a gold-standard data management system, this patient could upload high-quality photos to their medical record which could be quickly reviewed by pertinent medical professionals to determine which follow-up steps need to be implemented.

14.8   The Future Direction

In summary, the field of digital health and drug allergy management continues to evolve, with ongoing technological advancements and innovations. Some potential future directions include [24–28]:

- Artificial Intelligence and Machine Learning: AI-driven algorithms can analyze vast amounts of medical data to predict and prevent adverse reactions, improving drug allergy management.
- Blockchain for Data Integrity: Blockchain technology holds promise in ensuring the integrity and security of patient data, enhancing trust in digital health systems.
- Interoperability: Efforts to improve the interoperability of different digital health tools and systems will enable seamless sharing of allergy information across various healthcare settings.

The future of digitalizing drug allergies holds exciting possibilities. As technology continues to evolve, several trends are likely to shape this domain such as AI algorithms can help identify complex patterns within patient data, leading to more accurate allergy predictions and personalized treatment recommendations. This can aid healthcare providers in avoiding potentially allergenic medications; empowering patients to manage their own allergy profiles through secure digital platforms that could enhance patient engagement and reduce errors resulting from miscommunication. Patients could easily share allergy information with different healthcare providers as needed in a secure and tamper-proof method of storing and sharing allergy data which would build a trust among patients and healthcare providers.

The creation of comprehensive global databases could provide insights into regional and global trends in drug allergies. Such databases could aid researchers in understanding the factors contributing to allergies and developing preventive measures.

14.9 Conclusion

The integration of digital health technologies has substantially improved the management of drug allergies by offering innovative solutions for tracking, monitoring, and education. Wearable devices, AI-powered decision support systems, and telemedicine platforms empower patients to actively participate in their healthcare journey, while allergy tracking apps and online educational resources provide critical information and alerts. As technology continues to advance, the intersection of digital health and drug allergies holds great promise for enhancing patient outcomes and safety.

Declaration of All Sources of Funding SE is chairing the Scientific Committee of the 3rd Emirate Allergy and Clinical Immunology Conference, none of the funds received related to this article.

References

1. Blumenthal KG, Park MA, Macy EM. Redesigning the allergy module of the electronic health record. Ann Allergy Asthma Immunol. 2016;117:126–31.
2. Inglis JM, Caughey GE, Smith W, Shakib S. Documentation of adverse drug reactions to opioids in an electronic health record. Intern Med J. 2021;51(9):1490–6. https://doi.org/10.1111/imj.15209.
3. Deng F, Li MD, Wong A, Kowalski LT, Lai KH, Digumarthy SR, Zhou L. Quality of documentation of contrast agent allergies in electronic health records. J Am Coll Radiol. 2019;16(8):1027–35. https://doi.org/10.1016/j.jacr.2019.01.027. Epub 2019 Mar 4.
4. Kuperman GJ, Bobb A, Payne TH, Avery AJ, Gandhi TK, Burns G, Classen DC, Bates DW. Medication-related clinical decision support in computerized provider order entry systems: a review. J Am Med Inform Assoc. 2007;14(1):29–40. https://doi.org/10.1197/jamia.M2170.
5. Carspecken CW, Sharek PJ, Longhurst C, Pageler NM. A clinical case of electronic health record drug alert fatigue: consequences for patient outcome. Pediatrics. 2013;131(6):e1970–3.
6. Guyer AC, et al. Allergy electronic health record documentation: a 2022 work group report of the AAAAI adverse reactions to drugs, biologicals, and latex committee. J Allergy Clin Immunol Pract. 2022;10(11):2854–67. https://doi.org/10.1016/j.jaip.2022.08.020. Epub 2022 Sep 21.
7. Brockow K, et al. Drug allergy passport and other documentation for patients with drug hypersensitivity—an ENDA/EAACI drug allergy interest group position paper. Allergy. 2016;71(11):1533–9. https://doi.org/10.1111/all.12929. Epub 2016 Aug 14.
8. Adler-Milstein J, Jha AK. HITECH act drove large gains in hospital electronic health record adoption. Health Aff. 2016;35(4):698–706. https://doi.org/10.1377/hlthaff.2015.1258.

9. Li L, Fu X, Lin J, et al. The role of mHealth apps in improving medication adherence for drug allergy patients. J Am Med Inform Assoc. 2020;27(7):1021–6.

10. Shah A, Rakhmanina N. Wearable devices in allergic diseases: opportunities and challenges. Curr Allergy Asthma Rep. 2020;20(8):25.

11. Ghassemian A, Sadi G, Mak R, Erdle S, Wong T, Jeimy S. Virtually supported penicillin allergy de-labelling during COVID-19. Allergy Asthma Clin Immunol. 2023;19(1):17.

12. Shenoy ME, Rowe T, Blumenthal KG. Evaluation and management of penicillin allergy: a review. JAMA J Am Med Assoc. 2019;321(2):188–99.

13. Powell N, West R, Sandoe JAT. The impact of penicillin allergy de-labelling on the WHO AWaRe antibiotic categories: a retrospective cohort study. J Hosp Infect. 2021;115:10–6.

14. Zhou L, Dhopeshwarkar N, Blumenthal KG, Goss F, Topaz M, Slight SP, et al. Drug allergies documented in electronic health records of a large healthcare system. Allergy. 2016;71(9):1305–13.

15. Excellence NIfHac. Drug allergy: diagnosis and management Clinical guideline [CG183] 2014. 2014. https://www.nice.org.uk/guidance/cg183.

16. West RM, Smith CJ, Pavitt SH, Butler CC, Howard P, Bates C, et al. Warning: allergic to penicillin': association between penicillin allergy status in 2.3 million NHS general practice electronic health records, antibiotic prescribing and health outcomes. J Antimicrob Chemother. 2019;74(7):2075–82.

17. DesBiens M, Scalia P, Ravikumar S, Glick A, Newton H, Erinne O, et al. A closer look at penicillin allergy history: systematic review and meta-analysis of tolerance to drug challenge. Am J Med. 2020;133(4):452.

18. Powell N, Elkhalifa S, Guyer A, Garcez T, Sandoe J, Zhou L. Addressing the challenges of penicillin allergy Delabeling with electronic health records and Mobile applications. J Allergy Clin Immunol Pract. 2023;11(2):414–21.

19. Elkhalifa S, Bhana R, Blaga A, Joshi S, Svejda M, Kasilingam V, Garcez T, Calisti G. Development and validation of a Mobile clinical decision support tool for the diagnosis of drug allergy in adults: the drug allergy app. J Allergy Clin Immunol Pract. 2021;9(12):4410–4418.e4.

20. Krishna MT, Huissoon AP, Li M, Richter A, Pillay DG, Sambanthan D, Raman SC, Nasser S, Misbah SA. Enhancing antibiotic stewardship by tackling "spurious" penicillin allergy. Clin Exp Allergy. 2017;47(11):1362–73.

21. Cooper L, Harbour J, Jacqueline Sneddon R, Seaton A. Safety and efficacy of de-labelling penicillin allergy in adults using direct oral challenge: a systematic review. JAC Antimicrob Resist. 2021;3(1):dlaa123.

22. Chen JR, Tarver SA, Alvarez KS, Tran T, Khan DA. A proactive approach to penicillin allergy testing in hospitalized patients. J Allergy Clin Immunol Pract. 2017;5(3):686–93.

23. Lee RU. Penicillin allergy Delabeling can decrease antibiotic resistance, reduce costs, and optimize patient outcomes. Fed Pract. 2020;37(10):460–5.

24. Smith A, et al. Digitalization of drug allergies: benefits and challenges. J Health Inform. 2022;12(3):167–80.

25. Johnson RH. AI-powered predictive models for drug allergy management. HealthTech Innov. 2023;8(2):45–52.

26. Williams EK, et al. Blockchain Technology in Healthcare: enhancing data security for allergy information. J Med Data Security. 2023;15(4):320–35.

27. Global Healthcare Alliance. Trends in digital health: focus on drug allergy management. 2024. https://www.gha.org/research.

28. World Health Research Institute. Global allergy database: insights into allergy prevalence and patterns. 2025. https://www.whri.org/allergy-database.

Chapter 15
Smart Devices and Digital Therapeutics for Asthma Care: Regulatory Challenges

Francesca Cefaloni, Luca Passantino, Mario Di Stasio, and Matteo Bonini

Contents

Abstract Mobile health technologies, remote care, and digital therapeutics are finding their way into clinical care for patients with chronic respiratory diseases like asthma. A trend that gained momentum during preventative contact restrictions due to the COVID-19 pandemic, has shown its potential to continuously improve (home) care for patients, particularly in underserved or remote areas also afterward. However, many solutions like smart inhalers, connective spirometers, apps, and comprehensive monitoring platforms haven't found their way into clinical routines yet, despite their potential to improve symptom control, quality of life, treatment adherence, and

F. Cefaloni (✉) · L. Passantino · M. Di Stasio
Department of Cardiovascular and Pulmonary Sciences, Università Cattolica del Sacro Cuore, Rome, Italy
e-mail: francesca.cefaloni@unicatt.it

M. Bonini
Department of Public Health and Infectious Diseases, Sapienza University of Rome, Rome, Italy

National Heart and Lung Institute (NHLI), Imperial College London, London, UK
e-mail: matteo.bonini@uniroma1.it

© The Author(s), under exclusive license to Springer Nature
Switzerland AG 2025
P. M. Matricardi, S. Dramburg, *Digital Allergology*, Health Informatics,
https://doi.org/10.1007/978-3-031-71021-6_15

patient satisfaction in the field of asthma and allergies. This may be in part due to the current lack of standardization across different countries. As more and more apps and devices are being developed, regulatory guidance, and standardized quality criteria become essential. The present manuscript aims to summarize current knowledge and challenges related to the process of digital health device standardization and data integration. It further provides an update on ongoing research projects designed to optimize home care solutions for asthmatic and atopic patients.

Abbreviations

RCT	Randomized Clinical Trial
WHO	World Health Organization
EAACI	European Academy of Allergy and Clinical Immunology
PROM	Patient-Reported Outcome Measure
DHT	Digital Health Technology
ACT	Asthma Control Test
ACQ	Asthma Control Questionnaire
AQLQ	Asthma Quality of Life Questionnaire
ATS	American Association of Thoracic Society
ERS	European Respiratory Academy
FeNO	Fractional exhaled Nitric Oxide
ICS	Inhaled corticosteroids
pMDI	Pressurized Metered-Dose Inhaler
FDA	Food and Drug Administration
ACM	Asthma Control Measure
ACQ5	5-items Asthma Control Questionnaire
MASK	Mobile Airways Sentinel networK
VAS	Visual analog scale
CARAT	Control of Allergic Rhinitis and Asthma Test
e-DASTHMA	Electronic DAily control Score for aSTHMA
INCA	INhaler Compliance Assessment
WAO	World Allergy Organization
GDPR	General Data Protection Regulation
IMPACT	Improving Asthma Care Together

15.1 Smart Devices for Remote Monitoring of Respiratory Diseases

Over the past years, with a particular boost during the COVID-19 pandemic, the use of telemedicine has exponentially increased, leading to the need of keeping healthcare systems and professionals up to date on this matter [1]. In both adults and children, mobile phones and electronic devices allow 24/7 real-time connectivity

[2]. Hence, digital health devices have assumed a crucial role in monitoring and treating acute and chronic diseases [3]. Despite the lack of consistent data, digital health might offer a great opportunity for facing the challenge of improving patient care by making it more efficient, tailored, and cost-effective. Indeed, the World Health Organization (WHO) [4], the European Union [5], national governments [6, 7], and medical associations [8] are particularly attracted by this exciting opportunity [2]. WHO has made important steps in that direction by promoting the "Be He@lthy, Be Mobile" initiative for several chronic noncommunicable diseases like cancer, diabetes, and cardiovascular diseases, as well as for the prevention and control of respiratory diseases, such as asthma and chronic obstructive pulmonary disease (COPD). Also, WHO implemented a mobile Health (mHealth) Technical Evidence Review Group, including a panel of external experts to improve and standardize digital health approaches [9].

As an example of the abovementioned entities, asthma represents a relevant burden, in terms of quality of life, productivity, morbidity, and mortality. Considering the variability in symptom frequency and severity, digital health technology (DHT) may have a pivotal role in improving disease control, treatment adherence, and satisfaction of patients over time [10]. Teleassistance in asthma bares great potential in quickly detecting disease deterioration via patient-reported outcome measures (PROM, i.e., Asthma Control Test (ACT) [11], the Asthma Control Questionnaire (ACQ) The Asthma Quality of Life Questionnaire (AQLQ) [12]), together with clinical and functional data, such as pulmonary function parameters, or markers of eosinophilic airway inflammation.

15.2   Remote Lung Function Assessment

Home spirometers and peak expiratory flow (PEF) meters represent the key tools for detecting early modifications of functional parameters in asthmatic patients. Digital home spirometers aim to ameliorate disease awareness and Quality of Life (QoL), also by providing technical maneuver performance feedback. When necessary, clinical suggestions are provided to patients in simple and comprehensible terms, as well as more accurate information is sent to attending healthcare professionals. Ideally, spirometers for home testing should meet ATS/ERS criteria and should not require frequent calibrations. To optimally match these requirements, the use of ultrasonic or vertical turbine systems has been suggested [13].

15.3   Home Oximetry for Remote Monitoring

Oximeters to measure peripheral oxygen saturation (spO_2) are probably the most widely diffused digital health devices in home care settings, particularly since the COVID-19 pandemic brought one of these easy-to-use devices to almost every household. Quality controls are performed by manufacturers and are well-defined in international regulatory certifications (e.g., ISO 80601-2-61 for FDA in the USA). The need for data integration from oximeters is little to none, as self-reported measurements represent a valid, cheap, and time-sparing alternative to data sharing via Bluetooth or Wi-Fi connections. The use of oximeters only requires brief training (by healthcare professionals and/or audio-visual material) on the correct use, possible confounders, and result interpretation. Despite their handiness, oximetry results can be tricky to interpret in some individuals: while the results of current smokers could be slightly overestimated, the presence of a reduced cardiac output or peripheral arteriopathies can lead to an underestimation of the peripheral oxygenation [14]. To be noted, oximeters overestimate SpO_2 by a 5–10% factor in people with darker skin tones (phototypes 5–6) [15].

15.4   Remote Monitoring of Exhaled Nitric Oxide

The FeNO evaluation represents a valid and helpful marker of eosinophilic airway inflammation. Some studies tested the reliability of FeNO measurement devices (e.g., NIOX Vero) in a home setting. Data provided by measurements are useful but not quite ready to be integrated into clinical practice yet. Poor adherence to correct usage technique and wide variability of results, influenced by patient conditions (i.e., fasting status, smoking habit, chewing-gum use) currently make solid evidence for a domiciliary setting impossible [16]. Given the intrinsic variability of the test, several studies highlighted that neither the mean nor the absolute value of FeNO (parts per billion; ppb) are useful in evaluating asthma control or exacerbation risk. However, greater potential has been attributed to the fluctuation over time, for example, measured twice daily, daily [17] or even randomly [18]. By note, FeNO measurement in children seems to be more sensitive than home spirometry in assessing response to ICS, application which led the authors to propose the titration of ICS in this setting. Another limitation to the application of at home FeNO measurements in the real world are the relatively high costs of the devices [19].

15.5   Sensor Technology and Wearables for Asthma Monitoring

Further remote tools in asthma care include cough frequency detectors, breath composition analysis, lung sound, and sleep monitors. In the field of wearable technologies, smartwatches, fitness trackers, smart rings, and smart clothing are designed to identify clinical deterioration at an early stage, but currently without consistent standardized cut-offs [20]. In a cohort study of children with controlled asthma, the recording of lung sounds allowed investigators to better identify nocturnal wheezing in the majority of subjects, differently from the traditional respiratory function tests [21]. For example, skin contact microphones can detect the flow and respiratory rates, tidal volumes, wheezing, and cough [22]. In addition, several smartwatches include the possibility of the self-triggered oximetry, which are usually prompted in relation to alarms for tachycardia or arrhythmias. Independently from their monitoring functions, smartwatches and their reminder functions could be useful to motivate patients to take their therapy [23].

15.6   Digital Therapeutics in Asthma Care

Low treatment adherence and incorrect inhaler technique are a significant challenge for asthma management. The amount of emerging digital tools addressing these topics demonstrates the effort to improve inhaler technique and adherence support to improve disease control.

Digital inhalers (smart inhalers, smarthalers) are electronic sensors attached to or integrated into traditional inhalers, with the potential of improving medication adherence and, consequently, asthma control [24]. They have been available since the early 2000s but remain variably diffused in clinical practice. Most available tools are based on the following key features:

1. logging of performed inhalations.
2. reminders to ensure patients adhere to their therapeutic regimen.
3. quality feedback about the inhalation technique.
4. sensors quantifying the delivered dose, ensuring that patients receive the correct dose of medication.
5. remote monitoring of real-life asthma control, accessible even by healthcare providers and allowing a proactive intervention.

Unfortunately, despite several innovative approaches based on machine learning and neural networks, there is great heterogeneity regarding clinical outcomes in clinical studies [25, 26].

A valid example is Teva's Digihaler™, approved by the FDA for the combined use with the inhalers ProAir® (albuterol sulfate 117 mcg), AirDuo® (fluticasone propionate and salmeterol), and ArmonAir® (fluticasone propionate). Teva's Digihaler™ relies on a sensor that allows checking the timing of use. With this information on reliever medication use, it was possible to predict asthma exacerbations within 12 weeks. The Hailie™ solution (previously known as the SmartInhaler™ platform) allows recording the number of dispensed inhaled doses and the time at which they are taken. This system has been shown to improve adherence to therapy compared to traditional methods [25, 26]. Smart inhalers provide real-time data on medication adherence to both patients and healthcare professionals, supporting clinical decision-making. They can be connected to other devices, such as smartphones, combining them with an application (app) and therefore increasing the possibility of self-management of asthma [27]. The overall satisfaction of patients with eHealth tools appears to be very high in young people though more studies are needed to understand which population could benefit more from the use of smart inhalers [28].

Smart spacers are also available for pMDI inhalers; they have been developed to provide feedback on the quality of inhalation, reducing up to 30% of errors in inhalation techniques. These devices, which are particularly relevant when treating children, evaluate the quality of inhalations through a flow sensor [29].

Another area of digital therapeutics is covered by apps which can be installed directly on patients' smartphones (Table 15.1) [30]. Following a comprehensive review of interactive mobile allergy and asthma apps available within the USA in 2018, they should be: easy to use; reliable; technically supported; no time consuming (short questionnaires); no too low costs; validated [31]. For instance, the ACM is a 5-item questionnaire developed for being suitable in asthma digital health symptom monitoring with a weekly lookback (a shorter period than commonly considered in RCTs) and promoting a fast recognition of clinical modifications. Compared with the ACQ5 questionnaire, it demonstrated a sensitivity of 0.99 in identifying uncontrolled asthma [32]. The Mobile Airways Sentinel networK (MASK) of Allergic Rhinitis and its Impact on Asthma (ARIA) initiative (MASK-air) app is available in 29 countries and 20 languages and collects information about allergic rhinitis and asthma symptoms addressing unmet needs in the field of digital health [33]. The validated PROMs used in the program (i.e., VAS, self-reported asthma medication, CARAT score) assess clinical asthma control over a week or more. However, a recent data-driven electronic daily control score for asthma (e-DASTHMA) has been validated using the MASK-air app, with the potential to assess disease control in patients with fluctuating symptoms. The results, retrospectively derived from the validated scores, offer a new tool to assess patient conditions in a shorter timeframe [34]. The "Inhaler Compliance Assessment (INCA)" study matched clinical digital data with digital PROMs resulting in an improvement in medication adherence of the asthmatic patients and a reduction of the treatment burden [35]. Similarly, the MyAirCoach project proposed an innovative monitoring

Table 15.1 The most downloaded asthma apps available on the App Store and Play Store [30]

APP	Symptoms monitoring	Parameter recording (i.e., vital signs or PEF)	Environmental notices	Education	Medication tracker or management
AsthmaTrack®	√	√	√	×	×
Asthma-Diary®	√	√	×	×	√
Asthma Manager®	√	×	×	√	√
Propeller Health®	√	×	√	√	√
SaniQ Asthma®	√	×	√	√	√
FindAir®	√	√	×	√	√

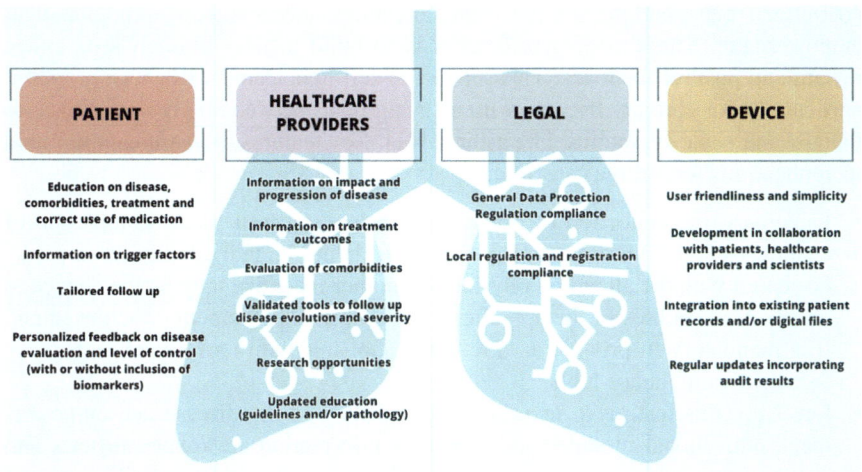

Fig. 15.1 Quality criteria for e-health in allergy and respiratory care from WAO proposal [4]

system aimed at predicting clinical deterioration or asthma exacerbations by using proprietary devices [36, 37].

As health applications deliver data and/or recommendations directly related to decisions and actions on the user's health, it is essential for the apps to meet standards in quality and usability. Therefore, several quality measures have been proposed:

- "The Mobile Application Rating Scale (MARS)": a comprehensive way to evaluate an mHealth app considering four domains: engagement, functionality, esthetics, and information. All users are invited to use the app for at least 10 min daily and encouraged to give an overall subjective evaluation [38].
- "The patient empowerment index through mobile technology": an endpoint entirely based on the concept of patient empowerment. Three key elements have been used to evaluate the apps: self-monitoring, personalized feedback, and patient education [39].
- "The WAO Upper Airway Diseases Committee proposal": a quality assurance flow-chart for allergy and asthma apps, including a total of 16 criteria, divided into four different domains. This proposal could be considered a guide for the future development of digital health tools (Fig. 15.1) [4].

15.7 Gamification to Improve Adherence and Disease-Related Knowledge

Gamification, defined as "the craft of deriving all the fun and addicting elements found in games and applying them to the real-world or productive activities" [40], is an increasingly hot topic in health management thanks to the high cost-effectiveness and the ability to maintain compliance and focus through patient empowerment. The aim of gamification is to build a habit through progressive reward and positive feedback. This support of self-management has been proposed particularly for chronic diseases with a strong bond between daily compliance to therapy and acute symptoms, like asthma [41]. Key features of gamification, found in applications for asthma care, are:

- Incentives: the collection of points, and badges, as well as the completion of challenges and achievement of goals: these should be individually set and may be shared with the attending physician. Another incentive may be the chance to unlock new features of the app after a noticeable improvement or achievement. It is mandatory to provide a variety and short-medium term renewals to keep focus and compliance high.
- Level up: this feature to increase understanding of the disease and empowerment, educational modules and pieces of information are related to tests and challenges to enhance problem-solving related to asthma self-care. This feature increases knowledge in a playful way and could be a game changer in pediatric care. Customizable avatars may increase personal identification.
- Constraints: time dependency for completing tasks, goals, challenges, etc. may increase the feeling of challenge and competition.
- Teamwork: forming groups with similar objectives and characteristics. This feature should be carefully managed in healthcare settings due to healthcare-related privacy.
- Positive feedback: giving clear proof of improvement is a key component of gamification. In digital asthma care, this feedback could be achieved using PROMs and other instruments, such as spirometers or smart inhalers, tracking daily or weekly variations or stability (Fig. 15.2) [41].

Fig. 15.2 Key features of gamification

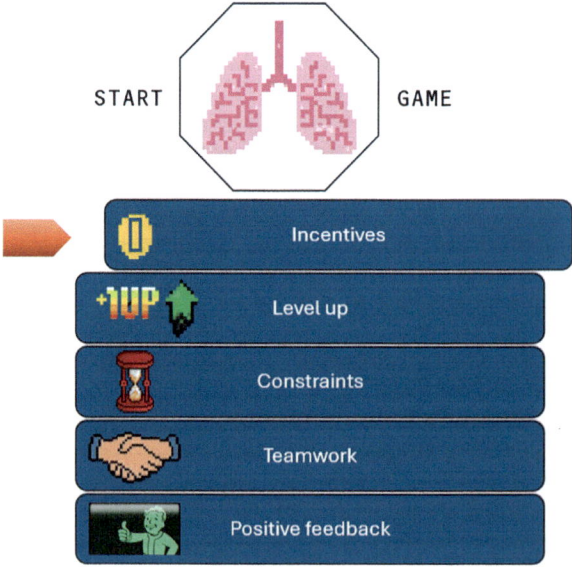

Other key features, like leaderboards and competition, may be included, but they should be carefully managed, due to their potential to demotivate the patient to keep on improving [41].

A valid example of gamification designed for digital asthma care is the Cohero® health mobile platform, by Aptar Digital Health (New York, US—Suresnes, France). The Cohero® connects an mHealth app (BreatheSMART), a spirometer (mSpirometer™), and a smart inhaler and provide users with daily logs of inhalation technique, spirometry values modifications, allowing clinicians to access data through a cloud-based platform [42]. Overall, studies showed that gamification is well-tolerated and appreciated by patients [43, 44].

15.8   Quality Criteria and Regulatory Aspects

The development of digital health is incredibly fast and dynamic. However, the clinical validation of a telehealth approach requires standardized outcome evaluation systems. For this reason, establishing criteria that guarantee the efficiency of remote monitoring is essential. To be available for purchase, digital inhalers must respect the Medical Device Regulation, EU 2017/745-746 for EU countries and should undergo FDA approval for the USA. The Health Insurance Portability and Accountability Act indicates that data from digital health should be shared only for health-related purposes; any other actor, such as insurance companies or marketing agencies, should be authorized by the patient [45]. The US Department of Health and Human Services further provides indications for health app developers, and the Federal Trade Commission enlists in the Mobile Health App Interactive Tool [46] the respective laws and regulations, such as the FTC's Health Breach Notification Rule and Children's Online Privacy Protection Act. All societies legitimately involved in data and personal information use, for health-related reasons, should respect the HIPAA and respond legally in cases of violations. In Europe, the same role is covered by the GDPR EU regulation 2016/679 on April 27th, 2016 [47–49].

In the field of archiving data, the preferred digital platforms for storage and service delivery are cloud services. Their use is controversial as some authors believe in their usefulness, while others consider the risk of exposure to cyberattacks and privacy violations too high [50]. Consequently, no available databases are completely capable of guaranteeing privacy and data security protection. However, four pillars which make it possible to safeguard data privacy and accessibility have been identified in literature:

- Open source code.
- Zero Knowledge-STARK: a cryptographic solution aimed at resolving the potential conflict between personal privacy and institutional integrity.
- Federated learning, to send computational models instead of data.
- Use of differential privacy algorithms when sensitive data are aggregated [51, 52].

15.9   Integration of Patient-Generated Data in Remote Care

Digital health in atopy and asthma includes the detection of acute symptoms which could request clinical advice in specific situations (e.g., environmental exposure to pollen or pollutants detected by GPS), the adherence assessment to therapy, and the re-training of inhalator technique when needed [53, 54]. The aim of digital health is not only to support patients in self-monitoring but also to offer a novel assessment method of adherence to therapy (including push notification reminders) and to evaluate the need for a reliever therapy [10]. This approach may be tailored by identifying the most suitable monitoring tool for each asthmatic patient. For these reasons, the availability of platforms aimed at clinical practice such as call visits as well as for data storage is crucial [55]. Data should always be transmitted with a minimum level of encryption (i.e., the operation which translates data into code nearly impossible to understand, unless the reader possesses a "key" to translate them back) and can be managed through:

- Apps, which allow patients to choose which information to share with individually selected physicians or third parties.
- Cloud networks, which constitute the best option for research purposes by supporting a robust data analysis (nonetheless, they require anonymization and a major cost in data storage).
- Clinician reserved portal dashboards [35, 36].

Once the data has been collected via platforms, there are different possibilities to integrate them into the workflow of patient care. For example, the first level of response could involve allied healthcare professionals (e.g., pharmacists/nurses) capable of assessing symptoms and/or other tests to classify the severity of symptoms and address relevant cases to a medical evaluation. The medical management could include video call visits, as in the "IMPACT" study, where children (7–11 year-old) perform weekly video calls (integrated with their parents through the IMPACT app) with healthcare to assess their asthma control. As the study is ongoing, results have not been shared yet [56]. The teleassistance approach, requires, more than traditional face-to-face visits, constant patient collaboration, and a strong relationship between healthcare and patients, to guarantee the achievement of the shared clinical goals [30, 57].

15.10   Future Potential

Alongside the increased use of digital devices, the awareness of remote healthcare in the management of respiratory and allergic diseases is rising. In this light, it is essential to ensure the quality, usability, and safety of digital health technologies. Regulatory authorities are providing and increasing guidance for this matter. However, widespread use may also be limited by legal constraints. As the regulation and implementation of remote care is still heterogeneous at national levels, international standardization seems currently not achievable. Despite that, clinical studies and real-life experience have shown encouraging outcomes for digital health technologies in remote asthma management, reducing geographical barriers and burden of disease. In the future, a more routine integration of validated virtual care and digital therapeutics into asthma care could enhance patient engagement, improve medication adherence, and ultimately lead to better outcomes and reduced healthcare costs.

References

1. Elliott T, Shih J, Dinakar C, Portnoy J, Fineman S. American College of Allergy, Asthma & Immunology Position Paper on the use of telemedicine for allergists. Ann Allergy Asthma Immunol. 2017;119(6):512–7. https://pubmed.ncbi.nlm.nih.gov/29103799/.
2. Matricardi PM, Dramburg S, Alvarez-Perea A, Antolín-Amérigo D, Apfelbacher C, Atanaskovic-Markovic M, et al. The role of mobile health technologies in allergy care: an EAACI position paper. Allergy. 2020;75(2):259–72. https://pubmed.ncbi.nlm.nih.gov/31230373/.
3. Kvedarienė V, Burzdikaitė P, Česnavičiūtė I. mHealth and telemedicine utility in the monitoring of allergic diseases. Front Allergy. 2022;3:919746. http://www.ncbi.nlm.nih.gov/pubmed/36118170.
4. Verhoeven E, Rouadi P, Abou Jaoude E, Abouzakouk M, Ansotegui I, Al-Ahmad M, et al. Digital tools in allergy and respiratory care. World Allergy Organization J. 2022;15:100661. https://doi.org/10.1016/j.waojou.2022.100661.
5. Market study on telemedicine. 2018. http://europa.eu.
6. Benjamin K, Potts HW. Digital transformation in government: lessons for digital health? Digit Health. 2018;4:205520761895916. http://nhsalpha.herokuapp.com/.
7. (Enabling Environment) Advancing National Digital Health Strategies.
8. Proceedings of the 2014 Annual Meeting of the House of Delegates | American Medical Association. https://www.ama-assn.org/house-delegates/annual-meeting/proceedings-2014-annual-meeting-house-delegates.
9. Hui CY, Walton R, McKinstry B, Jackson T, Parker R, Pinnock H. The use of mobile applications to support self-management for people with asthma: a systematic review of controlled studies to identify features associated with clinical effectiveness and adherence. J Am Med Inform Assoc. 2017;24(3):619–32. https://pubmed.ncbi.nlm.nih.gov/27694279/.
10. Bonini M. Electronic health (e-Health): emerging role in asthma. Curr Opin Pulm Med. 2017;23(1):21–6. https://pubmed.ncbi.nlm.nih.gov/27763999/.
11. Przybyszowski M, Polczyk R, Sliwka A, Pilinski R, Wloch T, Nowobilski R, et al. Asthma control test (ACT) result as a predictor of asthma exacerbations. Eur Respir J. 2017;50(suppl 61):PA1124. https://erj.ersjournals.com/content/50/suppl_61/PA1124.
12. Khusial RJ, Honkoop PJ, van der Meer V, Snoeck-Stroband JB, Sont JK. Validation of online asthma control questionnaire and asthma quality of life questionnaire. ERJ Open Res. 2020;6(1). https://openres.ersjournals.com/content/6/1/00289-2019.
13. Graham BL, Steenbruggen I, Barjaktarevic IZ, Cooper BG, Hall GL, Hallstrand TS, et al. Standardization of spirometry 2019 update. An official American Thoracic Society and European Respiratory Society technical statement. Am J Respir Crit Care Med. 2019;200(8):E70–88. https://pubmed.ncbi.nlm.nih.gov/31613151/.
14. Jensen LA, Onyskiw JE, Prasad NGN. Meta-analysis of arterial oxygen saturation monitoring by pulse oximetry in adults. Heart Lung. 1998;27(6):387–408. https://pubmed.ncbi.nlm.nih.gov/9835670/.

15. Sjoding MW, Dickson RP, Iwashyna TJ, Gay SE, Valley TS. Racial bias in pulse oximetry measurement. N Engl J Med. 2020;383(25):2477–8. https://pubmed.ncbi.nlm.nih.gov/33326721/.
16. Wang R, Usmani OS, Chung KF, Sont J, Simpson A, Bonini M, et al. Domiciliary fractional exhaled nitric oxide and spirometry in monitoring asthma control and exacerbations. J Allergy Clin Immunol Pract. 2023;11(6):1787–1795.e5. https://pubmed.ncbi.nlm.nih.gov/36801491/.
17. Saito J, Gibeon D, Macedo P, Menzies-Gow A, Bhavsar PK, Chung KF. Domiciliary diurnal variation of exhaled nitric oxide fraction for asthma control. Eur Respir J. 2014;43(2):474–84. https://pubmed.ncbi.nlm.nih.gov/23949962/.
18. Stern G, De Jongste J, Van Der Valk R, Baraldi E, Carraro S, Thamrin C, et al. Fluctuation phenotyping based on daily fraction of exhaled nitric oxide values in asthmatic children. J Allergy Clin Immunol. 2011;128(2):293–300. https://pubmed.ncbi.nlm.nih.gov/21489612/.
19. Anderson WJ, Short PM, Williamson PA, Lipworth BJ. Inhaled corticosteroid dose response using domiciliary exhaled nitric oxide in persistent asthma: the FENOtype trial. Chest. 2012;142(6):1553–61. https://pubmed.ncbi.nlm.nih.gov/23364390/.
20. Dunn J, Coravos A, Fanarjian M, Ginsburg GS, Steinhubl SR. Remote digital health technologies for improving the care of people with respiratory disorders. Lancet digit. Health. 2024;6(4):e291. https://pubmed.ncbi.nlm.nih.gov/38402128/.
21. Boner AL, Piacentini GL, Peroni DG, Irving CS, Goldstein D, Gavriely N, et al. Children with nocturnal asthma wheeze intermittently during sleep. J Asthma. 2010;47(3):290–4. https://pubmed.ncbi.nlm.nih.gov/20394513/.
22. Greiwe J, Nyenhuis SM. Wearable technology and how this can be implemented into clinical practice. Curr Allergy Asthma Rep. 2020;20(8):1–10. https://doi.org/10.1007/s11882-020-00927-3.
23. Huang N, Bian D, Zhou M, Mehta P, Shah M, Rajput KS, et al. Pulse rate guided oxygen saturation monitoring using a wearable armband sensor. Annu Int Conf IEEE Eng Med Biol Soc. 2022;2022:4303–7. https://pubmed.ncbi.nlm.nih.gov/36086022/.
24. van de Hei SJ, Stoker N, Flokstra-de Blok BMJ, Poot CC, Meijer E, Postma MJ, et al. Anticipated barriers and facilitators for implementing smart inhalers in asthma medication adherence management. NPJ Prim Care Respir Med. 2023;33(1).
25. O'Dwyer S, Greene G, MacHale E, Cushen B, Sulaiman I, Boland F, et al. Personalized biofeedback on inhaler adherence and technique by community pharmacists: a cluster randomized clinical trial. J Allergy Clin Immunol Pract. 2020;8(2):635–44. https://pubmed.ncbi.nlm.nih.gov/31568927/.
26. Chan AHY, Pleasants RA, Dhand R, Tilley SL, Schworer SA, Costello RW, et al. Digital inhalers for asthma or chronic obstructive pulmonary disease: a scientific perspective. Pulm Ther. 2021;7(2):345–76. https://pubmed.ncbi.nlm.nih.gov/34379316/.
27. Van De Hei SJ, Poot CC, Van Den Berg LN, Meijer E, Van Boven JFM, Flokstra-De Blok BMJ, et al. Effectiveness, usability and acceptability of a smart inhaler programme in patients with asthma: protocol of the multicentre, pragmatic, open-label, cluster randomised controlled ACCEPTANCE trial. BMJ Open Respir Res. 2022;9(1).
28. Merchant R, Inamdar R, Henderson K, Barrett M, Su JG, Riley J, et al. Digital Health intervention for asthma: patient-reported value and usability. JMIR Mhealth Uhealth. 2018;6(6):e133. https://pubmed.ncbi.nlm.nih.gov/29866644/.
29. Dierick BJH, Achterbosch M, Eikholt AA, Been-Buck S, Klemmeier T, van de Hei SJ, et al. Electronic monitoring with a digital smart spacer to support personalized inhaler use education tion in patients with asthma: the randomized controlled OUTERSPACE trial. Respir Med. 2023;218. https://pubmed.ncbi.nlm.nih.gov/37549796/.
30. Gaynor M, Schneider D, Seltzer M, Crannage E, Barron ML, Waterman J, et al. A user-centered, learning asthma smartphone application for patients and providers. Learn Health Syst. 2020;4(3):e10217. https://pubmed.ncbi.nlm.nih.gov/32685685/.
31. Kagen S, Garland A. Asthma and Allergy Mobile Apps in 2018. 2019:19. https://doi.org/10.1007/s11882-019-0840-z.
32. Rudin RS, Qureshi N, Foer D, Dalal AK, Edelen MO. Toward an asthma patient-reported outcome measure for use in digital remote monitoring. J Asthma. 2022;59(8):1697–702. https://pubmed.ncbi.nlm.nih.gov/34279179/.

33. Bousquet J, Anto JM, Sousa-Pinto B, Czarlewski W, Bedbrook A, Haahtela T, et al. Digitally-enabled, patient-centred care in rhinitis and asthma multimorbidity: the ARIA-MASK-air® approach. Clin Transl Allergy. 2023;13(1). https://pubmed.ncbi.nlm.nih.gov/36705508/.

34. Sousa-Pinto B, Jácome C, Pereira AM, Almeida R, Vieira RJ, Amaral R, et al. Development and validation of an electronic daily control score for asthma (e-DASTHMA): a real-world direct patient data study. Articles Lancet Digit Health. 2023;5:227–65. www.thelancet.com/.

35. Hale EM, Greene G, Mulvey C, Mokoka MC, van Boven JFM, Cushen B, et al. Use of digital measurement of medication adherence and lung function to guide the management of uncontrolled asthma (INCA sun): a multicentre, single-blinded, randomised clinical trial. Lancet Respir Med. 2023;11(7):591–601. https://pubmed.ncbi.nlm.nih.gov/36963417/.

36. Khusial RJ, Honkoop PJ, Usmani O, Soares M, Simpson A, Biddiscombe M, et al. Effectiveness of myAirCoach: a mHealth self-management system in asthma. J Allergy Clin Immunol Pract. 2020;8(6):1972–1979.e8.

37. Honkoop PJ, Simpson A, Bonini M, Snoeck-Stroband JB, Meah S, Fan Chung K, et al. MyAirCoach: the use of home-monitoring and mHealth systems to predict deterioration in asthma control and the occurrence of asthma exacerbations; study protocol of an observational study. BMJ Open. 2017;7(1):e013935. https://pubmed.ncbi.nlm.nih.gov/28119390/.

38. Stoyanov SR, Hides L, Kavanagh DJ, Wilson H. Development and validation of the user version of the Mobile application rating scale (uMARS). JMIR Mhealth Uhealth. 2016;4(2):e72. https://pubmed.ncbi.nlm.nih.gov/27287964/.

39. Sleurs K, Seys SF, Bousquet J, Fokkens WJ, Gorris S, Pugin B, et al. Mobile health tools for the management of chronic respiratory diseases. Allergy. 2019;74(7):1292–306. https://pubmed.ncbi.nlm.nih.gov/30644567/.

40. What is Gamification—Yu-kai Chou. https://yukaichou.com/gamification-examples/what-is-gamification/.

41. Gamified Health. How can gamification and technology… I by Jemma Eagleson I Medium. https://medium.com/@jemmaeagleson/gamified-health-8c98f6574e88.

42. Melvin E, Cushing A, Tam A, Kitada R, Manice M. Assessing the use of BreatheSmart® mobile technology in adult patients with asthma: a remote observational study. BMJ Open Respir Res. 2017;4(1)

43. Jácome C, Almeida R, Pereira AM, Amaral R, Mendes S, Alves-Correia M, et al. Feasibility and acceptability of an asthma app to monitor medication adherence: mixed methods study. JMIR Mhealth Uhealth. 2021;9(5):e26442. https://pubmed.ncbi.nlm.nih.gov/34032576/.

44. Huang X, Xiang X, Liu Y, Wang Z, Jiang Z, Huang L. The use of gamification in the self-management of patients with chronic diseases: scoping review. JMIR Serious Games. 2023;11. https://pubmed.ncbi.nlm.nih.gov/38133907/.

45. HIPAA Home I HHS.gov. https://www.hhs.gov/hipaa/index.html.

46. Mobile Health App Interactive Tool I Federal Trade Commission. https://www.ftc.gov/business-guidance/resources/mobile-health-apps-interactive-tool#lawsandregs.

47. EUR-Lex - L:2017:117:TOC - EN - EUR-Lex. https://eur-lex.europa.eu/legal-content/EN/TXT/?uri=OJ:L:2017:117:TOC.

48. EUROPEAN COMMISSION DIRECTORATE-GENERAL FOR HEALTH AND FOOD SAFETY Health systems and products Medical products-quality, safety and innovation Question and Answers on the interplay between the Clinical Trials Regulation and the General Data Protection Regulation. http://ec.europa.eu/newsroom/article29/item-detail.cfm?item_id=611235.

49. EDPB Document on response to the request from the European Commission for clarifications on the consistent application of the GDPR, focusing on health research I European Data Protection Board. https://edpb.europa.eu/our-work-tools/our-documents/other-guidance/edpb-document-response-request-european-commission_en.

50. Galvin HK, DeMuro PR. Developments in privacy and data ownership in Mobile Health technologies, 2016-2019. Yearb Med Inform. 2020;29(1):32–43. https://pubmed.ncbi.nlm.nih.gov/32823298/.

51. Ben-Sasson E, Bentov I, Horesh Y, Riabzev M. Scalable, transparent, and post-quantum secure computational integrity. Cryptology ePrint Arch. 2018.

52. Yazijy S, Schölly R, Kellmeyer P. Towards a toolbox for privacy-preserving computation on Health data. Stud Health Technol Inform. 2022;290:234–7. https://pubmed.ncbi.nlm.nih.gov/35673008/.
53. Tsang KCH, Pinnock H, Wilson AM, Salvi D, Shah SA. Home monitoring with connected mobile devices for asthma attack prediction with machine learning. Sci Data. 2023;10(1):370. http://www.ncbi.nlm.nih.gov/pubmed/37291158.
54. Tsang KCH, Pinnock H, Wilson AM, Salvi D, Shah SA. Predicting asthma attacks using connected mobile devices and machine learning: the AAMOS-00 observational study protocol. BMJ Open. 2022;12(10):e064166.
55. Persaud YK, Portnoy JM. Ten rules for implementation of a telemedicine program to Care for Patients with asthma. J Allergy Clin Immunol Pract. 2021;9(1):13–21. https://pubmed.ncbi.nlm.nih.gov/33039648/.
56. Sonney J, Ward T, Thompson HJ, Kientz JA, Segrin C. Improving asthma care together (IMPACT) mobile health intervention for school-age children with asthma and their parents: a pilot randomised controlled trial study protocol. BMJ Open. 2022;12(2):e059791. https://pubmed.ncbi.nlm.nih.gov/35144958/.
57. Saleh S, Farah A, Dimassi H, El Arnaout N, Constantin J, Osman M, et al. Using Mobile Health to enhance outcomes of noncommunicable diseases Care in Rural Settings and Refugee Camps: randomized controlled trial. JMIR Mhealth Uhealth. 2018;6(7):e137. https://pubmed.ncbi.nlm.nih.gov/30006326/.

Chapter 16
Wearables and Sensor Technology for Allergy Care

Justin Greiwe, Anil Nanda, and Sharmilee M. Nyenhuis

Contents

Abstract The increasing adoption of smart, wearable technology and remote patient monitoring (RPM) has the potential to revolutionize the way healthcare is provided, giving personal insights into various health metrics including heart rate, VO2 max, sleep, glucose levels, calorie expenditure, and step tracking just to name a few. Most commercial applications of this technology appeal to fastidious athletes and health-conscious consumers, but with continually improving sensors, real-time

J. Greiwe (✉)
Bernstein Allergy Group, Inc., Cincinnati, OH, USA

Division of Immunology/Allergy Section, Department of Internal Medicine, The University of Cincinnati College of Medicine, Cincinnati, OH, USA

A. Nanda
Asthma and Allergy Center, Lewisville, TX, USA

Division of Allergy and Immunology, University of Texas Southwestern Medical Center, Dallas, TX, USA

S. M. Nyenhuis
Section of Allergy, Immunology, and Pediatric Pulmonary, Department of Pediatrics, University of Chicago, Chicago, IL, USA
e-mail: snyenhuis@bsd.uchicago.edu

© The Author(s), under exclusive license to Springer Nature Switzerland AG 2025
P. M. Matricardi, S. Dramburg, *Digital Allergology*, Health Informatics, https://doi.org/10.1007/978-3-031-71021-6_16

health monitoring of vitals in sick patients and earlier detection of insidious disease in patients suffering from chronic illnesses are just some of the many possibilities this technology can offer. Wearables like the Apple Watch introduced in 2015 popularized health tracking, but initial poor battery life and limited functions hampered their use as a reliable health device. Now wearables can collect both active and passive data more accurately, enabling digital phenotyping and artificial intelligence (AI)-based risk prediction for various health conditions. As wearable technology and RPM improves, these devices have expanded their reach and are now being utilized in the asthma space with limited applications in patients suffering from rhinitis, primary immunodeficiency, and atopic dermatitis as well. These metrics are giving consumers and their physicians an increasingly nuanced awareness of general health and well-being, compelling users to make wearables an integral part of their everyday lives.

16.1 Transformational Potential of Wearable and Sensor Technology in Healthcare

By harnessing this technology, healthcare professionals have a growing opportunity to extend their reach outside of the office and connect with patients in their homes and workplaces. Capturing individual health metrics in real-time over extended periods can provide a wealth of previously inaccessible data that can influence clinical decision-making, especially in those suffering from chronic diseases like asthma. Prior to wearables and other RPM devices, an asthmatic might suffer from untreated symptoms at home before requiring emergency room treatment for an acute attack. With wearable sensors, acute changes such as forced expiratory volume in 1 s (FEV1) can be recognized right away by an informed patient and physician, allowing preventative steps to be taken to treat the flare effectively at home and reduce reliance on emergency services. RPM models have been shown to improve patient outcomes, reduce healthcare costs, and increase profitability for practices as these services qualify for reimbursements [1, 2]. According to a study evaluating the cost-effectiveness of an RPM program that included lifestyle education software for Type 2 diabetes, the telemonitoring group trended to a 21% cost decrease for the patient over 1 and 2 years of follow-up [3].

The COVID-19 pandemic uncovered weaknesses in the US healthcare system forcing many private practices and large hospital systems to quickly adopt new technologies including RPM and telemedicine to accommodate the growing demand for remote services. Medicare visits conducted through telehealth in 2020, for example, increased 63-fold, from approximately 840,000 in 2019 to 52.7 million [4]. RPM has been widely used in patients with cardiovascular diseases, hypertension, and diabetes but when it comes to allergic disease, the use of RPM remains negligible. Asthma stands out as the main condition in the allergy space that seems best suited for this technology, with some studies suggesting RPM reduces asthma morbidity and improves treatment outcomes, although these effects might be small and are not well described [5, 6]. To meet the needs of an aging and increasingly unhealthy population, RPM and wearable devices should play a more prominent role in preventative care, providing real-time data to objectively monitor patients with various chronic medical conditions, including those who suffer from asthma and allergies.

16.2 Wearables and Sensor Technology for Asthmatic Conditions

As mentioned previously, of all the allergic diseases, asthma has been the main disease of focus in the wearable tech space. The study populations of focus have been mainly in children with asthma, but two studies have used wearables in women with asthma. Castner et al. used the Fitbit Charge™ to validate sleep measures in women with asthma [7]. The Fitbit sleep measures were compared to a validated device (i.e., Actigraph GT3X +) and found that the Fitbit device overestimated sleep efficiency [8, 9]. Additionally, the Fitbit underestimated wake counts compared to actigraphy. Nyenhuis and colleagues used Fitbit Charge™ as an intervention tool to promote physical activity as part of a lifestyle intervention for Black women with asthma [10]. They found that women in the intervention group were able to increase moderate physical activity and saw clinically significant improvements in asthma quality of life.

In children, wearables have been used to correlate Fitbit-derived sleep measures to asthma control and asthma impact [11, 12]. Bian and colleagues assessed the association between self-reported asthma impact and Fitbit-derived sleep quality (the ratio of minutes asleep to minutes in bed) and physical activity measures (daily minutes of moderate and vigorous activity) in adolescents with asthma [11]. Fitbit-derived sleep quality was moderately correlated with Patient-Reported Outcomes Measurement Information System (PROMIS) sleep disturbance score ($r = -0.31$, $P = 0.01$) and had a weak but significant correlation with the PROMIS pediatric asthma impact score (average $r = -0.18$, $P = 0.02$). Fitbit-derived physical activity levels were not associated with PROMIS pediatric asthma impact ($r = 0.04$, $P = 0.62$). These findings suggest that measurement of sleep quality, using the Fitbit device, may help develop personalized asthma management strategies for children and their caregivers in real time.

Another study, measured several mobile metrics of asthma such as Fitbits to measure physical activity and sleep, FEV1 and peak expiratory flow, an indoor air quality monitor using Foobot (https://foobot.io/), and a mobile app that collected information on asthma control (symptoms, physical limitations due to asthma, nighttime awakenings, and medication intake). These metrics were used together to digitally phenotype children with asthma and provide a better measure of the patient's asthma control to their clinician when compared with the Asthma Control Test scores taken infrequently during clinic visits. Additional work using this ecological metric of asthma control is needed and may be used in the future to generate insights on the relationship between a patient's asthma symptoms and triggers across different seasons [13]. Other mobile health technologies to improve self-management of asthma have been investigated including the myAirCoach support system. This self-management tool consisted of an inhaler adapter, an indoor air-quality monitor, a physical activity tracker, a portable spirometer, a fraction exhaled nitric oxide device, and an app that was used in addition to standard of care for asthma in 42 patients. Using the myAirCoach support system improved both asthma control and quality of life, with a reduction in severe asthma exacerbations. Based on these findings, it seems that well-validated mobile health technologies should be further studied [14].

As symptoms of asthma (e.g., wheezing, cough) may be audible, acoustic monitoring has been studied in asthma. Breathing sounds are measured by microphones over human skin and can detect breathing patterns (i.e., respiratory rate, flow rate, tidal volume) and symptoms that may be due to asthma. One such device was tested on 374 children with a history of asthma and was found to identify wheeze remotely with high accuracy. The sensitivity, specificity, positive predictive value, and negative predictive value of the wheeze recognition algorithm device was 96.6%, 98.5%, 98.3%, and 97.0%, respectively [15]. In addition to wheeze, chest movement signals can be acquired using an accelerometer or belt-shaped device [16, 17]. One study, measured the nocturnal wheeze in children with asthma using an acoustic respiratory monitor and found that among children with apparently well-controlled asthma, 57% had considerable amounts of night wheezing that was unrelated to conventional measures of lung function [18]. More recently, an AI-powered wearable stethoscope, AeviceMD, was developed and recently approved for use in Singapore (March 2023) [19]. The device is worn on the chest, continuously detects and records abnormal breath sounds, such as wheezing, and monitors vital signs including heart rate and respiratory rate. As this area of wearable is still developing, future research needs to examine the clinical impact of these devices in asthma populations across the lifespan.

16.3   Wearables and Sensor Technology for Non-asthmatic Conditions

Newer technologies for allergic rhinitis include wearable devices, short message service (SMS) reminders, and mobile applications [20]. Mobile health technologies for rhinitis have included smartphones applications, social media messengers, and web-based applications [21]. These have been used to improve adherence to nasal corticosteroids, with improved symptoms and quality of life [21]. The POPET (physician on call engagement trial) assessed mobile applications on reminding patients to use intranasal corticosteroids and enabled them to communicate directly with their physicians, leading to improved rhinitis symptom scores [21, 22]. The WeChat mobile application was used to educate patients on chronic rhinosinusitis and nasal spray techniques, with improved adherence rates in the WeChat group [21, 23]. The Allergy Monitor (AM) internet web-based application recorded rhinitis symptoms and nasal steroid adherence as well as pollen counts in a pediatrics study with improved adherence to nasal corticosteroids [21, 24]. Another study evaluated adherence to nasal corticosteroid treatment after a short message service reminders (SMS) by mobile phone with improved medication adherence [25]. Wearable devices are being developed which can classify common allergic rhinitis gestures, including nose, eye, and ear movements [26].

Wearable technologies have been used for other allergy and immunology conditions also. For patients with primary immunodeficiency and on immunoglobulin replacement therapy, a new investigational wearable infusor (IWI) was compared with an infusion pump for subcutaneous therapy [27]. The wearable infusor therapy allowed similar levels of immunoglobulin to be administered [27]. Another study looked at a wearable sensor on the hand for evaluating scratching movements in adult patients with atopic dermatitis [28]. This study quantified scratching movements and other sleep metrics accurately in these patients [28]. For food allergy, affecting about 2–5% of adults and 6–8% of children worldwide, electrochemical sensors have been developed for food allergen detection, including the Allergy Amulet and the integrated exogenous antigen testing (iEAT) device [29, 30].

While multiple asthma wearable technologies, as discussed previously, have been devised, measuring inhalations, timing of inhalations, and medication adherence [31], there is a substantial gap in innovations in the rhinitis space. Feasibility and difficulty in measuring rhinitis symptoms including nasal congestion likely make developing sensor technology in this space more challenging.

16.4 Integration of Wearables and Sensor Technology in Clinical Practice

While we have highlighted the nascent state of wearable research in asthma and allergies, it is important to understand how data from wearables might be integrated into practice and used to improve healthcare delivery. Wearable data may be most useful in its ability to inform individuals or caregivers of the effects of patient actions or treatments or underlying clinical status [32]. The data could then be used to offer decision support for clinicians and/or patients and even offer built-in therapies. Despite, the potential to transform patient care, issues such as patient privacy, system interoperability, and the immense amount of patient data pose a challenge to the adoption of wearables by healthcare professionals [33, 34].

While users have instant access to the health data gleaned from their wearable devices, physicians interested in reviewing this information have a much more difficult time gaining access. Barriers including HIPAA compliance, incompatibility with electronic health records (EHR), as well as concerns about privacy and data sharing continue to be an issue hampering efforts for these devices to be truly interactive and sharable. First and foremost, if wearable data is being used in a healthcare setting the privacy and security of that health information must be addressed to meet HIPAA standards [35]. Hospitals and private practices must ensure that devices are connected to a secure network and there should be protections in place to monitor network data continuously to protect against potential cybersecurity attacks and missing or stolen patient records [36]. To prioritize data privacy, health systems are likely to be required to set up another secure network for wearable devices, separate from the main network [37]. Additionally, wearable device and EHR vendors use a range of methods that include distinct, proprietary, and closed communication methods to integrate wearable data into EHR [38, 39]. These differences in methods make it difficult for various devices and EHR systems to communicate and transfer data streams, leading to the lack of system interoperability. Finally, to implement wearable technology data widely, clinicians need to have an easy way to extract and view the data from wearables. As it is, clinicians experience alert fatigue in their daily clinical decision support systems. Successful solutions to patient data integration in EHR should be able to sift through the immense amount of data and automatically deliver meaningful and actionable items to clinicians [40]. Machine learning and AI algorithms are potential solutions to this issue. These challenges are important to consider for future wearable use to deliver safe and quality care for patients. Although there are potential solutions for these implementation issues, more innovative work is required for wide-scale adoption of wearable health technology.

16.5 Quality and Reproducibility of Wearables and Sensor Technology

When thinking about utilizing wearables or other RPM devices, first it must be determined if the proposed device provides value. This will of course depend on the quality and reproducibility of the data the device provides. It is also important to consider if the information gleaned is actionable and relevant for the condition or habit being treated. Real-time, actionable feedback is of vital importance if the device is going to lead to symptom improvement or lasting change. Recent studies investigating the utility of wearable sensors indicate that the information provided by these devices is physiologically meaningful and actionable [41]. Tracking health metrics outside of regularly scheduled office visits is rare in the allergy space, and physicians are often relying on patients with chronic health conditions to consistently self-report progress and medication compliance which is inefficient and unpredictable at best [42]. Self-reported inhaled corticosteroid (ICS) use in asthmatics, for example, showed significant inconsistencies compared to objective ICS use measured by electronic medication monitoring (EMM). These observations suggest that EMM provides clinicians with more accurate information with which to base treatment decisions on vs. relying on self-reporting which is notoriously inaccurate due to potential recall bias [43]. There are a lot of wearables on the market that propose to measure certain parameters, but their accuracy is often questionable. Take VO2 max testing for example. VO2 max, the maximum amount of oxygen that your body can use during intense exercise, was previously something that only serious athletes considered measuring. Clinical grade testing is cumbersome and involves fastening an oxygen mask over the face along with heart monitors on the chest all while running on a treadmill or pedaling on a bike with the goal of gradually building to maximum effort over 10–20 min. It is a physically demanding test that is very different from the way wearables like the Apple Watch and Garmin estimate VO2 max. These devices use an algorithm to examine the users' heart rate and movement while walking or running for at least 10 min and tally a score. These devices aren't measuring oxygen intake and therefore aren't really measuring VO2max, it's just an estimate based on an algorithm. A medical literature search revealed very little data on quality control or standardization of many of the wearable devices on the market today although efforts have been made by some companies to compare to standard-of-care testing. For example, the portable Aluna spirometer has been shown to be as accurate as the in-office nSpire KoKo spirometer and obtained FDA approval for their asthma management platform in 2020. Unfortunately, there is substantial heterogeneity among various wearable device studies making comparisons difficult [44]. There are several potential intrinsic data quality challenges that can occur when analyzing wearable device data and poor data quality can compromise the reliability and accuracy of research results [45]. It is apparent that further high-quality studies are needed to address the data quality challenges of wearable devices, and these shortcomings should be discussed with patients on a case-by-case basis when discussing the utility of wearable devices.

16.6   The Future of Wearables and Sensor Technology

By leveraging wearable technology and RPM to improve outcomes for patients suffering from chronic disease, the healthcare community has a unique opportunity to change the way chronic disease is managed. Instead of reacting to a medical condition after it already presents, these devices provide early warning signs of disease progression allowing physicians to be proactive and to act before symptoms get out of control. This has the potential to reduce healthcare costs by decreasing reliance on urgent care and emergency room visits and keeping patients out of the hospital [46]. The first seeds of this technological medical revolution have already been planted, and the COVID-19 pandemic provided fertile ground to test new innovations and drive investment into this burgeoning industry. Next-generation wearables are entering the commercial market including epidermal skin technology (wearable electronic skin), smart jewelry like the Oura Ring, AI hearing aids, and smart clothing like Google's Project Jacquard whose threads are composed of electric fibers that enable the user to control their devices right from their sleeves. These devices are getting smaller, smarter, and more seamlessly integrated into our everyday lives. Machine learning algorithms are continually improving, transforming sensor input into more actionable health data allowing users and prescribers to gain a better understanding of how wearables can and will be used in the future. There are conflicting views on whether digital technologies can reduce health disparities and improve access to care. Some view these devices as transformational giving marginal populations access to health information that was previously inaccessible [47]. Others point to cost as a barrier to entry, limiting this technology to only those that can afford it. As technology improves and competition increases, the hope is that price points will continue to drop in the coming years. Clinicians must carefully weigh the potential risks and benefits of implementing wearables and RPM in their practice, considering various factors including device selection, patient comfort and ease of use, data security and privacy, as well as the potential impact on patient outcomes and resource utilization. No matter how this topic is discussed with patients, it is becoming more and more apparent that wearables and sensor technology are here to stay. The only question is how clinicians will utilize this technology for the management of chronic disease now and in the future.

References

1. Farias FAC, Dagostini CM, Bicca YA, Falavigna VF, Falavigna A. Remote patient monitoring: a systematic review. Telemed J E Health. 2020;26(5):576–83.
2. Leo DG, Buckley BJR, Chowdhury M, Harrison SL, Isanejad M, Lip GYH, Wright DJ, Lane DA, TAILOR investigators. Interactive remote patient monitoring devices for managing chronic health conditions: systematic review and meta-analysis. J Med Internet Res. 2022;24(11):e35508.
3. Mounié M, Costa N, Gourdy P, et al. Cost-effectiveness evaluation of a remote monitoring Programme including lifestyle education software in type 2 diabetes: results of the Educ@dom study. Diabetes Ther. 2022;13(4):693–708.
4. Samson L, Tarazi W, Turrini G, et al. Medicare Beneficiaries' Use of Telehealth Services in 2020: Trends by Beneficiary Characteristics and Location (Issue Brief No. HP-2021-27). Office of the Assistant Secretary for Planning and Evaluation, U.S. Department of Health and Human Services; 2021.
5. Steel S, Lock S, Johnson N, Martinez Y, Marquilles E, Bayford R. A feasibility study of remote monitoring of asthmatic patients. J Telemed Telecare. 2002;8(5):290–6.
6. Snoswell CL, Rahja M, Lalor AF. A systematic review and meta-analysis of change in health-related quality of life for interactive telehealth interventions for patients with asthma. Value Health. 2021;24(2):291–302.
7. Castner J, Mammen MJ, Jungquist CR, Licata O, Pender JJ, Wilding GE, et al. Validation of fitness tracker for sleep measures in women with asthma. J Asthma. 2019;56(7):719–30.
8. Koinis-Mitchell D, Kopel SJ, Seifer R, LeBourgeois M, McQuaid EL, Esteban CA, et al. Asthma-related lung function, sleep quality, and sleep duration in urban children. Sleep Health. 2017;3(3):148–56.

9. Rosenberger ME, Buman MP, Haskell WL, McConnell MV, Carstensen LL. Twenty-four hours of sleep, sedentary behavior, and physical activity with nine wearable devices. Med Sci Sports Exerc. 2016;48(3):457–65.

10. Nyenhuis SM, Shah N, Kim H, Marquez DX, Wilbur J, Sharp LK. The feasibility of a lifestyle physical activity intervention for black women with asthma. J Allergy Clin Immunol Pract. 2021;9:4312.

11. Bian J, Guo Y, Xie M, Parish AE, Wardlaw I, Brown R, et al. Exploring the association between self-reported asthma impact and Fitbit-derived sleep quality and physical activity measures in adolescents. JMIR Mhealth Uhealth. 2017;5(7):e105.

12. Jaimini U, Thirunarayan K, Kalra M, Venkataraman R, Kadariya D, Sheth A. "How is my child's asthma?" digital phenotype and actionable insights for pediatric asthma. JMIR Pediatr Parent. 2018;1(2):e11988.

13. Venkataramanan R, Thirunarayan K, Jaimini U, Kadariya D, Yip HY, Kalra M, et al. Determination of personalized asthma triggers from multimodal sensing and a mobile app: observational study. JMIR Pediatr Parent. 2019;2(1):e14300.

14. Khusial RJ, Honkoop PJ, Usmani O, Soares M, Simpson A, Biddiscombe M, Meah S, Bonini M, Lalas A, Polychronidou E, Koopmans JG, Moustakas K, Snoeck-Stroband JB, Ortmann S, Votis K, Tzovaras D, Chung KF, Fowler S, Sont JK, myAirCoach study group. Effectiveness of myAirCoach: a mHealth self-management system in asthma. J Allergy Clin Immunol Pract. 2020;8(6):1972–1979.e8.

15. Habukawa C, Ohgami N, Arai T, Makata H, Tomikawa M, Fujino T, Manabe T, Ogihara Y, Ohtani K, Shirao K, Sugai K, Asai K, Sato T, Murakami K. Wheeze recognition algorithm for remote medical care device in children: validation study. JMIR Pediatr Parent. 2021;4(2):e28865.

16. Anusha AR, Soodi AL, Kumar SP. Design of low-cost hardware for lung sound acquisition and determination of inspiratory-expiratory phase using respiratory waveform. In: 2012 third international conference on computing, communication and networking technologies (ICCCNT'12). 2012:1–5.

17. Liu GZ, Guo YW, Zhu QS, Huang BY, Wang L. Estimation of respiration rate from three-dimensional acceleration data based on body sensor network. Telemed J E Health. 2011;17(9):705–11.

18. Boner AL, Piacentini GL, Peroni DG, Irving CS, Goldstein D, Gavriely N, et al. Children with nocturnal asthma wheeze intermittently during sleep. J Asthma. 2010;47(3):290–4.

19. https://tmgpulse.com/singapore-approves-aevice-healths-wearable-stethoscope-for-respiratory-monitoring/.

20. Braido F, Baiardini I, Puggioni F, Garuti S, Pawankar R, Walter Canonica G. Rhinitis: adherence to treatment and new technologies. Curr Opin Allergy Clin Immunol. 2017;17(1):23–7.

21. Baxter M, Tibble H, Bush A, Sheikh A, Schwarze J. Effectiveness of mobile health interventions to improve nasal corticosteroid adherence in allergic rhinitis: a systematic review. Clin Transl Allergy. 2021:e12075.

22. Cingi C, Yorgancioglu A, Cingi CC, Oguzulgen K, Muluk N, Ulusoy S, et al. The "physician on call engagement trial" (POPET): measuring the impact of a mobile patient engagement application on health outcomes and quality of life in allergic rhinitis and asthma patients. Int Forum Allergy Rhinol. 2015;5:487–97.

23. Feng S, Liang Z, Zhang R, Liao W, Chen Y, Fan Y, et al. Effects of mobile phone WeChat services improve adherence to corticosteroid nasal spray treatment for chronic rhinosinusitis after functional endocscopic sinus surgery: a 3-month follow-up study. Eur Arch Otorrinolaringol. 2017;274:1477–85.

24. Pizzulli A, Perna S, Florack J, Pizzulli A, Giordani P, Tripodi S, et al. The impact of tele-monitoring on adherence to nasal corticosteroid treatment in children with seasonal allergic rhinoconjunctivitis. Clin Exp Allergy. 2014;44:1246–54.

25. Wang K, Wang C, Xi L, Zhang Y, Ouyang Y, Lou H, et al. A randomized controlled trial to assess adherence to allergic rhinitis treatment following a daily short message service (SMS) via the mobile phone. Int Arch Allergy Immunol. 2014;163:51–8.
26. Aggelides X, Bardoutsos A, Nikoletseas S, Papadopoulos N, Raptopoulos C, Tzamalis P. A gesture recognition approach to classifying allergic rhinitis gestures using wrist worn devices 2020. In: 16th international conference on distributed computing in sensor systems (DCOSS).
27. Wasserman R, Cunningham-Rundles C, Anderson J, Lugar P, Palumbo M, Patel N, et al. Systemic IgG exposure and safety in patients with primary immunodeficiency: a randomized crossover study comparing a novel investigational wearable infusor versus the Crono pump. Immunotherapy. 2022;14:1315–28.
28. Yang A, Chun KS, Yu L, Walter J, Kim D, Lee JH, et al. Validation of hand-mounted wearable sensor for scratching movements in adults with atopic dermatitis. J Am Acad Dermatol. 2022;22:s0190–9622.
29. Sundhoro M, Agnihotra S, Khan N, Barnes A, BelBruno J, Mendecki L. Rapid and accurate electrochemical sensor for food allergen detection in complex foods. Sci Rep. 2021;11:20831.
30. Lin HY, Huang CH, Park J, Pathania D, Castro CM, Fasano A, Weissleder R, Lee H. Integrated magneto-chemical sensor for on-site food allergen detection. ACS Nano. 2017;11(10):10062–9.
31. Greiwe J, Nyenhuis S. Wearable technology and how this can be implemented into clinical practice. Curr Allergy Asthma Rep. 2020;20:36.
32. Pevnick JM, Birkeland K, Zimmer R, Elad Y, Kedan I. Wearable technology for cardiology: an update and framework for the future. Trends Cardiovasc Med. 2018;28(2):144–50.
33. L. E. 5 Challenges of integrating wearable data into electronic health records future health index. 2017. https://www.futurehealthindex.com/2017/10/23/challenges-wearable-data-health-records/.
34. Comstock J. Five barriers to wider clinical wearable adoption. Mobi Health News. 2017. https://www.mobihealthnews.com/content/five-barriers-wider-clinical-wearable-adoption.
35. Dinh-Le C, Chuang R, Chokshi S, Mann D. Wearable health technology and electronic health record integration: scoping review and future directions. JMIR Mhealth Uhealth. 2019;7(9):e12861.
36. Blau M. Health wearables raise new privacy concerns. The Boston Globe; 2017. https://www.bostonglobe.com/business/2017/08/09/health-wearables-raise-new-privacy-concerns/0W2X9iNuLttoa7dUTFTzLJ/story.html.
37. Greenstone P. HIPAA guidelines should evolve with wearable technology. The Hill; 2018. https://thehill.com/opinion/healthcare/378450-hipaa-guidelines-should-evolve-with-wearable-technology.
38. Clarke M, de Folter J, Verma V, Gokalp H. Interoperable end-to-end remote patient monitoring platform based on IEEE 11073 PHD and ZigBee health care profile. IEEE Trans Biomed Eng. 2018;65(5):1014–25.
39. The value of medical device interoperability: improving patient care with more than $30 billion in annual health care savings west health. 2013. https://www.westhealth.org/wp-content/uploads/2015/02/The-Value-of-Medical-Device-Interoperability.pdf.
40. Jacobson S, Wang T. The shifting center of care rock health. 2015. https://rockhealth.com/shifting-center-care.
41. Li X, Dunn J, Salins D, et al. Digital health: tracking physiomes and activity using wearable biosensors reveals useful health-related information. PLoS Biol. 2017;15(1):e2001402.
42. Brusco NK, Watts JJ. Empirical evidence of recall bias for primary health care visits. BMC Health Serv Res. 2015;15:381.
43. Mosnaim GS, Stempel DA, Gonzalez C, et al. Electronic medication monitoring versus self-reported use of inhaled corticosteroids and short-acting beta2-agonists in uncontrolled asthma. J Asthma. 2021:1–4.
44. Germini F, Noronha N, Borg Debono V, Abraham Philip B, Pete D, Navarro T, Keepanasseril A, Parpia S, de Wit K, Iorio A. Accuracy and acceptability of wrist-wearable activity-tracking devices: systematic review of the literature. J Med Internet Res. 2022;24(1):e30791.

45. Cho S, Ensari I, Weng C, Kahn MG, Natarajan K. Factors affecting the quality of person-generated wearable device data and associated challenges: rapid systematic review. JMIR Mhealth Uhealth. 2021;9(3):e20738.
46. Thompson JA, Hersch D, Miner MH, Melnik TE, Adam P. Remote patient monitoring for COVID-19: a retrospective study on health care utilization. Telemed J E Health. 2023.
47. Canali S, Schiaffonati V, Aliverti A. Challenges and recommendations for wearable devices in digital health: data quality, interoperability, health equity, fairness. PLOS Digit Health. 2022;1(10):e0000104.

Chapter 17
Unveiling the Potential of Social Media in Allergology: From Patient Education and Support to Advocacy and Activism

Florin-Dan Popescu and Stephanie Dramburg

Contents

Abstract Harnessing social media for enhanced patient support in managing allergic diseases has various perspectives and challenges. Healthcare professionals (HCPs) have a multifaceted role in leveraging social media platforms to sustain allergy patients effectively. The perspectives encompass providing allergy information and education, fostering patient engagement, facilitating disease monitoring, conducting patient surveys, and implementing public health interventions. Additionally, HCPs can function as allies, advocates, or activists for allergy patients. Patients can benefit from social media by joining dedicated online communities, accessing peer-to-peer support, crowdsourcing information, sharing resources, and participating in advocacy and fundraising campaigns. The unprecedented potential of artificial intelligence (AI) in enhancing patient support and disease management

F.-D. Popescu (✉)
Department of Allergology, "Nicolae Malaxa" Clinical Hospital, "Carol Davila" University of Medicine and Pharmacy, Bucharest, Romania

S. Dramburg
Department of Pediatric Respiratory Medicine, Immunology and Critical Care Medicine, Charité–Universitätsmedizin Berlin, a corporate member of Freie Universität Berlin and Humboldt–Universität zu Berlin, Berlin, Germany
e-mail: stephanie.dramburg@charite.de

through social media must be highlighted. It is essential to maximize the benefits of social media for patient support in allergy management while mitigating potential risks.

17.1 General Perspectives of Which Allergy Patients Benefit from Social Media

Allergy management may be improved by optimizing communication, with its motivational and behavioral modification components [1, 2]. Although web browsers are still used as conventional information and communication technologies to obtain health information [3], easy-to-use social media platforms may offer reliable educational content developed by HCPs, patient associations, and medical associations for patient support. Allergy-related social media content is created or co-created, accessed, shared or exchanged, endorsed, discussed, or modified by allergists or other HCPs, and patients or other users. Compared with traditional media, social media platforms are archived, searchable, and interactive [4]. There are several fundamental components of social media assistance for allergic patients (Fig. 17.1).

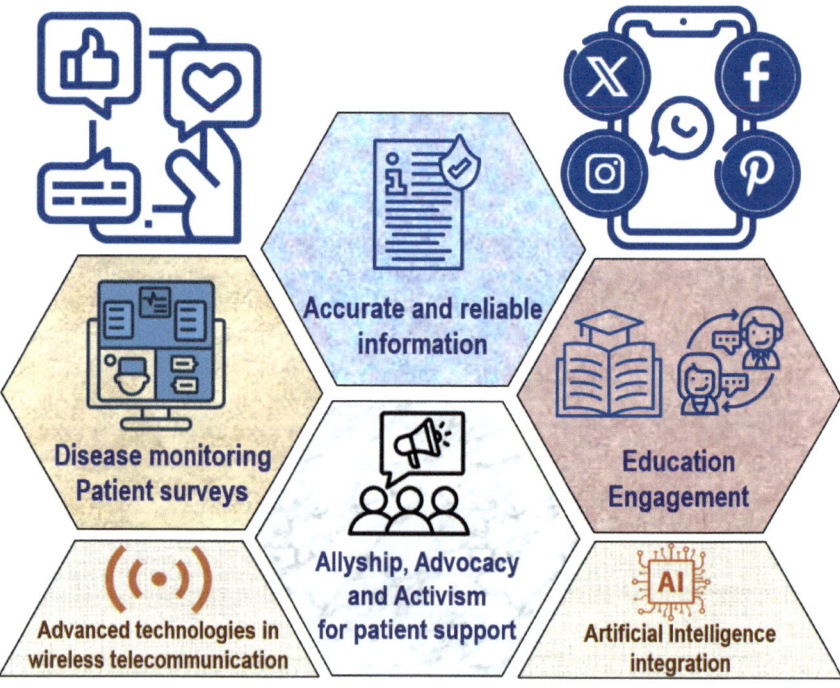

Fig. 17.1 The basic elements of social media support for allergic patients

The perspectives from which HCPs support patients to benefit from social media include being an allergy information and education *provider* and *generator* of patient engagement, acting as an online *operator* for disease monitoring, patient surveys, and public health interventions, and as an *ally*, *advocate* or *activist* for allergy patients. While the term "consumers" is sometimes used for people accessing healthcare information, it is crucial to acknowledge that the doctor-patient relationship goes far beyond such a simple transaction, even on social media. Healthcare is not a simple commodity to be sold and bought; it embodies the trust, care, and expertise that healthcare providers offer to patients in need. In this light, allergists play a crucial role in protecting the well-being of individuals and communities, and this responsibility transcends the market-driven terminology. Social networks may raise awareness about allergies, including triggers, prevention methods, and treatment options, and may be used to monitor and combat all aspects of online information disorder. Thus, they reduce the stigma associated with allergies and encourage more connections and support. By providing accurate and reliable educational information about allergies, HCPs can help patients understand their condition better and make informed decisions. Moreover, social networking can empower allergic patients to become more knowledgeable and engaged in disease management. In particular, social media can support allyship, advocacy, and activism for better policies and practices related to allergies, such as improved food labeling or increased funding for research [5–8]. Accessing health information via social networks correlates positively with perceived additional benefits, such as promoting *telemedicine* services for patient triage or second opinions and virtual visits [9, 10].

Crowdsourcing involves a collaborative approach where a collective endeavors to tackle a problem, sharing their solutions with a broader audience. This method is increasingly leveraged to enrich training by creating educational resources and fostering mentorship opportunities [11]. Using crowdsourcing on social media can effectively reach a broad audience and engage patients. Patient support may benefit from creating or joining online communities with dedicated support groups and peer-to-peer support, crowdsourcing information and resource sharing, assessing allergy-associated factors, advocacy and fundraising campaigns, patient recruiting, patient-centered research, and obtaining financial aid. Social media communication complements traditional strategies and web-based advertising to recruit participants in allergy *research* trials [4, 12, 13].

17.2 Providing Allergy Information, Education, and Engagement on Social Media

The diverse influences of social media on health information, education, and engagement are increasingly understood and recognized [14]. HCPs and medical organizations use social media platforms to disseminate allergy information, including disease prevention strategies, treatment options, and self-care tips, through high-quality content with validated resources and compressible language, sometimes with the support of influencers. Consequently, along with raising awareness about allergic diseases, they empower patients to take more proactive allergy management and contribute to the fight against misinformation [15, 16]. In addition, patients may benefit from selected high-quality instructional visual posts on social media for the correct self-administration of medication (intranasal sprays, asthma inhalers, epinephrine autoinjectors) [17–19]. Moreover, Facebook groups and Twitter chats allow topic-focused, text-based discussions important for allergy information, education, and patient engagement [15].

Facebook is a dominant socializing network that HCPs may use for patients' education in many powerful ways, including creating and sharing health-related pages and posts, hosting live streams for teaching and engaging with followers through comments, likes, and shares [15, 20]. Specific posts may familiarize allergic patients with the office settings, waiting areas, consultation rooms, physicians and support personnel, with staff photos on location; release announcements and news about the working hours and pollen counts; and raise awareness about allergy news and health concerns [15, 16]. To sustain patients using topic-focused text-based discussions on this platform, HCPs and organizations may create non-commercial private Facebook *groups* to support patients by providing a sense of community, help, along with educational information and resources. It is essential to provide updated educational information, set ground rules for the group to create a safe and engaging virtual space, encourage members to participate in discussions and monitor feedback. Despite potential patient benefits and tremendous popularity, some HCPs often hesitate to take such actions due to privacy concerns when discussing health issues online. Invitation-only groups with clinicians acting as moderators are preferred to avoid misinformation, offensive content, inappropriate posts or concerns regarding potential medical emergencies. Patient support groups for several allergic diseases, for example, atopic dermatitis or allergic contact dermatitis were identified on this social network. Different Facebook groups, as assessed in a few studies, for patients' education, emotional support, and networking, had positive results for their care. However, further research is needed to determine the impact on quality of life and patient-centered care [21–24].

The famous microblogging platform X (formerly known as Twitter) is an effective tool for HCPs and organizations to upload instructive and useful posts (previously named tweets) using relevant hashtags and actively engage followers through actions like replies, reposts, and likes. In addition, allergists can use the X network to present allergy and asthma care practice, physician on-call information, and provide medical services, including telemedicine, vaccinations, and allergen immunotherapy to improve education and adherence. X posts related to regional weather and pollen forecasts may also be useful for patients [15, 16, 20, 25]. X chats (formerly known as TweetChats) are meaningful, real-time, topic-focused, text-based discussions for patient sustenance on social media. This free network tool recently gained widespread for online educational and informative talks using X posts, actively engaging patients and caregivers with organizers, including individual allergists, patient support, and professional organizations. Chats are designed to be structured as discussions on a predetermined topic or as informal education on allergy tips for distinct issues (e.g., specific allergy seasons, holidays or school time allergy tips, asthma and air quality). Formats include patient questions and their answers, as well as professionally developed posts to engage participants in targeted chats created to assess patients' experiences and needs in an atmosphere of psychological safety and comfort. Following the introduction of an allergy healthcare provider moderator, several practical tips are presented following a code of conduct and privacy policy, reminding participants to use the X platform chat hashtag in all posts. The start and end of the targeted chat (usually 60 min duration) is also communicated by the moderator. In addition, some technical tips relate to the use of online tools allowing messages to be effectively scheduled ahead, while registration of the dedicated hashtag supports the use of social media analytics (e.g., Symplur) to assess metrics after the chat and perform even more complex data analysis (e.g., Symplur Signals Sentiment Analysis) [15, 26–29].

The popular discussion platform Reddit is a social meta-forum for tracking, mining, and understanding public opinions and reactions to health issues and assessing patients' questions and perspectives. For example, it has been recently utilized to analyze patients' questions on atopic dermatitis and mine adverse events to allergen immunotherapy. There are several ways in which Reddit is used for patient education, for example, by creating and sharing educational content, participating in public subreddits (online communities) and hosting Ask Me Anything (AMA live question-and-answer) sessions dedicated to a specific topic. Patients with atopic dermatitis, especially younger ones, are known to increasingly engage on Reddit, forming subreddits, such as "r/eczema," an international community seeking emotional and medical support, "eczeMABs" subreddit, a forum dedicated to discussing monoclonal antibodies such as dupilumab for this condition, and "eczeJAKs," a group discussing Janus Kinase Inhibitors for Th2 dermatitis. False and inaccurate information can quickly be spread, given that healthcare professionals do not verify the posts and the presence of allergists, dermatologists, and atopic dermatitis organizations is extremely limited on this platform. There is also concern that it may create mistrust towards conventional medicine, as in topical steroid withdrawal syndrome. Moreover, many gaps in patient knowledge are found in such subreddits, revealing areas for future improvement [29–32].

Image-based social media such as Instagram or the visual curating platform Pinterest can be used for health education by sharing educational pictures and infographics, encouraging visually appealing content and hosting campaigns related to specific health topics or events. Such image-based platforms may be specifically useful to share and exchange information on diseases with a visible manifestation, for example, chronic spontaneous urticaria, atopic dermatitis or allergic contact dermatitis. Clinical practitioners can improve their engagement with young adults by using these networks. For example, hashtags # on Instagram may reveal the online presence of specialists, while pins on Pinterest may be used to assess the visual and textual medical-related information [33–35]. Although allergists and dermatologists maintain an essential but restricted presence on Instagram, it is noteworthy that individuals with minimal medical training often share the majority of skin-related content as "skinfluencers." Additionally, social media involvement poses ethical concerns, particularly regarding self-promotion and sponsorship [35]. Instagram has recently been considered a valuable social media platform for the online dissemination of medical information in the field of allergology. A recent pilot study examined the efficacy of allergy and immunology-focused video and audio content disseminated through Instagram. As anticipated, the video content outperformed the audio content, likely due to its higher engagement potential with the online audience [36]. Whether allergists opt to participate in such image-based social media or prefer to focus solely on clinical practice, it is imperative that they recognize the impact of these online networks on patients and acknowledge their inherent limitations [35].

Supporting patients through pre-recorded and live videos on social media represents a powerful approach to providing educational information, guidance, and motivating engagement while always encouraging viewers to consult with HCPs. Pre-recorded videos and real-time streaming are popular features on various social media platforms, including Facebook, Instagram, and TikTok. Each online network has its unique community and features. YouTube may be used to support allergic patients by creating educational videos to provide information about health topics in the form of tutorials, personal stories, or engaging scientific video content, partnering with organizations and influencers, hosting webinars or live streams, creating playlists and using closed captions and subtitles for people with hearing impairments and those speaking different languages. If looking to support patients with asthma and allergies using videos on Facebook, Instagram, and TikTok, HCPs must plan the content before posting, identify key topics to cover and prepare technical materials needed, engage with the audience for a sense of community and support, and monitor feedback from patients to understand their needs or concerns. Using relevant hashtags makes the online search easier for patients, and collaborations with organizations or influencers provide patients with more information and perspectives. Using animations, infographics, text overlays, and other visuals captures attention and conveys the educational message. Moreover, HCPs may post informative videos on healthcare services, present the allergy clinic to patients, provide tutorials, and provide information on what to expect from an upcoming appointment. When using Facebook Live, Instagram Live and IGTV (integrated into Instagram) or going live to followers on TikTok, HCPs should acknowledge their robust real-time engagement and the potential risks of sharing unedited content that may not always align with social media guidelines and etiquette [37–39]. Live communication via social media platforms can also support disease surveillance and result in new observations. For example, recently, TikTok was used to unveil an acrylate allergy epidemic with an analysis of dermatologic findings associated with at-home gel nails [40].

17.3   Disease Monitoring, Patient Surveys, and Public Health Interventions on Social Media

Social media can be used for asthma and allergy monitoring by providing real-time information, support, and resources. The diverse online platforms can serve as a valuable source of data for monitoring asthma and allergy trends, symptom tracking, awareness, education, and community support. Many social media networks integrate with mobile apps and wearable devices to track health data. For example, asthma and allergy management apps can connect with social media accounts to receive support, alerts, updates, and reminders related to disease management. Interesting information includes notifications about air quality, pollen forecasts, medication reminders, and public health announcements, but all these should not substitute professional medical advice in particular situations. In addition, social media can engage patients in their disease management through features like monitoring devices with sensors and reminders for appointment scheduling, medication administration, and refill reminders [15, 41–45]. Patients' right to have their health data protected is an essential issue in the context of patient-generated data from social media and wearable devices [4].

Recently, the importance of social media for patients with atopic eczema and allergic rhinitis was underlined [44, 45]. Moreover, an intelligent method (TopicS-ClusterREV) was constructed to identify risk factors of allergic rhinitis based on social media comments [46], and patient perspectives on new rhinology devices were assessed using social media posts [47].

Targeted data collection via different types of electronic patient *surveys* (e.g., SurveyMonkey) may also be shared on social media to increase the reach. These may include patient satisfaction surveys or surveys to evaluate patients' healthcare access, experiences, perspectives, and needs. The data collection may target specific patient groups (e.g., teenagers, those living in rural areas or inner cities) or particular clinical topics such as symptom severity, quality of life [48] and safety habits, feedback of adolescents and young adults on translational care [49], feedback regarding community outreach programs or healthcare questionnaires for relief efforts in case of an epidemic or disaster-affected areas [50]. Several factors influence the response rates to surveys distributed through social media, including the targeted population, questions' clarity, survey length, and social media reminders. The goals of such online questionnaires with patient-focused content are to analyze results and create and develop proper ways for allergy patient support, guidance, and information.

Social media can be used to investigate public health interventions, including disease surveillance (asthma and influenza), outbreak investigation (e.g., early alerts for acute disease events such as thunderstorm asthma), and health promotion campaigns [51–53]. In addition, by leveraging social media data, HCPs and public health officials can target specific populations with relevant messaging and information [54]. Social platforms are commonly utilized to disseminate information on asthma and allergies to increase public awareness and potentially reduce healthcare costs by improving disease management at many levels in a patient-friendly manner, including self-management, medication adherence, and disease control [7].

In addition, the ability to identify microblogging data during pregnancy for users who reported having a child with health problems, including asthma, suggests that social media, such as the X platform, could be a complementary tool for evaluating associations between pregnancy exposures and childhood health outcomes, with potential clinical implications for informing prenatal care [55].

17.4 Allyship, Advocacy, and Activism on Social Media for Patient Support

Although there are different levels of involvement and commitment in patient support on social media, it is imperative to mention that the ally-advocate-activist spectrum is not a hierarchy but a continuum in a fluid framework. Individuals and groups can move along the spectrum over time, and some advocates consider themselves activists and vice versa, these terms being intertwined (Fig. 17.2a). The allergy community needs all of them to create synergy. Moreover, allyship, advocacy, activism, and social media are strongly interlinked for successful campaigns to raise awareness. In addition, social media ambassadors are users with a robust online presence, preferably influencers, selected by professional allergy organizations, and

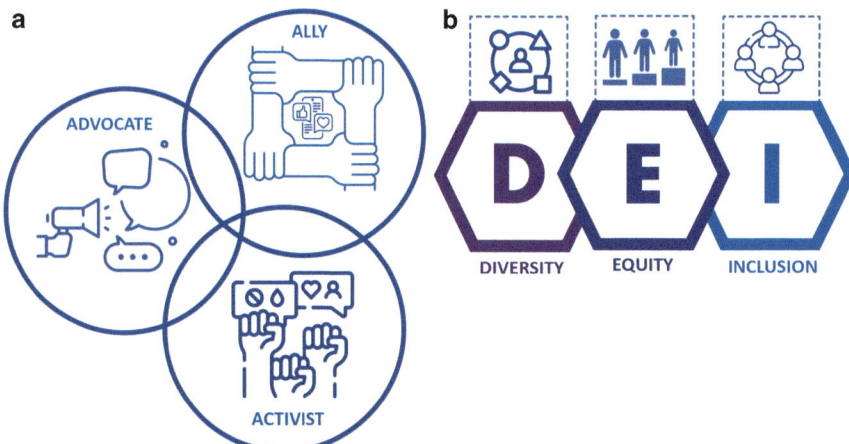

Fig. 17.2 (**a**) The ally-advocate-activist diagram to support allergic patients and the cause of allergy. (**b**) Diversity, equity, and inclusion are essential for a successful use of social media in the area of allergy care

support groups with similar values to represent them on dynamic social networks [56–62].

An *ally* is a social media user acting as a helper who connects and interacts with patients and others involved in the allergy community, listens and learns their values and aspirations, and expresses solidarity as well as support in online activities. A genuine ally is compassionate to the particular cause of allergy, is willing to use the power of personal identity and influence to promote and disseminate accurate information regarding it, and often provides support by speaking out on behalf of allergic patients and for allergy awareness [56, 57].

An *advocate* is a social media user who publicly supports, defends, and actively promotes the interests of the allergy cause, patients, and community. Advocates are more than allies who know specific aspirations and values; they openly endorse and care about informing and educating others about allergic patients on social networks, work to endorse a positive change and often take a more proactive and impactful approach, not only by speaking out to raise awareness but also by supporting events and lobbying actions for positively changing attitudes, policies, and laws [56].

An *activist* is an active and passionate social media user who energetically engages in direct actions to vigorously support and promote the allergy community's cause. An activist's organizational actions include public education and awareness-raising, mobilizing online supporters, and advocacy efforts by lobbying government officials or working with policymakers to bring about significant changes. Social media activism is the policy of direct actions, such as campaigning for such changes and fundraising for the cause of allergy [56–58].

For example, allergy allies and advocates participated in the so-called Tweetup meetings at Congresses of the European Academy of Allergy and Clinical Immunology (EAACI) for various social media actions using the *#AllergistsGetTogether* hashtag [59]. Moreover, EAACI representatives launched a European political Call to Action, *United Action for Allergy and Asthma*, promoted via a pan-European campaign on social media using the *#CallAllergyAsthma* hashtag [60]. In a collaboration between the European Federation of Allergy and Airways Diseases Patients' Associations (EFA) and a group of Members of the European Parliament with excellent online visibility, the European Parliament Interest Group on Allergy and Asthma and EAACI stand committed to fighting against allergy and asthma in Europe [61]. Other EAACI experts and social media activists campaigned in the European Parliament for proper food allergen labeling, allergy research, and food safety in memory of victims of anaphylaxis [62]. Moreover, orchestrated evidence-based activism is needed to overcome online manipulative inadequate information, while consistent, transparent messaging about scientific discoveries and clinical recommendations is critical for optimal patient support [63].

Table 17.1 Positive and negative aspects regarding social media in allergy healthcare

Major benefits and opportunities	Important risks and challenges
• Disseminating allergy information • Offering educational resources • Facilitating patient education	• Rapid spreading of misinformation, disinformation, and other forms of ID • Blurring differences between scientific evidence, anecdotes, and pseudoscience • Amplifying harmful effects of ID in conjunction with cognitive biases
• Encouraging patient engagement • Enhancing communication • Fostering community support	• Violating patient privacy and/or confidentiality • Distributing details of any specific patient without written consent[a] • Neglecting online security risks, copyrights, and trademarks
• Allergy and asthma patient monitoring • Allergic patient surveys • Telemedicine and virtual care support • Public health interventions	• Intended substitution of medical consultations, diagnosis, or treatments • Delaying the search for medical advice from qualified professional • Not maintaining boundaries between personal and professional communication • Not adhering to network service policies, ethical and professional conduct
• Allyship, advocacy, and activism for asthma, allergy, and patient support	• Garbage data collection and improper quality assessment for health research

Legend: ID = information disorder
[a] Even if protected personal health information is not included

17.5   Comments on the Present and Future of Social Media for Allergic Patients

Social media has transformed the healthcare landscape and represents a dual-edged sword with advantages, risks, and challenges (Table 17.1). Besides the multiple benefits for allergic patients previously detailed, social media networks pose many risks linked to misinformation, privacy, professional boundaries, and legal compliance. Allergists must navigate these challenges thoughtfully, leveraging the potential of social media while mitigating associated risks to ensure the proper high-quality support for their patients and the community at large [64–67].

The rapid spreading of misinformation and any other information disorder on social media generates inaccurate advice due to biased perspectives or unverified claims, pseudoscientific remedies or unproven treatments, even miracle cures, potentially compromising appropriate allergy healthcare and leading to potential harm or confusion. While it is true that not everyone can be reached, a significant part of the patient population seeks trustworthy information. Hence, combating misinformation on social media involves several strategies, including disseminating accurate information, explaining scientific data and developments using clear and accessible language, and crafting engaging, visually appealing and easy-to-understand shareable content. Utilizing narratives, citing credible sources, addressing discrepancies, prioritizing factual accuracy, and approaching discussions with politeness, authenticity, and empathy are also crucial to fight the information disorder present in online social platforms [14, 68, 69]. Before the COVID-19 pandemic, misinformation negatively affected patients with different chronic health conditions, while throughout the pandemic, numerous pitfalls emerged on social media, particularly regarding viral spread, protective masks, testing and, notably, vaccines [70, 71]. Recently, a study on social media use among parents of children with established diagnosis of food allergies revealed that the vast majority use social media platforms. The most common reasons are to access tips for school/travel, manifestations of allergic reactions, and food allergy support groups, mainly due to convenience, ease of information, and quick feedback. Other topics of interest include ways to treat allergic reactions and to test for food allergies [72]. Well-intended, evidence-based medical messages are sometimes met with disillusion, refusal or contradictory attitudes [73]. Online issues related to misinformation are those also present in real life regarding the diagnosis and treatment of IgE-mediated food allergy, including not understanding the difference between sensitization and allergy, unproven and not-scientific food allergy tests, improper allergy medication or unnecessary elimination diets, along with food-specific IgG testing offered by some practitioners and laboratories, particularly for patients with suspected food intolerance [74].

When using social media in a physician-patient setting, it is crucial not to delay or impede the seeking of medical advice, diagnosis, or treatments from a suitably qualified professional. Poor communication, erroneous medical guidance, or withholding conflicts of interest can expose healthcare providers to legal liability and even malpractice claims. Another risk healthcare providers, including allergists, face when using social media, is the potential violation of patient privacy and confidentiality. This may occur through inadvertently disclosing or sharing protected health information or patients' personal data in contravention of regulations such as the European General Data Protection Regulation (GDPR) or the US Health Insurance Portability and Accountability Act (HIPAA). Other risks are uploading/posting, discussing, distributing, or facilitating the distribution of information of any specific patient without written consent, even if protected health information is not included. Inappropriate use of social media blurs the boundaries between personal and professional communication, leading to breaches of professionalism, conflicts of interest, and reputational harm. Moreover, ethical concerns arise when healthcare professionals engage in self-promotion, endorsements, or commercial activities, exposing themselves to reputational risks stemming from negative feedback, complaints, or reviews on social media while neglecting security risks that jeopardize the integrity and security of healthcare information [14, 75–77].

Also in the context of research, certain risks need to be considered when working with data collected via social media platforms. Specifically, garbage data collection and improper quality assessment for health research, such as digital disease detection, infodemiology and infoveillance need to be considered [78]. If processed methodologically well (e.g., with a deep learning approach), highly unstructured social media streams, can provide important information to clinicians and patients alike. For example, the analysis of both syntactic (e.g., allergy, allergen) and semantic (e.g., pollen allergy, allergic rhinitis) associations between words, plus quantitative (volume of relevant posts per time/space), and qualitative analysis (text mining-based severity estimation) have been proven helpful for pollen allergy surveillance on the X platform [79]. In addition, data analysis of posts from X and Facebook may be used to assess allergic drug reactions [80].

Finally, the approach of diversity, equity, and inclusion (Fig. 17.2b) on social media involves actively addressing social and health inequities that disproportionately affect underrepresented populations [81, 82]. Understanding the multifaceted role of online social networks in allergy care and navigating the risks and challenges requires healthcare professionals and organizations to develop clear policies, guidelines, and training programs for the responsible use of social media [83].

In the future online social ecosystem, the platforms currently referred to as social media will continue to broaden their influence in everyday life, reshaping the search for information and selection of opinions and actions. In addition, there will be a rise of new creative AI tools, such as chatbots or text-to-text conversation, but such innovations will create not only exponential improvements in performance in the real world but also will escalate the debates around ethics, legal responsibilities, and potential risks, including inappropriate information [84, 85].

17.6 Conclusions

HCPs can support their allergy patients to benefit from social media as providers of allergy information and education, generating awareness and engagement on social media, acting for online support disease monitoring, patient surveys, and public health interventions. They can support patients' interests and needs by acting as social media allies, advocates, or activists. However, it is crucial to understand that social media should not be used as a substitute for medical advice, diagnosis, or treatments. No online content can be an alternative or replace consultations from suitably qualified HCPs, and it should not influence or delay seeking medical advice in any way. Social media has a great potential to improve allergic patient support and disease management, but potential risks and challenges must be carefully considered.

Disclosure F.D. Popescu reports serving as European Academy of Allergology and Clinical Immunology (EAACI) Social Media Editor 2019–2022 and oral presentation with no financial support at the EAACI Digital Congress 2020. FDP declares no conflict of interest. S. Dramburg reports serving as EAACI Scientific Communication Committee Chair 2020–2022. SD declares no conflict of interest.

References

1. Matricardi PM, Dramburg S, Alvarez-Perea A, Antolín-Amérigo D, Apfelbacher C, Atanaskovic-Markovic M, Berger U, Blaiss MS, Blank S, Boni E, Bonini M, Bousquet J, Brockow K, Buters J, Cardona V, Caubet JC, Cavkaytar Ö, Elliott T, Esteban-Gorgojo I, Fonseca JA, Gardner J, Gevaert P, Ghiordanescu I, Hellings P, Hoffmann-Sommergruber K, Fusun Kalpaklioglu A, Marmouz F, Meijide Calderón Á, Mösges R, Nakonechna A, Ollert M, Oteros J, Pajno G, Panaitescu C, Perez-Formigo D, Pfaar O, Pitsios C, Rudenko M, Ryan D, Sánchez-García S, Shih J, Tripodi S, Van der Poel LA, van Os-Medendorp H, Varricchi G, Wittmann J, Worm M, Agache I. The role of mobile health technologies in allergy care: an EAACI position paper. Allergy. 2020;75(2):259–72. https://doi.org/10.1111/all.13953.
2. Demoly P, Passalacqua G, Pfaar O, Sastre J, Wahn U. Patient engagement and patient support programs in allergy immunotherapy: a call to action for improving long-term adherence. Allergy Asthma Clin Immunol. 2016;12:34. https://doi.org/10.1186/s13223-016-0140-2.
3. Maurer M, Weller K, Magerl M, Maurer RR, Vanegas E, Felix M, Cherrez A, Mata VL, Kasperska-Zajac A, Sikora A, Fomina D, Kovalkova E, Godse K, Rao ND, Khoshkhui M, Rastgoo S, Criado RFJ, Abuzakouk M, Grandon D, van Doorn M, Valle SOR, de Souza Lima EM, Thomsen SF, Ramón GD, Matos Benavides EE, Bauer A, Giménez-Arnau AM, Kocatürk E, Guillet C, Ignacio Larco J, Zhao ZT, Makris M, Ritchie C, Xepapadaki P, Ensina LF, Cherrez S, Cherrez-Ojeda I. The usage, quality and relevance of information and communications technologies in patients with chronic urticaria: a UCARE study. World Allergy Organ J. 2020;13(11):100475. https://doi.org/10.1016/j.waojou.2020.100475.
4. Antolín-Amérigo D, Popescu FD, Alvarez-Perea A. Patient-friendly HIT tools and the advent of crowdsourcing clinical trials. In: Hellings PW, Agache I, editors. Implementing precision medicine in best practices of chronic AirwayDiseases. London: Elsevier; 2018. p. 135–44.
5. Moreira A, Mendes FC, Rama T, Mota D, Silva D, Pádua I, Abreu C, Vasconcelos MJ, Farraia M, Paciência I, Rufo J, Barros R, Padrão P, Moreira P, Seabra D, Barros H. AlergiaPT: a Portuguese media campaign to inspire people with allergies to make a positive change in their life. Porto Biomed J. 2022;7(1):e169. https://doi.org/10.1097/j.pbj.0000000000000169.
6. Alvarez-Perea A, Sánchez-García S, Muñoz Cano R, Antolín-Amérigo D, Tsilochristou O, Stukus DR. Impact of "ehealth" in allergic diseases and allergic patients. J Investig Allergol Clin Immunol. 2019;29(2):94–102. https://doi.org/10.18176/jiaci.0354.
7. Poowuttikul P, Seth D. New concepts and technological resources in patient education and asthma self-management. Clin Rev Allergy Immunol. 2020;59(1):19–37. https://doi.org/10.1007/s12016-020-08782-w.
8. Grajales FJ 3rd, Sheps S, Ho K, Novak-Lauscher H, Eysenbach G. Social media: a review and tutorial of applications in medicine and health care. J Med Internet Res. 2014;16(2):e13. https://doi.org/10.2196/jmir.2912.
9. Gong W, Liu J. Investigating the predictors of telemedicine service usage intention in China during the COVID-19 pandemic: an extended technology acceptance perspective. Telemed J E Health. 2023;29:1390. https://doi.org/10.1089/tmj.2022.0352.
10. Portnoy JM, Pandya A, Waller M, Elliott T. Telemedicine and emerging technologies for health care in allergy/immunology. J Allergy Clin Immunol. 2020;145(2):445–54. https://doi.org/10.1016/j.jaci.2019.12.903.
11. Tahlil KM, Nwaozuru U, Conserve DF, Onyeama UF, Ojo V, Day S, Ong JJ, Tang W, Rosenberg NE, Gbajabiamila T, Nkengasong S, Obiezu-Umeh C, Oladele D, Iwelunmor J, Ezechi O, Tucker JD. Crowdsourcing to support training for public health: a scoping review. PLOS Glob Public Health. 2023;3(7):e0002202. https://doi.org/10.1371/journal.pgph.0002202.
12. Aramaki E, Shikata S, Ayaya S, Kumagaya SI. Crowdsourced identification of possible allergy-associated factors: automated hypothesis generation and validation using crowdsourcing services. JMIR Res Protoc. 2017;6(5):e83. https://doi.org/10.2196/resprot.5851.

13. Weisblum M, Trussell E, Schwinn T, Pacheco AR, Nurkin P. Screening and retaining adolescents recruited through social media: secondary analysis from a longitudinal clinical trial. JMIR Pediatr Parent. 2024;7:e47984. https://doi.org/10.2196/47984.
14. Patrick M, Venkatesh RD, Stukus DR. Social media and its impact on health care. Ann Allergy Asthma Immunol. 2022;128(2):139–45. https://doi.org/10.1016/j.anai.2021.09.014.
15. Dimov V, Eidelman F. Utilizing social networks, blogging and YouTube in allergy and immunology practices. Expert Rev Clin Immunol. 2015;11(10):1065–8. https://doi.org/10.1586/1744666X.2015.1065731.
16. Joshi S, Dimov V. Use of new technology to improve utilization and adherence to immunotherapy. World Allergy Organ J. 2014;7(1):29. https://doi.org/10.1186/1939-4551-7-29.
17. Peters-Geven MM, Rollema C, Metting EI, van Roon EN, de Vries TW. The quality of instructional YouTube videos for the administration of intranasal spray: observational study. JMIR Med Educ. 2020;6(2):e23668. https://doi.org/10.2196/23668.
18. Rosenzweig D, Nickels AS. #Asthma #Inhaler: evaluation of visual social media depictions of inhalers and spacers. J Allergy Clin Immunol Pract. 2017;5(6):1787–8. https://doi.org/10.1016/j.jaip.2017.04.029.
19. Alvarez-Perea A, Cabrera-Freitag P, Fuentes-Aparicio V, Infante S. Advancements in anaphylaxis management. Curr Pharm Des. 2023;29(3):185–95. https://doi.org/10.2174/1381612829666221021150946.
20. Alvarez-Perea A, Cabrera-Freitag P, Fuentes-Aparicio V, Infante S, Zapatero L, Zubeldia JM. Social media as a tool for the management of food allergy in children. J Investig Allergol Clin Immunol. 2018;28(4):233–40. https://doi.org/10.18176/jiaci.0235.
21. Howell WL, Patient education. Facebook isn't just for status updates or playing games anymore. Hosp Health Netw. 2011;85(4):13.
22. Dhar VK, Kim Y, Graff JT, Jung AD, Garrett J, Dick LE, Harris J, Shah SA. Benefit of social media on patient engagement and satisfaction: results of a 9-month, qualitative pilot study using Facebook. Surgery. 2018;163(3):565–70. https://doi.org/10.1016/j.surg.2017.09.056.
23. Nguyen M, Case S, Botto N, Liszewski W. The use of social media platforms to discuss and educate the public on allergic contact dermatitis. Contact Derm. 2022;86(3):196–203. https://doi.org/10.1111/cod.14004.
24. Titgemeyer SC, Schaaf CP. Facebook support groups for pediatric rare diseases: cross-sectional study to investigate opportunities, limitations, and privacy concerns. JMIR Pediatr Parent. 2022;5(1):e31411. https://doi.org/10.2196/31411.
25. Wakamiya S, Matsune S, Okubo K, Aramaki E. Causal relationships among pollen counts, tweet numbers, and patient numbers for seasonal allergic rhinitis surveillance: retrospective analysis. J Med Internet Res. 2019;21(2):e10450. https://doi.org/10.2196/10450.
26. Thomas TH, Nauth-Shelley K, Thompson MA, Attai DJ, Katz MS, Graham D, Sparacio D, Lizaso C, Utengen A, Dizon DS. The needs of women treated for ovarian cancer: results from a #gyncsm twitter chat. J Patient Cent Res Rev. 2018;5(2):149–57. https://doi.org/10.17294/2330-0698.1592.
27. Popescu FD. Thank you @AAAAI_org and Great Social Media #Allergy Activists Dr. Dave Stukus @AllergyKidsDoc & Gerald Lee @DrGerryLee for the very interesting and useful #AsthmaAirQuality Twitter Chat! @EAACI_HQ @eaaci_patients. Twitter. 2018. https://twitter.com/FlorinDanPopesc/status/1045360234506715136. Accessed 4 Apr 2024.
28. Admon AJ, Kaul V, Cribbs SK, Guzman E, Jimenez O, Richards JB. Twelve tips for developing and implementing a medical education twitter chat. Med Teach. 2020;42(5):500–6. https://doi.org/10.1080/0142159X.2019.1598553.
29. Blumenthal KG, Topaz M, Zhou L, Harkness T, Sa'adon R, Bar-Bachar O, Long AA. Mining social media data to assess the risk of skin and soft tissue infections from allergen immunotherapy. J Allergy Clin Immunol. 2019;144(1):129–34. https://doi.org/10.1016/j.jaci.2019.01.029.
30. Joly-Chevrier M, Aly S, Bahous K, Lefrançois P. Atopic dermatitis patient needs assessed through the largest online patient community: a cross-sectional Reddit analysis. J Cutan Med Surg. 2024;28(1):75–7. https://doi.org/10.1177/12034754231221988.

31. Kurtti A, Cohen M, Jagdeo J. Analysis of Reddit reveals Dupilumab questions among atopic dermatitis patients. J Drugs Dermatol. 2022;21(3):292–4. https://doi.org/10.36849/JDD.5942.
32. Ahuja K, DeSena G, Lio P. Analysis of Reddit reveals JAK inhibitor questions among atopic dermatitis patients. J Drugs Dermatol. 2024;23(4):e121–3. https://doi.org/10.36849/JDD.7787.
33. Whitsitt J, Mattis D, Hernandez M, Kollipara R, Dellavalle RP. Dermatology on Pinterest. Dermatol Online J. 2015;21(1):13030/qt7dj4267p.
34. Chen JY, Gardner JM, Chen SC, McMichael JR. Instagram for dermatology education. J Am Acad Dermatol. 2020;83(4):1175–6. https://doi.org/10.1016/j.jaad.2020.02.001.
35. Johnson H, Herzog C, Shaver RL, Hylwa SA. A deep dive into Instagram's top Skinfluencers. JMIR Dermatol. 2023;6:e49653. https://doi.org/10.2196/49653.
36. Cinquantasei M, Albanesi M. Allergy and immunology diffusion via social media: performance of video and audio contents on Instagram. Postepy Dermatol Alergol. 2023;40(6):817–9. https://doi.org/10.5114/ada.2023.133607.
37. Fuller MY, Allen TC. Let's have a tweetup: the case for using twitter professionally. Arch Pathol Lab Med. 2016;140(9):956–7. https://doi.org/10.5858/arpa.2016-0172-SA.
38. Gómez Rivas J, Rodríguez-Socarras ME, Cacciamani G, Dourado Meneses A, Okhunov Z, van Gurp M, Bloemberg J, Porpiglia F, Liatsikos E, Veneziano D. Live videos shared on social media during urological conferences are increasing: time to reflect on advantages and potential harms. An ESUT-YAU study. Actas Urol Esp (Engl Ed). 2019;43(10):551–6.
39. Mao E. How live stream content types impact viewers' support behaviors? Mediational analysis on psychological and social gratifications. Front Psychol. 2022;13:951055. https://doi.org/10.3389/fpsyg.2022.951055.
40. Axler EN, Lipner SR. Unveiling an acrylate allergy epidemic: analysis of dermatologic findings associated with at-home gel nails on TikTok. J Cutan Med Surg. 2024;28(1):92–4. https://doi.org/10.1177/12034754231220930.
41. Greiwe J, Nyenhuis SM. Wearable technology and how this can be implemented into clinical practice. Curr Allergy Asthma Rep. 2020;20(8):36. https://doi.org/10.1007/s11882-020-00927-3.
42. Nickels A, Dimov V. Innovations in technology: social media and mobile technology in the care of adolescents with asthma. Curr Allergy Asthma Rep. 2012;12(6):607–12. https://doi.org/10.1007/s11882-012-0299-7.
43. Ramsey RR, Carmody JK, Holbein CE, Guilbert TW, Hommel KA. Examination of the uses, needs, and preferences for health technology use in adolescents with asthma. J Asthma. 2019;56(9):964–72. https://doi.org/10.1080/02770903.2018.1514048.
44. Walter-Leitzgen T. Social Media bei medizinischen problemen: einfluss und bedeutung für patienten beim atopischen ekzem [Using social media for medical issues: influence and importance for patients with atopic eczema]. Dermatologie (Heidelb). 2023;74(9):733–5. German. https://doi.org/10.1007/s00105-023-05194-7.
45. Sitaru S, Wecker H, Buters J, Biedermann T, Zink A. Social media to monitor prevalent diseases: hay fever and twitter activity in Germany. Allergy. 2023;78(10):2777–80. https://doi.org/10.1111/all.15787.
46. Gu D, Wang Q, Chai Y, Yang X, Zhao W, Li M, Zolotarev O, Xu Z, Zhang G. Identifying the risk factors of allergic rhinitis based on Zhihu comment data using a topic-enhanced word-embedding model: mixed method study and cluster analysis. J Med Internet Res. 2024;26:e48324. https://doi.org/10.2196/48324.
47. LaHaye JJ, Moffatt DC, Dunmire A, Corona KK, Rossi NA, Siddiqui FN. A social media analysis examining new-age devices of the rhinology industry. Int Forum Allergy Rhinol. 2023;13(11):2092–5. https://doi.org/10.1002/alr.23176.
48. Banjar SA, Assiri RA, Alshehri GA, Binyousef FH, Alaudah TI, Alawam AS, Aloriney AM. The impact of allergic rhinitis on asthma and its effect on the quality of life of asthmatic patients. Cureus. 2023;15(3):e35714. https://doi.org/10.7759/cureus.35714.
49. Khaleva E, Knibb R, DunnGalvin A, Vazquez-Ortiz M, Comberiati P, Alviani C, Garriga-Baraut T, Gowland MH, Gore C, Angier E, Blumchen K, Duca B, Hox V, Jensen B, Mortz

CG, Pite H, Pfaar O, Santos AF, Sanchez-Garcia S, Timmermans F, Roberts G. Perceptions of adolescents and young adults with allergy and/or asthma and their parents on EAACI guideline recommendations about transitional care: a European survey. Allergy. 2022;77(4):1094–104. https://doi.org/10.1111/all.15109.

50. Tashkandi E, Zeeneldin A, AlAbdulwahab A, Elemam O, Elsamany S, Jastaniah W, Abdullah S, Alfayez M, Jazieh AR, Al-Shamsi HO. Virtual management of patients with cancer during the COVID-19 pandemic: web-based questionnaire study. J Med Internet Res. 2020;22(6):e19691. https://doi.org/10.2196/19691.

51. Aiello AE, Renson A, Zivich PN. Social media- and internet-based disease surveillance for public health. Annu Rev Public Health. 2020;41:101–18. https://doi.org/10.1146/annurev-pub lhealth-040119-094402.

52. Koppeschaar CE, Colizza V, Guerrisi C, Turbelin C, Duggan J, Edmunds WJ, Kjelsø C, Mexia R, Moreno Y, Meloni S, Paolotti D, Perrotta D, van Straten E, Franco AO. Influenzanet: citizens among 10 countries collaborating to monitor influenza in Europe. JMIR Public Health Surveill. 2017;3(3):e66. https://doi.org/10.2196/publichealth.7429.

53. Joshi A, Sparks R, McHugh J, Karimi S, Paris C, MacIntyre CR. Harnessing tweets for early detection of an acute disease event. Epidemiology. 2020;31(1):90–7. https://doi.org/10.1097/EDE.0000000000001133.

54. Jones CJ, Sommereux LA, Smith HE. Exploring what motivates and sustains support group engagement amongst young people with allergies: a qualitative study. Clin Exp Allergy. 2018;48(9):1195–205. https://doi.org/10.1111/cea.13193.

55. Klein AZ, Gutiérrez Gómez JA, Levine LD, Gonzalez-Hernandez G. Using longitudinal twitter data for digital epidemiology of childhood health outcomes: an annotated data set and deep neural network classifiers. J Med Internet Res. 2024;26:e50652. https://doi.org/10.2196/50652.

56. Zuzelo PR. Ally, advocate, activist, and adversary: rocking the status quo. Holist Nurs Pract. 2020;34(3):190–2. https://doi.org/10.1097/HNP.0000000000000389.

57. Wang JTH, Power CJ, Kahler CM, Lyras D, Young PR, Iredell J, Robins-Browne R. Communication ambassadors—an Australian social media initiative to develop communication skills in early career scientists. J Microbiol Biol Educ. 2018;19(1):19.1.25. https://doi.org/10.1128/jmbe.v19i1.1428.

58. Kerr A, Chekar CK, Swallow J, Ross E, Cunningham-Burley S. Accessing targeted therapies for cancer: self and collective advocacy alongside and beyond mainstream cancer charities. New Genet Soc. 2021;40(1):112–31. https://doi.org/10.1080/14636778.2020.1868986.

59. Popescu FD. Remembering the enthusiastic #AllergistsGetTogether Tweetup event at the great #EAACl2018 Congress. X/Twitter. 2018, https://twitter.com/FlorinDanPopesc/status/1002917076556746753. Accessed 4 Apr 2024.

60. Popescu FD. EAACI_HQ: support the "united action for allergy and asthma" campaign by signing online #CallAllergyAsthma. X/Twitter. 2017. https://twitter.com/FlorinDanPopesc/status/876681638247370753. Accessed 4 Apr 2024.

61. Popescu FD. Read in the latest #EAACINewsletter the #EPAllergyAsthma social media review on European Parliament interest group on allergy and asthma first meeting of 2019–2024 legislature "a new direction for #allergy and #asthma health in Europe" #EAACI_Newsletter #eaaci2020 X/twitter. 2020. https://twitter.com/FlorinDanPopesc/status/1267063000927698944. Accessed 4 Apr 2024.

62. Brough H. Honoured to represent #EAACI in #EU parliament to present the #DetectiveFood report by @EFA_Patients; proper food allergen labelling and future research to protect people with #foodallergy. Twitter. 2019. https://twitter.com/broughallergy/status/1205411291977965569. Accessed 4 Apr 2024.

63. Haberer JE, van der Straten A, Safren SA, Johnson MO, Amico KR, Del Rio C, Andrasik M, Wilson IB, Simoni JM. Individual health behaviours to combat the COVID-19 pandemic: lessons from HIV socio-behavioural science. J Int AIDS Soc. 2021;24(8):e25771. https://doi.org/10.1002/jia2.25771.

64. Dimov V, Gonzalez-Estrada A, Eidelman F. Social media and allergy. Curr Allergy Asthma Rep. 2018;18(12):76. https://doi.org/10.1007/s11882-018-0822-6.
65. Alvarez-Perea A, Dimov V, Popescu FD, Zubeldia JM. The applications of eHealth technologies in the management of asthma and allergic diseases. Clin Transl Allergy. 2021;11(7):e12061. https://doi.org/10.1002/clt2.12061.
66. Muhammed TS, Mathew SK. The disaster of misinformation: a review of research in social media. Int J Data Sci Anal. 2022;13(4):271–85. https://doi.org/10.1007/s41060-022-00311-6.
67. WHO Press release. Infodemics and misinformation negatively affect people's health behaviours, new WHO review finds. 2022. www.who.int/europe/news/item/01-09-2022-infodemics-and-misinformation-negatively-affect-people-s-health-behaviours%2D%2Dnew-who-review-finds. Accessed 4 Apr 2024.
68. Anagnostou A, Lieberman J, Greenhawt M, Mack DP, Santos AF, Venter C, Stukus D, Turner PJ, Brough HA. The future of food allergy: challenging existing paradigms of clinical practice. Allergy. 2023;78(7):1847–65. https://doi.org/10.1111/all.15757.
69. Suarez-Lledo V, Alvarez-Galvez J. Prevalence of health misinformation on social media: systematic review. J Med Internet Res. 2021;23(1):e17187. https://doi.org/10.2196/17187.
70. Alanazi A, Aldosari H, Aldosari B. Pitfalls of social media in the era of COVID-19 pandemics. Stud Health Technol Inform. 2022;289:473–6. https://doi.org/10.3233/SHTI210960.
71. Lu Q, Schulz PJ, Chang A. Medication safety perceptions in China: media exposure, healthcare experiences, and trusted information sources. Patient Educ Couns. 2024;123:108209. https://doi.org/10.1016/j.pec.2024.108209.
72. Anagnostou A, Hearrell M, Timberlake D, Huang X, Staggers KA, Stukus D. Social media use among parents of children with food allergies. Ann Allergy Asthma Immunol. 2024;S1081-1206(24):00208–4. https://doi.org/10.1016/j.anai.2024.03.025.
73. Stukus DR. Tackling medical misinformation in allergy and immunology practice. Expert Rev Clin Immunol. 2022;18(10):995–6. https://doi.org/10.1080/1744666X.2022.2108016.
74. Stukus DR, Mikhail I. Pearls and pitfalls in diagnosing IgE-mediated food allergy. Curr Allergy Asthma Rep. 2016;16(5):34. https://doi.org/10.1007/s11882-016-0611-z.
75. Markopoulou V, Nieri A, Liaskos J, Zoulias E, Mantas J. Nursing Staff's awareness of processing personal data according to GDPR. Stud Health Technol Inform. 2020;272:237–40. https://doi.org/10.3233/SHTI200538.
76. EAACI. European Academy of Allergy and Clinical Immunology. EAACI Social Media Disclaimer. https://www.eaaci.org/images/EAACI_Social_Media_Disclaimer.pdf. Accessed 4 Apr 2024.
77. Popescu FD. Basic rules when using #SocialMedia in the great #EAACI_Newsletter 50th issue! To be active on social media, create meaningful content & post new content frequently for maximum visibility! X/Twitter. 2018. https://twitter.com/FlorinDanPopesc/status/982565722474807296. Accessed 4 Apr 2024.
78. Kim Y, Huang J, Emery S. Garbage in, garbage out: data collection, quality assessment and reporting standards for Social Media data use in Health Research, Infodemiology and digital disease detection. J Med Internet Res. 2016;18(2):e41. https://doi.org/10.2196/jmir.4738.
79. Rong J, Michalska S, Subramani S, Du J, Wang H. Deep learning for pollen allergy surveillance from twitter in Australia. BMC Med Inform Decis Mak. 2019;19(1):208. https://doi.org/10.1186/s12911-019-0921-x.
80. Zhou Z, Hultgren KE. Complementing the US Food and Drug Administration adverse event reporting system with adverse drug reaction reporting from social media: comparative analysis. JMIR Public Health Surveill. 2020;6(3):e19266. https://doi.org/10.2196/19266.
81. Florez N, Karmo M, Beltrán Ponce S, Barry MM, Henry E, Katz MS, Dizon DS, Hylton HM, Collaboration for Outcomes Using Social Media in Oncology (COSMO). Social Media and the quest for equity and diversity in oncology: on safe spaces and the concept of the public physician. JCO Oncol Pract. 2022;18(8):572–7. https://doi.org/10.1200/OP.21.00762.

82. Nyariro M, Emami E, Caidor P, Abbasgholizadeh Rahimi S. Integrating equity, diversity and inclusion throughout the lifecycle of AI within healthcare: a scoping review protocol. BMJ Open. 2023;13(9):e072069. https://doi.org/10.1136/bmjopen-2023-072069.
83. Jeyaraman M, Ramasubramanian S, Kumar S, Jeyaraman N, Selvaraj P, Nallakumarasamy A, Bondili SK, Yadav S. Multifaceted role of Social Media in Healthcare: opportunities, challenges, and the need for quality control. Cureus. 2023;15(5):e39111. https://doi.org/10.7759/cureus.39111.
84. Rebelo M. The best AI productivity tools in 2024. 2024. https://zapier.com/blog/best-ai-productivity-tools. Accessed 4 Apr 2024.
85. Offiah AC, Khanna G. ChatGPT: an editor's perspective. Pediatr Radiol. 2023;53(5):816–7. https://doi.org/10.1007/s00247-023-05668-9.

Chapter 18
A Practical Guide to Social Media in Allergic Disease Management: Background, Tools, Tips, and Tactics

Florin-Dan Popescu and Stephanie Dramburg

Contents

Abstract Social media platforms are increasingly utilized to support allergy patients in diverse forms. Popular socializing and microblogging networks are valuable online tools for patient education and information, allowing the creation and sharing of various types of content and active involvement with followers. Image-

F.-D. Popescu (✉)
Department of Allergology, "Nicolae Malaxa" Clinical Hospital, "Carol Davila" University of Medicine and Pharmacy, Bucharest, Romania

S. Dramburg
Department of Pediatric Respiratory Medicine, Immunology and Critical Care Medicine, Charité–Universitätsmedizin Berlin, a corporate member of Freie Universität Berlin and Humboldt–Universität zu Berlin, Berlin, Germany
e-mail: stephanie.dramburg@charite.de

© The Author(s), under exclusive license to Springer Nature Switzerland AG 2025
P. M. Matricardi, S. Dramburg, *Digital Allergology*, Health Informatics, https://doi.org/10.1007/978-3-031-71021-6_18

and video-based social media services are also helpful in supporting allergic disease management via visually appealing and engaging content. At the same time, forum-style networking is advantageous in text-based education on various topics. However, social media platforms may be utilized also to spread misinformation and disinformation on health topics, which is a particular threat to susceptible subjects, for example, with lower emotional intelligence and education. Independently from the used technology, user may promote products or services unsupported by scientific guidelines. Therefore, healthcare providers on social media need to perform as contributors to information and education. In this role, it is essential to combat all forms of online information disorder and to respect basic rules as well as guiding principles when using social media.

18.1 Background

Digital healthcare technologies have witnessed significant growth and development in recent years. Mobile health utilizes modern mobile communication devices such as smartphones, phablets (mobile devices larger than a phone but smaller than a tablet), and tablet computers to support and improve patient support and disease management [1]. Digital health approaches educate patients about diseases, treatments, self-management options, and medical circumstances. These save valuable medical working time, boost accuracy and efficiency, and allow patients to access information anytime and anywhere [2].

Mobile communication device use has increased dramatically in the last decade, moving a significant part of the world to our fingertips. Recent data reveals that over 97% of internet users aged 16–64 in many of the world's largest economies use at least one social media platform monthly. There are 5.04 billion social media users worldwide, currently equating to 62.3% of the global population. Furthermore, the number of global social media users has increased significantly since the start of the COVID-19 pandemic, with 266 million new users in 2023, equating to an average increase of 8.4 new users every single second [3]. The typical working-age internet user spends over 2.5 h daily on social platforms [4]. Compared with traditional media, social media platforms work faster and farther in spreading information while being archived, searchable, and interactive [5].

A brief presentation of the social media ecosystem must start by mentioning that there were no such online platforms before 1997, when the first modern social network, SixDegrees, was launched. From 2003 onward, many new social networking sites appeared, such as LinkedIn (2003), Facebook (2004), Twitter (2006), and Instagram (2010). Although there is an increasing tendency of patients to rely on online content and social networks for health-related information [6], the credibility and accuracy of information found in this way can be variable, and patients need to be very cautious when evaluating information from these sources [7, 8, 9].

Online interactions between patients with chronic conditions and peers can influence their communication and relationships with healthcare professionals (HCPs), as they may wish to discuss obtained medical information referring to their relationships on social networks [10]. Besides one-to-one and one-to-many technologies such as email, instant messaging, and web browsers, patients use many-to-many online technologies, including platforms such as Facebook, Twitter, Instagram, and LinkedIn [6]. Interestingly, it has been shown that some groups of adolescents tend to be skeptical towards social media platforms for medical information, mainly due to privacy concerns [10]. On the other hand, adolescents and young adults may be interested in offering feedback regarding recommendations on transitional care [11].

Social networks have fundamentally changed how people share and receive information, becoming a widespread source of health information for allergy patients and the general population. As a result, there is growing recognition of how social media impacts patient-centered management. Therefore, HCPs must increase their understanding of such complex interactions for better disease management and should consider active social media engagement to support their patients. Moreover, professional organizations in allergy and immunology use social networks for individual members, public advocacy and continuous online education during annual congresses and focused meetings with dedicated hashtags [12].

If properly used, modern social media can be a powerful tool to improve allergic disease management due to its influence on health education and awareness, patient engagement and support, disease monitoring, and public health interventions [13–15]. However, online disinformation and non-evidence-based content can also lead to harmful behavior and wrong assumptions regarding important health topics. Additionally, it is necessary to remember that only some adults have proficient health literacy [16], suggesting that patients may need additional support in understanding basic medical information and properly engaging in chronic disease management. Persons with greater eHealth literacy searching for health information on popular social networking sites are younger and more educated [17]. New versatile elements of social media and the support of artificial intelligence (AI) provide patients with helpful outlets to comprehend their health conditions and improve communication and engagement [18].

18.2 Definitions and Basic Terminology to Work with Social Media Tools

Social media is defined as dynamic computer-mediated communication tools *based* on mobile and internet technologies to generate highly interactive online *platforms* in which individuals or groups create *user-specific profiles* for a site or application designed and maintained by a social media service. The users are *connected* in online social networks or virtual communities, in which *user-generated content* is created or co-created, accessed, shared, or exchanged, possibly discussed or modified. Social media content is produced in various formats, such as text, images, audio, and/or video digital recordings, with or without the use of filters or other inventive tools. Users have unique identifiers and can interact with each other on social media and engage in many activities, such as *sharing, liking, commenting,* and *favoriting* content, along with *messaging, following* or *friending.* Social networks are a specific type of social media platform designed to facilitate connections and interactions between individuals, while social media is a general term for online tools that allow people to create, share, or exchange information and content with others. The user-specific profiles represent the sustaining *structural component* of a social media service, while the user-generated content is its indispensable *functional constituent.* Social media platforms can serve various purposes, including communication, information sharing, networking, entertainment, social allyship or advocacy and social activism [19].

18.3 Catalogue of Relevant Social Media Platforms for Patient Engagement and Disease Management

Due to the rapid development of social media, there are many ways to categorize social media platforms based on different criteria. Social media can be classified by the type of content, including text-based content such as microblogging (e.g., Twitter), image-based content (e.g., Instagram), and video-based content (e.g., YouTube), by their purpose or function, being designed primarily for communication and networking (e.g., LinkedIn) or focused on content sharing and discovery (e.g., Pinterest), or by the audience, some being designed especially for younger users, such as TikTok and Snapchat, while others cater to older users (e.g., Facebook). Based on the business model, some social media may be considered advertising-driven or subscription-based. The most popular social networks dominate the social media landscape, but other services also play an important role in specific groups, regions, or user settings. Social media platforms are registered trademarks or service marks, and most use AI to improve users' experience and provide personalized content [8].

Social media has facilitated a new culture of connectivity, where people can connect and interact in new and unprecedented ways. They allow HCPs to have interactive and real-time communication with patients, set goals, improve patient care and disease management, and create bonds of confidence that consolidate their relationship. Relevant examples of online social networks potentially supporting the management of allergic patients are presented in Table 18.1. In January 2024, the list of the world's most-used social platforms according to a ranking by global active user figures included Facebook, YouTube, Instagram, TikTok, Snapchat, X (formerly known as Twitter), and Pinterest. The online encyclopedia project Wikipedia is not typically considered a social media platform. Although the wiki-based website (a wiki being an online hypertext publication collaboratively edited and managed by its audience) allows users to communicate with each other through discussion

Table 18.1 Social media and social networks which may be used in allergic disease management

Social media platforms[a]	Example (Owner[b])	Founded	Current statistics[c]	Web address (URL)
Popular online social networks				
Socializing and content dissemination	Facebook (Meta)	2004	3049	www.facebook.com
Photo and video hosting and sharing	Instagram (Meta)	2010	2000	www.instagram.com
Microblogging and social networking	X (fka Twitter) (X Corp)	2006	619	www.x.com
Video hosting and sharing	YouTube (Google)	2005	2421	www.youtube.com
Short-form video hosting and sharing	TikTok (ByteDance)	2017	1562	www.tiktok.com
Visual search and curation	Pinterest (public)	2009	482	www.pinterest.com
Multimedia instant messaging	Snapchat (Snap Inc)	2011	750	www.spapchat.com
Other online networks and social services				
Professional and business-oriented	LinkedIn (Microsoft)	2003	922	www.linkedin.com
Collaborative filtering	Reddit (Advance)	2005	1224	www.reddit.com
Microblogging and social networking	Tumblr (Automattic)	2007	198	www.tumblr.com

Notes: General information and indicative statistics
Sources: January 2024 data from https://datareportal.com; www.statista.com; www.wikipedia.org
[a] Available in Latin alphabet
[b] Current owner (2023); fka (formerly known as); URL = Uniform Resource Locator
[c] Global active user figures in millions (note: users may not represent unique individuals)

pages, it is not primarily designed for social networking. Platforms in the Chinese language include Douyin (counterpart of TikTok), the short-form video platform Kuaishou and Weibo (previously known as Sina Weibo), a popular Chinese microblogging website. Worldwide, WhatsApp and Weixin (known as WeChat outside of China) dominate the instant messaging market, while Line is currently the messenger of choice in Japan. Notably, there's a large audience overlap, with almost 90% of X and Snapchat users and about 80% of the people active on TikTok also using Instagram [3]. An increase in the time people spend online is associated with a decline in TV viewership [4]. Over the years, several social media platforms have faced controversies and criticism related to privacy and security issues, particularly related to the collection and use of user data [3, 20].

The following paragraphs will overview the most-used social media platforms and their functionalities.

18.3.1 Socializing and Microblogging Tools

Among the widely embraced socializing and microblogging platforms, Facebook and X reign are the most often used channels for millions worldwide.

Facebook is an online social media and networking service that allows users to create personal profiles, connect with friends and family, and share content. When creating a post on Facebook, users can include text, images, videos, and links. They can post up to 63,206 characters in length. However, many keep their posts relatively short, similar to microblogging. Facebook offers a variety of interactions such as following, commenting, sharing, liking, sending private messages and tagging (marking) other users to notify someone mentioned. The platform also offers various features, such as events, groups, and pages allowing users to organize, join, or follow activities and communities based on shared interests. In addition, it offers a wide range of advertising options for organizations to reach their target audiences. In 2023, Facebook users spent almost 20 h/month on this platform [4]. Facebook uses AI to power the news feed algorithm, which determines what content to show users based on their interests, activity, and behavior on the network. It also uses AI for image and speech recognition and natural language processing. Facebook supports allergy patients and caregivers of all ages in various ways. Some groups and pages dedicate their content to allergies, including rare ones, where users can connect, share tips and advice, and find support.. Many professional societies, allergy organizations, and advocacy groups also have Facebook pages to engage with patients, share up-to-date information, and provide education for different medical conditions. Allergy services may also use it to share visual information about the clinic location, examination rooms, allergy immunotherapy waiting room, staff members, and announcements about specific clinic work hours and events. Patient support groups use Facebook to connect and share experiences, resources, and information about different health conditions [13, 21]. Some HCPs may also use Facebook to share health tips and answer common questions from patients [4, 21, 22].

Facebook analytics helps to determine popularity, but professional organizations and clinics compete with friends for attention in the news feed, and only a limited percentage sees content posted by followers due to its algorithm. Like other social media platforms, Facebook may be utilized sometimes to spread misinformation and disinformation on health issues. Subjects with lower emotional intelligence and high school or less education are likelier to fall for fake news on the platform. Therefore, in recent years, social networks have implemented several AI-powered tools to detect and remove false or misleading health information and to promote accurate information from trusted sources [7, 23].

X (former: Twitter) is an online social media and networking service allowing users to post short messages (microblogging) called X posts or *tweets* of up to 280 characters. It is a popular platform for sharing news, opinions, discussions, ideas, and updates in real-time, connecting with others who share similar interests, engaging in public conversations on current events or other topics, and staying up-to-date with the latest news and trends. X users were formerly called *tweeps* or *twitterati*. They can follow others to notice their X posts in the home feed. The interactions include reposts (previously named *retweets*), *likes*, *replies*, and *mentions* in X posts, including usernames preceded by the @ symbol and *direct messages*. Hashtags (*#* symbol followed by a word or phrase) are usually used to categorize tweets and to make them more discoverable. Promoting products and services is also possible. In 2023, people spent about 4.5 h/month on Twitter [4]. This platform uses AI to detect and filter spam or abusive posts and promote relevant content. Twitter is increasingly used to sustain allergy management [8]. Patients share information, seek support and connect with others, while many individual HCPs, professional organizations and support groups engage with them, share accurate information, and provide resources and support for different allergies. Hospitals and allergy clinics may use this network to distribute news and updates about their services for informative purposes. Various accounts and hashtags are dedicated to discussing allergies and providing information, resources, and support for those with allergies. Moreover, the X platform allows easy, quick updates and real-time engagement with hashtags and chats, is helpful with live events, and can be very fast-paced in content [8, 10, 12].

Allergies and asthma are commonly discussed on the X platform by clinicians, patients, and the interested public, including caretakers and various (patient) organizations. Although the online analytic tool Symplur (Part of Real Chemistry) is more frequently used to extract and analyze data related to specific hashtags from this social media network, the accuracy of the information on a particular profile online is only sometimes verifiable. Moreover, objective scores such as the HONcode (a Health On the Net certification) and DISCERN scores (an instrument designed to measure the quality of written health information) are not disease-specific. Highly shared X posts and links on the X platform are only sometimes a good source of information on medical topics and may facilitate the spread of disinformation. Therefore, and because disinformation can penetrate deeper and faster than evidence-based truth, healthcare professionals and medical organizations need to play an active role in providing reliable health information on the platform X. A thorough assessment of ongoing microblogging conversations may support HCPs and organizations in the efficient dissemination of accurate content and practical updates regarding their practice [24].

18.3.2 Image-Based Social Media

Instagram and Pinterest mainly represent image-based social media. Static digital images are commonly stored and distributed in popular file formats on social media, including JPEG (Joint Photographic Experts Group), PNG (Portable Network Graphics), and GIF (Graphics Interchange Format), among others.

Instagram is a social medium that allows users to share photos and videos, follow others, and engage with content through *likes*, *comments*, and *direct messaging*. It is mainly a visual platform focusing on good-quality photos and videos. Users can edit visual posts with stickers, filters, and other creative tools. Commonly used for photos related to personal and social purposes, it also offers features such as *stories* (temporary photos and short videos), *reels* (short-form videos), and *Instagram TV* (IGTV long-form videos) for more engaging and dynamic content. Influencers also use it to promote products and services. In 2023, people spent almost 16 h/month on Instagram [4]. Its AI provides personalized user recommendations based on image and video recognition and aims to detect and block inappropriate content [25–27]. Instagram may be used to support allergy patients in various ways. Many patients connect for similar experiences and to share resources and information on managing their allergies. Many accounts are dedicated to different types of allergies, where users can find information about allergy-friendly foods, products, and lifestyle tips. In addition, some allergy organizations, advocacy groups, HCPs, and allergy journals utilize this channel to provide visual information and educational resources. Allergy clinics and hospitals may use it to share photos and videos of their services, staff, and facilities, promote safe choices, and provide updates on news and events. Hashtags related to specific topics help find relevant content [12, 24, 28]. Unfortunately, some Instagram posts promote products or services unsupported by scientific guidelines, and health misinformation may quickly be disseminated on the platform. Therefore, further research is needed into its use as an intervention tool for ethical issues, patient education, and to reduce stigmatization. In addition, it is essential to highlight the opportunities for HCPs to promote online evidence-based approaches, including self-management pieces of advice [29–31].

Pinterest is a bookmarking-type network enabling individuals and organizations to discover, share, save, comment, and organize visual content, mainly images, related to their interests and projects, emphasizing inspirational imagery, new ideas, and valuable and creative information. *Pins* are visual bookmarks that users, referred to as *pinners*, can save to their personalized collections called *boards* themed around specific topics. An additional visual search tool represented by *Pinterest Lens* may be utilized for online searches using images instead of keywords. When saving a *pin*, it links to the original online source, allowing other users to discover and save it [32]. In 2023, people spent almost 2 h/month on Pinterest [4]. Pinterest is not explicitly designed to support patients and may not have as much allergy content as other social media networks. Nevertheless, some HCPs and patient organizations use Pinterest to share content related to specific health conditions with patients and their followers, such as educational photos, pictograms, infographics, and even short videos. Patients may use Pinterest to curate visual information on allergy-friendly products and food recipes, home remedies, and tips for managing allergies. However, some of these are not posted by HCPs or professional organizations and may be risky, not regulated or adequately tested [33, 34]. Informative and advocacy pins dominate the landscape of posts related to allergy and dermatology. However, more research is needed to assess how social media users discuss health through sharing visual content online and how health professionals can more effectively communicate using image-sharing social media [35].

18.3.3   Video-Based Social Media Platforms

The main representatives of video-based social media are YouTube and TikTok. Frequently used video formats on these social media are MP4 (Moving Picture Experts Group-4) and MOV (QuickTime Movie) [55].

YouTube is a social media platform utilized mainly for entertainment visual content, with users (*YouTubers*) discovering and sharing various types of videos. In 2023, people spent about 28 h/month on YouTube [4]. It is popular among teenagers with allergies. Trends detected using YouTube may notice geographic hot spots and treatment strategies for atopic disorders [22, 36]. In recent years, YouTube has become a recognized source of medical information for healthcare consumers. However, there are potential dangers as videos may contain non-scientific, misleading, or even harmful information. A formal analysis of YouTube videos found that the medical information presented on this online platform was heterogeneous, with room for improvement [37]. For example, only a few selected YouTube videos on allergic rhinitis and asthma can be used as a source of accurate information for patient education. In addition, only some videos reflect correct nasal spray or asthma inhaler use [38, 39]. Moreover, many videos are below acceptable medical quality standards regarding atopic dermatitis and anaphylaxis [37, 40]. Because subjective and anecdotal content may be overrepresented, and viewers do not distinguish between high- and low-quality videos, valid and reliable instruments to help standardize evaluations of YouTube-based medical videos covering a variety of subjects, including asthma and allergy are needed, such as the Medical Quality Video Evaluation Tool (MQ-VET) [41]. There is a need for high-quality, evidence-based, educational videos on allergies from HCPs and professional medical organizations [42], such as the appealing animated infographic entitled "EAACI explains food allergy" [43].

Ideally, allergic patients should be supported via hosted channels and videos providing accurate information on allergies, including tips for dealing with symptoms, nutritional approaches to atopic diseases, and management of allergic and atopic disorders, including new treatments [44–46]. By avoiding videos uploaded by individual users who were not HCPs or some for-profit companies, there is an increased chance of finding pertinent health information on YouTube. Many HCPs and professional organizations share educational videos about allergies and treatments on YouTube. It is essential to consider more videos describing patients' personal experiences and engaging, concise, easy-to-understand video content to reach more patients.

TikTok is a social media platform based on short-form videos or *TikToks* with many tools and effects, usually related to fun and interacting with others through *comments*, *likes*, and *shares*. It is popular with teenagers and young adult users (*TikTokers*) and utilizes AI to power its content recommendation algorithm based on interests, activity, and viewing history. In 2023, people spent 34 h/month on this platform [3]. Although some HCPs and organizations have started using TikTok to share health information and engage with patients, there are significant concerns about the accuracy and reliability of other health information content shared on the network. Some TikTok accounts are specifically dedicated to sharing allergy-related content, such as allergy-friendly recipes, tips for managing allergies, and discussions about living with allergies. Health information videos may be classified as educational, personal, or product/treatment-related. Allergists should be aware that especially adolescents may use TikTok to gather information about allergic and atopic disorders and post their personal experiences; therefore, they should prioritize appropriate education in this patient group due to the generally low-quality scientific content of such posts [47, 48].

The allergy community should be vigilant of misinformation regarding approved and safe allergy drugs and actively counteract it with evidence-based advice [49]. Although TikTok is a powerful tool for information distribution, the educational value of health-related videos entered public attention because of scientific misunderstandings [49]. Teenagers are a particularly susceptible group that needs to be informed of the risks associated with videos related to life-threatening challenges, such as those suggesting the misuse of over-the-counter-medication such as diphenhydramine [50]. TikTok is a far-reaching opportunity for HCPs to address allergies, and specialists should know that multiple interrelated conditions are required to produce an influential account on this platform [51]. Few allergists already use TikTok for high-quality allergy information, explanatory reactions, and comments to different posts from young TikTokers [47]. Moreover, using TikTok to display health journeys can facilitate engagement by patients, family members, and loved ones interested in information about challenging conditions [52].

18.3.4   Professional and Forum-Style Networking Platforms

LinkedIn is a professional networking platform that allows users to share personal updates and work-related content. The tool supports business networking, professional development, and the search for job opportunities. It is not commonly used to support allergy patients. However, some allergists and organizations may use it to connect with other professionals in the healthcare industry, share news and updates, and promote their services for patients [7, 53].

Reddit is a social media platform structured as a forum-style discussion website featuring a collection of topic-based mini-communities called *subreddits* (with unique URLs and names beginning with r/) where users can submit links, texts/discussion posts, images, and videos to their chosen *subreddits*, and other users can upvote or downvote them based on their relevance, quality, or popularity. It focuses on sharing information and fostering discussions around various issues, from news to personal interests. Registered users (*redditors*) have a social media karma defined by their net upvote score. While Reddit is not specifically designed for patients, it has subreddits dedicated to health conditions, including allergies, where patients can connect, share information, and provide support. However, it is essential to note that the information on Reddit may not always be accurate or reliable, so patients should exercise caution and consult their HCPs for medical advice [54, 55].

18.3.5 Other Social Networking Services

Snapchat is a multimedia messaging service that may be considered a social media for sharing and receiving spontaneous, ephemeral disappearing visual content and messages and for exploring various creative and entertaining posts. Its core feature is the ability to send *snaps*, which are photos or videos customizable with text, stickers, and other effects using filters and lenses. In early 2023, Snapchat launched *My AI*, a custom chatbot offering users access to a mobile version of the AI chatbot ChatGPT. Snapchat is not usually used for patient or healthcare-related purposes, being primarily a social media for informal communication with friends. However, some healthcare organizations may use Snapchat to reach youth audiences or share health education or awareness content creatively and engagingly [56]. In addition, young allergic patients may use Snapchat to connect with others with similar conditions and share experiences or tips. A study on American adolescents recruited from regularly scheduled asthma clinic appointments in 2016 revealed that 90% used social media, with Snapchat and Instagram being the most frequently endorsed. Some expressed the desire to obtain general asthma knowledge, including asthma-related news and symptom management tips, via social media posts [57].

Tumblr is a hybrid website structured as a mycelial-like network, depicted by features of visual social media and, in other regards, similar to conventional blogs. This highly customizable microblogging platform shares photos, audio and video content, links, quotes, and text. Tumblr short-form blogs may be followed via the dashboard. However, each has its own RSS (*Really Simple Syndication*) feed, similar to other internet blogs, and interaction between users involves functions such as *reblog, share, reply,* and *like.* Young patients may use Tumblr to share health-related content and interact with others. Since Tumblr is a general-purpose social media not specifically focused on health or medical topics, it is less used for this purpose [58–60]. While Tumblr allows audio content, other platforms like X and Facebook are more frequently used to share links to podcasts and promote social audio [61–64].

18.4 Communication with Allergic Patients in the Social Media Era

In digital times, communication with allergic patients and their caregivers is an important topic, as social media networks have become increasingly popular for rapidly sharing health-related information and seeking support from online communities. It should start by recalling that as many as eight out of ten Internet users access health information online, and about three-quarters of patients with chronic illnesses are influenced by online information in making decisions for their condition. Moreover, patients and physicians have different perceptions of social media for health care, mainly due to miscommunication [63]. Nevertheless, social media can act as a community and support network, promoting information-seeking behaviors and enabling health data access, allowing patients to assess information on appropriate care. HCPs must be cognizant of several factors for effective communication with allergic patients on social media. These include using clear, concise language with visual aids to provide individualized and up-to-date information. In addition, by sharing accurate resources and information to help patients manage their allergies, such as educational materials and support groups, HCPs may help patients feel more connected, informed, and able to use practical tools and strategies for better disease management. HCPs should also monitor social media platforms for patients' concerns, respect their privacy, and encourage them to seek medical advice from qualified personnel, including disclaimers [12, 64, 65].

The time is now to combine traditional methods of information dissemination with communication on social media. However, the main limitation of social media regarding medical purposes is content reliability; therefore, it is fundamental for allergists to engage in online networking and tackle medical misinformation related to their practice [12, 66]. With a world of information at their fingertips, patients seek advice through social media, but the information needs to be constantly updated, corrected, or completed. Besides inaccurate information, social media's potential as an unfavorable health mediator may also be related to personalization algorithms of social platforms that can polarize available information through "recommended" or "suggested" content. The way information spreads on these online networks does not reflect the accuracy of evidence-based medicine and clinical guidelines. Information overload on social media and the possibility of inaccuracy represent challenges when validating information. HCPs need to be aware of the multiple cognitive biases that can affect communication with patients on social media and negatively impact medical decision-making to put effort into counteracting them. They can actively interrogate biases and assumptions and be empathetic and open-minded to others' experiences and perspectives. Moreover, the risks associated with harmful or incorrect advice on social media from non-professional users add to concerns regarding patient confidentiality and privacy breaches. In a worst-case scenario, wrong advice spread on social media may even prevent patients from seeking appropriate medical care. Allergists should discuss these negative influences of health-related online content with their patients and consider integrating social media into their clinical practice [12, 66–68].

The social media landscape for professional organizations is also constantly evolving and expanding. For example, many allergy associations and societies have social media accounts to post evidence-based and up-to-date information for patients and HCPs. In the last 5 years, the European Academy of Allergy and Clinical Immunology (EAACI), an association of clinicians, researchers, and allied health professionals dedicated to improving the health of people affected by allergic diseases, held a distinguished position between large professional allergy organizations by having active accounts on the most popular social media platforms: Facebook, Instagram, Twitter, YouTube, LinkedIn and Pinterest. In addition, EAACI experts developed a series of interactive resources that may adequately assist and inform patients and their families about allergic diseases and asthma. The academy also partners with patient organizations using their social media channels to communicate directly with patients worldwide [69].

18.5   Practical Guidelines When Using Social Media in the Allergy Care Setting

Basic rules and core guiding principles when using social media by HCPs were suggested in the last decade as practical guidelines (Fig. 18.1). HCPs should be ethical and vigilant in respecting social media networking rules while complying with legal restrictions and obligations. Patient privacy, confidentiality, and data protection standards should always be respected. At the same time, freedom of expression should be granted, avoiding non-inclusive, disrespectful, stigmatizing, hateful or discriminatory language in postings, and any other type of inappropriate, inaccurate, or illegal content. It is important to respect copyright and intellectual property while combating all forms of information disorder, including misinterpreting non-peer-reviewed data. HCPs should post in their capacity, being professional, objective, and unbiased while staying authentic and credible without excessive self-disclosure. They should post trusted, verified, updated, evidence-based content

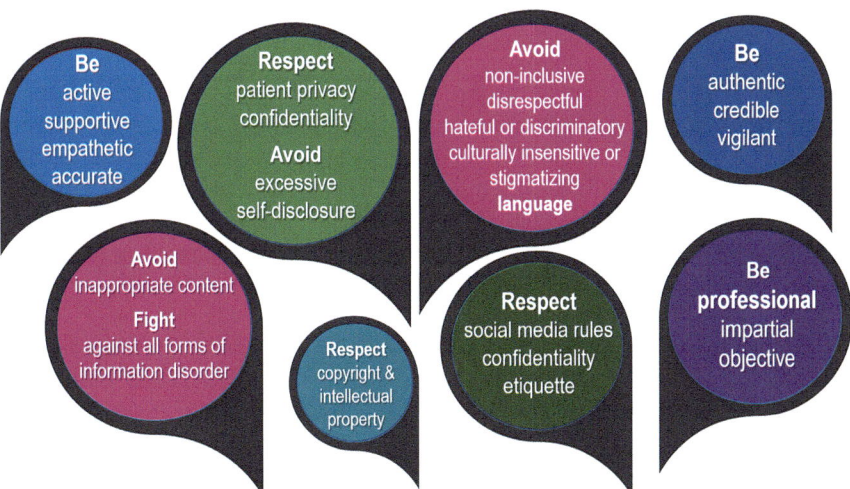

Fig. 18.1 General practical guidelines when using social media by HCPs. (Adapted from [64, 69–72])

without blurring professional and social boundaries. Other basic principles are being active, accurate, and supportive, creating constantly useful, sharing wisely, reacting timely, and differentiating opinions from facts. Complying with advertising regulations by clearly labeling sponsored content or advertisements is also essential. Moreover, everyone must always remember that content posted online is usually permanent. Further, HCPs should act responsibly on social media to avoid possible negative consequences concerning accepted standards of medical practice [8, 64, 70, 71].

Conversely, all social media users must understand that online content is not necessarily comprehensive, complete, accurate, suitable, valid, optimal, cognizant, constant, or available. Moreover, being culturally sensitive, empathetic, respectful, and kind does not mean that HCPs should accept requests for specific medical advice because content on social media platforms is not intended nor recommended as an alternative, substitute, or influencing factor for professional medical advice, diagnosis, or treatment, in any way and under no circumstances [72].

18.6 Tips and Tactics for a Social Media Approach to Patient-Centered Care

Developing a patient-centered approach to online social networks involves several tips and tactics. However, no universally recommended social media plan for such an approach exists. When considering digital forms of information therapy by "prescribing" the right information to the right patient at the right time, HCPs must provide trustworthy resources and create valuable content that educates, informs, and encourages patients, being mindful of their privacy and confidentiality and empowering them to take an active part of their disease management. HCPs build their social media strategy by choosing the best channels and optimizing their profiles according to the targeted patients, the content intended to be created, and online suggestions and opinions. The central focus is on providing accurate health information by regularly sharing valuable content in a practical, compact and credible manner, with hashtags and visual impacts such as images, infographics, Graphics Interchange Formats or GIFs, and short videos [18, 73, 74].

HCPs must act professionally, honestly and with good judgment in their communications, and need to practice social media detection and listening to online patient voices from posts, comments, conversations or chats relevant to allergy, patient feedback on clinical practice and allergy services, tracking and understanding patients' opinions and reactions to health issues, unreported health trends form specific diseases (e.g., pollen allergies), by monitoring dedicated accounts, keywords, and hashtags or using patient surveys on social media. They should regularly seek opportunities to collaborate, ensure an interactive approach, and create opportunities for an environment of networked care to complement the role of face-to-face patient education and information [74, 75].

18.7 Relationship Between Patients and Social Media

The association between HCPs and allergic patients on social media changed along-side the progress of these online platforms. The *informational value* of social net-working for disease management includes promoting access to valid science-based information to patients by offering high-quality, easy-to-understand, reliable data and fighting the different forms of information disorder. In addition, patients pro-vide valuable information by expressing their *feelings* with various sentiment sig-nals, sharing *experiences* and voicing *perspectives* related to allergy management. Health-related interventions on social media are therefore significant to help empower patients through information and education, via support groups and non-profit patient organizations for advocacy, and by initiating and participating in microblogging campaigns (e.g., #ContinuousAllergyAwareness with ribbon for support on Twitter) [76–79].

Potential negative psychosocial impacts, especially in young persons and sensi-tive individuals using social media, include falsifying age and identity, cyberbully-ing (online actions to deliberately produce harassment, intimidation, threatening, denigration and insults, impersonation, or public humiliation), and cyberostracism (online intentionally marginalization, exclusion, discrimination, or socially rejec-tion). Cyberbullying can be more damaging than traditional bullying because of online accessibility and anonymity, privacy issues such as identity theft, sharing psychosocial information that others may misuse, and re-sharing pirated informa-tion. Moreover, excessive gamification (application of game elements and princi-ples in non-game contexts to enhance overall user experience) may be associated with addictive behaviors, neglect of real-world responsibilities, and decreased offline social interactions. It can exacerbate anxiety and self-esteem, while unneces-sary glamorization may induce shallow engagement and superficiality [78]. Asthma and food allergy-related cyberbullying behaviors include being teased about the disease, being made fun of or called mean names due to it, being threatened with allergen exposure, and other online actions to make others dislike patients, mainly due to preventive measures and carrying medication [77, 79].

Bullying on social media can have serious consequences, such as negative impacts on self-esteem and social relationships. Online social bullying negatively impacts young patients with asthma. Mainly when associated with depression, psy-chological stress triggers on socializing online platforms may be of particular con-cern as risk factors for exacerbations [80–82]. Allergists should recognize and address such problems; therefore, bullying-specific questions and algorithms are needed to assist in identifying and addressing bullying in cyberspace for young patients [77]. Moreover, it is vital to create safe spaces on social media, encourage individuals to report and block any bullying behaviors encountered online, engage in bystander interventions and involve the authorities, parents and the school because confrontations are not usually productive. Another intervention is using specific hashtags to stimulate reports (e.g., #StopAllergyBullying on Twitter) [82, 83].

18.8   Fighting Against All Forms of Information Disorder on Social Media

Understanding the role of social media in spreading unreliable, poor-quality health-related information and its magnitude during health emergencies, humanitarian crises pandemics, represents a first step in mitigating its harmful effects, such as wrong interpretation of scientific knowledge, polarization of opinions, intensifying fear and reduced access to proper health care. Many social media platforms have a global reach. Because they are not bound to journalistic standards, relevant legislation and deontological ethics the way professional media is supposed to be, they have an essential role in the origination and development of the *information disorder*. In addition, some online users or accounts, such as automated (bots) and human (trolls), have augmentation roles. Due to the volume and velocity of information on social media, it has the characteristics of an infodemic. Therefore, infoveillance is needed to monitor and analyze such digital data [84–87].

Information disorder applies to all cases of inaccurate information and is not limited to a particular topic. There are many landscapes related to health, such as textual representation, linguistic-stylistic, linguistic-emotional, linguistic-medical, propagation-network, and user-profile features [87]. Different forms of information disorder are presented in Table 18.2, including misinformation, misconception, disinformation, fake news, rumors, conspiracy theories, and malinformation [86–89]. All these have harmful outcomes if not recognized and adequately addressed.

Because information shared on social media is often presented in pieces that lack perspective or context, the conjunction between social media and *cognitive biases* can amplify the harmful effects of information disorder. Many cognitive biases can

Table 18.2 Different categories of the information disorder [86–89]

Forms/aspects	Definition and comments
Misinformation	Inaccurate information with false connections and misleading content that is spread unintentionally and may be the result of a mistake or a lack of understanding of the facts
Misconception	Belief or idea not based on accurate or complete information, often a result of a lack of knowledge or misunderstanding of a particular topic
Disinformation	Intentionally spread of false or misleading information for deceiving or manipulating purposes, usually with a specific agenda or motive
Fake news	Type of fabricated disinformation to have a significant impact on public opinion and beliefs, presented as legitimate news, in the form of an entirely fictional story or distorted actual news
Rumors	Unverified or unofficial pieces of information or stories without credible sources or evidence
Conspiracy theories	Explanations or narratives that propose secret plots or hidden agendas
Malinformation	True information that is shared with the intention of causing harm, spreading of negative stories or sharing of private or sensitive information, some leaks, harassment, and hate speech

influence how people process and understand information, making them susceptible to misconceptions, misinformation, disinformation, and the propagation of fake news. Numerous significant biases are related to the processing of information, including *confirmation bias* (tendency to search and prioritize information that confirms previous beliefs regardless of the strength of contradictory evidence), *availability bias* (tendency to rely on easily accessible information decisions), *anchoring bias* (over-reliance on initial information, even if it is inaccurate), and *recency bias* (tendency to place more emphasis on most recent experiences or knowledge). Further, the misinformation effect is a *memory bias* related to misleading details after an event that can lead to distortions in the memory of that event. The *bandwagon effect* is a social cognitive bias involved in the rapid spread and acceptance of false information. It describes the tendency to adopt beliefs or behaviors simply because others embrace them. Since social media supports networking and interest groups, the *group attribution error* must be mentioned. It describes the tendency to overgeneralize how a group will behave based on interacting with only one person from that group. Other cognitive biases that should be mentioned include the *Dunning-Kruger* effect, related *ultracrepidarianism* behavior, and *overconfidence* bias. On the other hand, social cognition biases need to be considered, like the *false consensus effect*, describing individuals' tendency to overestimate the extent to which others share their beliefs, behaviors, attitudes, or preferences [66, 90, 91].

The mentioned examples of skewed perception represent only a part of the scientifically described biases. However, understanding them can help individuals become more critical information consumers and develop strategies to mitigate their impact.

Medical information disorder is still a complex, unresolved issue. The combat against it has several general action rules, such as engagement on social media using fact-checks, accurate, and up-to-date information from trusted sources to educate patients and their families, and awareness of the information landscape while considering the controversies and debates [92].

All HCPs are responsible for this fight, and collaboration between them and various organizations is essential. In addition, AI approaches to detect fake news automatically still need to be more capable of overcoming the challenge of crafting content to closely mimic truth, making it easier for AI to ascertain its veracity with supplementary information from external human sources. It is also essential to remember that AI techniques like machine learning and deep learning may also create and disseminate false and misleading posts. AI may also be used to create a dangerous form of disinformation, the deepfakes, namely highly realistic synthetically generated image, video, or audio representations. To be more treacherous, people who easily perceive the deepfakes as accurate are likelier to share them on social media [93–95].

Allergists must fight all aspects of allergy-related information disorder generated from not understanding the differences between *scientific evidence, anecdotes* (powerful and emotional stories with no proof of being true or highly subjected to multiple forms of bias) and *pseudoscience* (beliefs or practices mistakenly regarded as being based on scientific methods). When patients access inaccurate information, they can make harmful decisions; therefore, HCPs must educate others to discern and identify the various planes of the information disorder, blunt their effects and prevent their spread [96, 97].

Moreover, in the realm of social media, human influencers may play a critical role in shaping information disorder, both positively and negatively. These individuals, characterized by their substantial digital footprint and consumer engagement, wield significant power in disseminating content and shaping public opinion [98]. It is crucial to identify influencers renowned for their expertise in specific fields. Top medical professionals, including medical doctors, nurse practitioners, and informed responsible patients, may assume influential roles, amplifying their voices within specific domains. Their influence holds significant potential for positively impacting healthcare outcomes. Health e-mavens (individuals actively engaged in online health information-seeking and sharing) epitomize this vital category of influencers who combine expertise with significant online social influence [99]. Serving as essential health promotion practitioners, this group can enlist and galvanize various online health intervention contributors and campaigns [100]. Most influential voices originate from developed nations, primarily exhibiting higher social and academic influence. However, there is a pressing need for broader participation, emphasizing diversity, equity, and inclusion to ensure the dissemination of quality and relevant information [98–100].

18.9   Conclusions

In recent years, social media use has transformed healthcare communication, offering new pathways for patient engagement and disease management. Allergy HCPs can use such online networks to support patients in various ways. The ever-evolving landscape of online social networks and the patients' perspectives are complex and fluid. Popular socializing and microblogging social media are valuable platforms for patient education, permitting the creation and sharing of diverse, concise, and targeted information. Image-based social media can be used for educational purposes, allowing the creation and sharing of visually appealing and engaging content. Video-based social media represent useful platforms for health education, as they enable the creation and sharing of videos that can provide in-depth information and engage users in a more immersive way or short-form videos that can provide information in fun and engaging ways.

By leveraging the power of such online networks, HCPs and organizations can reach a large and diverse audience, potentially influencing disease management, behaviors, and lifestyles. Patients need to be supported to develop skills for selecting and comprehending accurate information available on social media. Moreover, HCPs need to be strategic and proactive when communicating with allergic patients on social media in their continuous effort to counteract the unwanted effects of all forms of online information disorder. Practical guidelines and the relationship between social media and allergy management must be emphasized from the patient's perspective. By providing a roadmap for navigating and integrating social media into allergic disease management, HCPs may be empowered to use the potential of social media platforms to improve patient care and outcomes.

Disclosure F.D. Popescu reports serving as European Academy of Allergology and Clinical Immunology (EAACI) Social Media Editor 2019–2022 and oral presentation with no financial support at the EAACI Digital Congress 2020. FDP declares no conflict of interest. S. Dramburg reports serving as EAACI Scientific Communication Committee Chair 2020–2022. SD declares no conflict of interest.

References

1. Matricardi PM, Dramburg S, Alvarez-Perea A, Antolín-Amérigo D, Apfelbacher C, Atanaskovic-Markovic M, Berger U, Blaiss MS, Blank S, Boni E, Bonini M, Bousquet J, Brockow K, Buters J, Cardona V, Caubet JC, Cavkaytar Ö, Elliott T, Esteban-Gorgojo I, Fonseca JA, Gardner J, Gevaert P, Ghiordanescu I, Hellings P, Hoffmann-Sommergruber K, Fusun Kalpaklioglu A, Marmouz F, Meijide Calderón Á, Mösges R, Nakonechna A, Ollert M, Oteros J, Pajno G, Panaitescu C, Perez-Formigo D, Pfaar O, Pitsios C, Rudenko M, Ryan D, Sánchez-García S, Shih J, Tripodi S, Van der Poel LA, van Os-Medendorp H, Varricchi G, Wittmann J, Worm M, Agache I. The role of mobile health technologies in allergy care: an EAACI position paper. Allergy. 2020;75(2):259–72. https://doi.org/10.1111/all.13953.
2. Dramburg S, Walter U, Becker S, Casper I, Röseler S, Schareina A, Wrede H, Klimek L. Telemedicine in allergology: practical aspects: a position paper of the Association of German Allergists (AeDA). Allergo J Int. 2021;30(4):119–29. https://doi.org/10.1007/s40629-021-00167-5.
3. Kemp S. DataReportal. Digital 2024: global overview report. 2024. https://datareportal.com/reports/digital-2024-global-overview-report. Accessed 4 Apr 2024.
4. Kemp S. DataReportal. Digital 2024 deep-dive: how much time do we spend on social media? https://datareportal.com/reports/digital-2024-deep-dive-the-time-we-spend-on-social-media. Accessed 4 Apr 2024.
5. Antolín-Amérigo D, Popescu FD, Alvarez-Perea A. Patient-friendly HIT tools and the advent of crowdsourcing clinical trials. In: Hellings PW, Agache I, editors. Implementing precision medicine in best practices of chronic AirwayDiseases. London: Elsevier; 2018. p. 135–44.
6. Cherrez-Ojeda I, Vanegas E, Cherrez A, Felix M, Weller K, Magerl M, Maurer RR, Mata VL, Kasperska-Zajac A, Sikora A, Fomina D, Kovalkova E, Godse K, Rao ND, Khoshkhui M, Rastgoo S, Criado RF, Abuzakouk M, Grandon D, Van Doorn MBA, Oliveira Rodrigues Valle S, De Souza Lima EM, Thomsen SF, Ramón GD, Matos Benavides EE, Bauer A, Giménez-Arnau AM, Kocatürk E, Guillet C, Larco JI, Zhao ZT, Makris M, Ritchie C, Xepapadaki P, Ensina LF, Cherrez S, Maurer M. How are patients with chronic urticaria interested in using information and communication technologies to guide their healthcare? A UCARE study. World Allergy Organ J. 2021;14(6):100542. https://doi.org/10.1016/j.waojou.2021.100542.
7. Dimov V, Eidelman F. Utilizing social networks, blogging and YouTube in allergy and immunology practices. Expert Rev Clin Immunol. 2015;11(10):1065–8. https://doi.org/10.1586/1744666X.2015.1065731.
8. Dimov V, Gonzalez-Estrada A, Eidelman F. Social media and allergy. Curr Allergy Asthma Rep. 2018;18(12):76. https://doi.org/10.1007/s11882-018-0822-6.
9. Kjærulff EM, Andersen TH, Kingod N, Nexø MA. When people with chronic conditions turn to peers on social media to obtain and share information: systematic review of the implications for relationships with health care professionals. J Med Internet Res. 2023;25:e41156. https://doi.org/10.2196/41156.

10. Applebaum MA, Lawson EF, von Scheven E. Perception of transition readiness and preferences for use of technology in transition programs: teens' ideas for the future. Int J Adolesc Med Health. 2013;25(2):119–25. https://doi.org/10.1515/ijamh-2013-0019.

11. Khaleva E, Knibb R, DunnGalvin A, Vazquez-Ortiz M, Comberiati P, Alviani C, Garriga-Baraut T, Gowland MH, Gore C, Angier E, Blumchen K, Duca B, Hox V, Jensen B, Mortz CG, Pite H, Pfaar O, Santos AF, Sanchez-Garcia S, Timmermans F, Roberts G. Perceptions of adolescents and young adults with allergy and/or asthma and their parents on EAACI guideline recommendations about transitional care: a European survey. Allergy. 2022;77(4):1094–104. https://doi.org/10.1111/all.15109.

12. Alvarez-Perea A, Dimov V, Popescu FD, Zubeldia JM. The applications of eHealth technologies in the management of asthma and allergic diseases. Clin Transl Allergy. 2021;11(7):e12061. https://doi.org/10.1002/clt2.12061.

13. Chirumamilla S, Gulati M. Patient education and engagement through social media. Curr Cardiol Rev. 2021;17(2):137–43. https://doi.org/10.2174/1573403X15666191120115107.

14. Charles-Smith LE, Reynolds TL, Cameron MA, Conway M, Lau EH, Olsen JM, Pavlin JA, Shigematsu M, Streichert LC, Suda KJ, Corley CD. Using social media for actionable disease surveillance and outbreak management: a systematic literature review. PLoS One. 2015;10(10):e0139701. https://doi.org/10.1371/journal.pone.0139701.

15. Kanchan S, Gaidhane A. Social media role and its impact on public health: a narrative review. Cureus. 2023;15(1):e33737. https://doi.org/10.7759/cureus.33737.

16. Leeman EJ, Loman L. Health literacy in adult patients with atopic dermatitis: a cross-sectional study. J Allergy Clin Immunol Glob. 2024;3(2):100218. https://doi.org/10.1016/j.jacig.2024.100218.

17. Tennant B, Stellefson M, Dodd V, Chaney B, Chaney D, Paige S, Alber J. eHealth literacy and Web 2.0 health information seeking behaviors among baby boomers and older adults. J Med Internet Res. 2015;17(3):e70. https://doi.org/10.2196/jmir.3992.

18. Chen J, Wang Y. Social media use for health purposes: systematic review. J Med Internet Res. 2021;23(5):e17917. https://doi.org/10.2196/17917.

19. Obar JA, Wildman SS. Social media definition and the governance challenge—an introduction to the special issue telecommunications policy. SSRN Electron J. 2015;39(9):745–50. https://doi.org/10.2139/ssrn.2663153.

20. Espino-Gaucin I, Rodríguez C, Ávila J, Soto J, Ruge C, Wagner R. Social networks and their role in current medicine: an indispensable tool for doctors. J Biosci Med. 2020;8:15–25. https://doi.org/10.4236/jbm.2020.88002.

21. Gaddy A, Topf J. Facebook groups can provide support for patients with rare diseases and reveal truths about the secret lives of patients. Kidney Int Rep. 2021;6(5):1205–7. https://doi.org/10.1016/j.ekir.2021.03.890.

22. Alvarez-Perea A, Cabrera-Freitag P, Fuentes-Aparicio V, Infante S, Zapatero L, Zubeldia JM. Social media as a tool for the management of food allergy in children. J Investig Allergol Clin Immunol. 2018;28(4):233–40. https://doi.org/10.18176/jiaci.0235.

23. Preston S, Anderson A, Robertson DJ, Shephard MP, Huhe N. Detecting fake news on Facebook: the role of emotional intelligence. PLoS One. 2021;16(3):e0246757. https://doi.org/10.1371/journal.pone.0246757.

24. Kaul V, Szakmany T, Peters JI, Stukus D, Sala KA, Dangayach N, Simpson SQ, Carroll CL. Quality of the discussion of asthma on twitter. J Asthma. 2022;59(2):325–32. https://doi.org/10.1080/02770903.2020.1847933.

25. Carpenter JP, Morrison SA, Craft M, Lee M. How and why are educators using Instagram? Teach Teach Educ. 2020;96:103149. https://doi.org/10.1016/j.tate.2020.103149.

26. Bhatia A, Gaur PS, Zimba O, Chatterjee T, Nikiphorou E, Gupta L. The untapped potential of Instagram to facilitate rheumatology academia. Clin Rheumatol. 2022;41(3):861–7. https://doi.org/10.1007/s10067-021-05947-6.

27. Faustino GPDS, Silva MOD, Almeida Filho AJ, Ferreira MA. Outline of a project for nursing health education on the Instagram social network. Rev Bras Enferm. 2023;76(2):e20220301. https://doi.org/10.1590/0034-7167-2022-0301.
28. Takao MMV, de Souza FS, Riccetto L, Evangelista-Poderoso R, Riccetto AGL, da Silva MTN. Pediatric allergy and immunology for patients and parents: challenges of developing website and social network during COVID-19 pandemic in Brazil. Rev Paul Pediatr. 2023;41:e2022032. https://doi.org/10.1590/1984-0462/2023/41/2022032.
29. Maurer M, Weller K, Magerl M, Maurer RR, Vanegas E, Felix M, Cherrez A, Mata VL, Kasperska-Zajac A, Sikora A, Fomina D, Kovalkova E, Godse K, Rao ND, Khoshkhui M, Rastgoo S, Criado RFJ, Abuzakouk M, Grandon D, van Doorn M, Valle SOR, de Souza Lima EM, Thomsen SF, Ramón GD, Matos Benavides EE, Bauer A, Giménez-Arnau AM, Kocatürk E, Guillet C, Ignacio Larco J, Zhao ZT, Makris M, Ritchie C, Xepapadaki P, Ensina LF, Cherrez S, Cherrez-Ojeda I. The usage, quality and relevance of information and communications technologies in patients with chronic urticaria: a UCARE study. World Allergy Organ J. 2020;13(11):100475. https://doi.org/10.1016/j.waojou.2020.100475.
30. Maspero S, Ebert C, Moser S, Zink A, Sichert P, Schielein M, Weis J, Ziehfreund S. The Potential of Instagram to reduce stigmatization of people with psoriasis: a randomized controlled pilot study. Acta Derm Venereol. 2023;103:adv3513. https://doi.org/10.2340/actadv.v103.3513.
31. Heineman B, Jewell M, Moran M, Bradley K, Spitzer KA, Lindenauer PK. Content analysis of promotional material for asthma-related products and therapies on Instagram. Allergy Asthma Clin Immunol. 2021;17(1):26. https://doi.org/10.1186/s13223-021-00528-3.
32. Whitsitt J, Mattis D, Hernandez M, Kollipara R, Dellavalle RP. Dermatology on Pinterest. Dermatol Online J. 2015;21(1):13030/qt7dj4267p.
33. Guidry JPD, Miller CA, Hayes R, Ksinan AJ, Carlyle KE, Fuemmeler BF. Reading, sharing, creating Pinterest recipes: parental engagement and feeding behaviors. Appetite. 2023;180:106287. https://doi.org/10.1016/j.appet.2022.106287.
34. Cheng X, Lin SY, Wang K, Hong YA, Zhao X, Gress D, Wojtusiak J, Cheskin LJ, Xue H. Healthfulness assessment of recipes shared on Pinterest: natural language processing and content analysis. J Med Internet Res. 2021;23(4):e25757. https://doi.org/10.2196/25757.
35. Fung IC, Blankenship EB, Ahweyevu JO, Cooper LK, Duke CH, Carswell SL, Jackson AM, Jenkins JC 3rd, Duncan EA, Liang H, Fu KW, Tse ZTH. Public health implications of image-based social media: a systematic review of Instagram, Pinterest, Tumblr, and Flickr. Perm J. 2020;24:18.307. https://doi.org/10.7812/TPP/18.307.
36. Hongler VNS, Navarini A, Brandt O, Goldust M, Mueller SM. Global trends in YouTube and Google search activity for psoriasis and atopic eczema: detecting geographic hot spots, blind spots and treatment strategies. Dermatol Ther. 2020;33(4):e13510. https://doi.org/10.1111/dth.13510.
37. Mueller SM, Hongler VNS, Jungo P, Cajacob L, Schwegler S, Steveling EH, Manjaly Thomas ZR, Fuchs O, Navarini A, Scherer K, Brandt O. Fiction, falsehoods, and few facts: cross-sectional study on the content-related quality of atopic eczema-related videos on YouTube. J Med Internet Res. 2020;22(4):e15599. https://doi.org/10.2196/15599.
38. Remvig CL, Diers CS, Meteran H, Thomsen SF, Sigsgaard T, Høj S, Meteran H. YouTube as a source of (mis)information on allergic rhinitis. Ann Allergy Asthma Immunol. 2022;129(5):612–7. https://doi.org/10.1016/j.anai.2022.06.031.
39. Diers CS, Remvig C, Meteran H, Thomsen SF, Sigsgaard T, Høj S, Meteran H. The usefulness of YouTube videos as a source of information in asthma. J Asthma. 2023;60(4):737–43. https://doi.org/10.1080/02770903.2022.2093218.
40. Carrillo-Martin I, Kallur L, Cuervo-Pardo L, Chavez J, Mahapatra SS, Mendiola-Jimenez J, Reddy K, Rammoha R, Mohn K, Gonzles-Estrada A, Iess S. 'What is anaphylaxis': a critical appraisal of the quality of anaphylaxis information on YouTube. J Allergy Clin Immunol. 2019;143:AB173. https://doi.org/10.1016/j.jaci.2018.12.530.

41. Guler MA, Aydın EO. Development and validation of a tool for evaluating YouTube-based medical videos. Ir J Med Sci. 2022;191(5):1985–90. https://doi.org/10.1007/s11845-021-02864-0.
42. Reddy K, Kearns M, Alvarez-Arango S, Carrillo-Martin I, Cuervo-Pardo N, Cuervo-Pardo L, Dimov V, Lang DM, Lopez-Alvarez S, Schroer B, Mohan K, Dula M, Zheng S, Kozinetz C, Gonzalez-Estrada A. YouTube and food allergy: an appraisal of the educational quality of information. Pediatr Allergy Immunol. 2018;29(4):410–6. https://doi.org/10.1111/pai.12885.
43. EAACI. EAACI explains food allergy. 2018. https://www.youtube.com/watch?v=iaQmGOYW5rg. Accessed 4 Apr 2024.
44. Høj S, Meteran H, Thomsen SF, Sigsgaard T, Meteran H. Nutritional treatment of atopic diseases according to YouTube videos. J Allergy Clin Immunol Pract. 2023;11(5):1552–3. https://doi.org/10.1016/j.jaip.2023.01.055.
45. Martin A, Thatiparthi A, Liu J, Wu JJ. Atopic dermatitis topical therapies: study of YouTube videos as a source of patient information. Cutis. 2021;108(3):139–41. https://doi.org/10.12788/cutis.0333.
46. Pithadia DJ, Reynolds KA, Lee EB, Wu JJ. Dupilumab for atopic dermatitis: what are patients learning on YouTube? J Dermatolog Treat. 2022;33(1):571–2. https://doi.org/10.1080/09546634.2020.1755418.
47. Oulee A, Ivanic M, Norden A, Javadi SS, Wu JJ. Atopic dermatitis on TikTok™: a cross-sectional study. Clin Exp Dermatol. 2022;47(11):2036–7. https://doi.org/10.1111/ced.15322.
48. Anastasio AT, Tabarestani TQ, Bagheri K, Bethell MA, Prado I, Taylor JR, Adams SB. A new trend in social media and medicine: the poor quality of videos related to ankle sprain exercises on TikTok. Foot Ankle Orthop. 2023;8(2):24730114231171117. https://doi.org/10.1177/24730114231171117.
49. Finnegan P, Murphy M, O'Connor C. #corticophobia: a review on online misinformation related to topical steroids. Clin Exp Dermatol. 2023;48(2):112–5. https://doi.org/10.1093/ced/llac019.
50. Elkhazeen A, Poulos C, Zhang X, Cavanaugh J, Cain M. A TikTok™ "Benadryl challenge" death-a case report and review of the literature. J Forensic Sci. 2023;68(1):339–42. https://doi.org/10.1111/1556-4029.15149.
51. Liu R, Yang T, Deng W, Liu X, Deng J. What drives the influence of health science communication accounts on TikTok? A fuzzy-set qualitative comparative analysis. Int J Environ Res Public Health. 2022;19(21):13815. https://doi.org/10.3390/ijerph192113815.
52. Basch CH, Hillyer GC, Yalamanchili B, Morris A. How TikTok is being used to help individuals cope with breast cancer: cross-sectional content analysis. JMIR Cancer. 2022;8(4):e42245. https://doi.org/10.2196/42245.
53. Wenner TA. Transitioning into professional practice with a LinkedIn assignment. J Nurs Educ. 2023;62(2):120. https://doi.org/10.3928/01484834-20221213-11.
54. Mahjoub H, Prabhu AV, Sikder S. What are ophthalmology patients asking online? An analysis of the eye triage subreddit. Clin Ophthalmol. 2020;14:3575–82. https://doi.org/10.2147/OPTH.S279607.
55. Dave AD, Zhu D. Ophthalmology inquiries on Reddit: what should physicians know? Clin Ophthalmol. 2022;16:2923–31. https://doi.org/10.2147/OPTH.S375822.
56. Kelly S. Snapchat rolls out chatbot powered by ChatGPT to all users | CNN Business. CNN; 2023. https://edition.cnn.com/2023/04/19/tech/snapchat-my-ai-bot-chatgpt/index.html. Accessed 4 Apr 2024.
57. Ramsey RR, Carmody JK, Holbein CE, Guilbert TW, Hommel KA. Examination of the uses, needs, and preferences for health technology use in adolescents with asthma. J Asthma. 2019;56(9):964–72. https://doi.org/10.1080/02770903.2018.1514048.
58. Duffy M. Microblogging: tumblr and pinterest. Am J Nurs. 2013;113(6):61–4. https://doi.org/10.1097/01.NAJ.0000431274.68030.90.

59. Bianchi M, Fabbricatore R, Caso D. Tumblr facts: antecedents of self-disclosure across different social networking sites. Eur J Investig Health Psychol Educ. 2022;12(9):1257–71. https://doi.org/10.3390/ejihpe12090087.
60. Hussain SA. Sharing visual narratives of diabetes on social media and its effects on mental health. Healthcare (Basel). 2022;10(9):1748. https://doi.org/10.3390/healthcare10091748.
61. Patrick MD, Stukus DR, Nuss KE. Using podcasts to deliver pediatric educational content: development and reach of PediaCast CME. Digit Health. 2019;5:2055207619834842. https://doi.org/10.1177/2055207619834842.
62. Kemp S. DataReportal. Digital 2023 Deep-Dive: Online Audio Captures More Of Our Attention. 2023. https://datareportal.com/reports/digital-2023-deep-dive-online-audio-captures-more-of-our-attention. Accessed 4 Apr 2024.
63. Forgie EME, Lai H, Cao B, Stroulia E, Greenshaw AJ, Goez H. Social media and the transformation of the physician-patient relationship: viewpoint. J Med Internet Res. 2021;23(12):e25230. https://doi.org/10.2196/25230.
64. Popescu FD. Basic rules when using #SocialMedia in the great #EAACI_Newsletter 50th issue! To be active on social media, create meaningful content & post new content frequently for maximum visibility! X/Twitter. 2018. https://twitter.com/FlorinDanPopesc/status/982565722474807296. Accessed 4 Apr 2024.
65. Dimov V, Gonzalez-Estrada A, Eidelman F. Social media and the allergy practice. Ann Allergy Asthma Immunol. 2016;116(6):484–90. https://doi.org/10.1016/j.anai.2016.01.021.
66. Stukus DR. Tackling medical misinformation in allergy and immunology practice. Expert Rev Clin Immunol. 2022;18(10):995–6. https://doi.org/10.1080/1744666X.2022.2108016.
67. Moorhead SA, Hazlett DE, Harrison L, Carroll JK, Irwin A, Hoving C. A new dimension of health care: systematic review of the uses, benefits, and limitations of social media for health communication. J Med Internet Res. 2013;15(4):e85. https://doi.org/10.2196/jmir.1933.
68. Anagnostou A, Lieberman J, Greenhawt M, Mack DP, Santos AF, Venter C, Stukus D, Turner PJ, Brough HA. The future of food allergy: challenging existing paradigms of clinical practice. Allergy. 2023;78(7):1847–65. https://doi.org/10.1111/all.15757.
69. EAACI. European Academy of Allergy and Clinical Immunology. Privacy notice. https://eaaci.org/privacy. Accessed 4 Apr 2024.
70. European Data Protection Board. Guidelines 8/2020 on the targeting of social media users Version 2.0. www.edpb.europa.eu/system/files/2021-04/edpb_guidelines_082020_on_the_targeting_of_social_media_users_en.pdf. Accessed 4 Apr 2024.
71. American Academy of Allergy, Asthma and Clinical Immunology. AAAAI social media guidelines. www.aaaai.org/Aaaai/media/MediaLibrary/PDF%20Documents/Global/Social-Media-Guidelines.pdf. Accessed 4 Apr 2024.
72. EAACI. European Academy of Allergy and Clinical Immunology. EAACI Social Media Disclaimer. https://www.eaaci.org/images/EAACI_Social_Media_Disclaimer.pdf. Accessed 4 Apr 2024.
73. Nickels AS, Wu AC, Stukus DR. Social media and the allergist: evidence supports increasing our engagement. J Allergy Clin Immunol Pract. 2018;6(1):313–4. https://doi.org/10.1016/j.jaip.2017.09.007.
74. Beveridge C. Strategy—how to use social media in healthcare: examples + tips 2022. https://blog.hootsuite.com/social-media-health-care. Accessed 4 Apr 2024.
75. Bornkessel A, Furberg R, Lefebvre RC. Social media: opportunities for quality improvement and lessons for providers-a networked model for patient-centered care through digital engagement. Curr Cardiol Rep. 2014;16(7):504. https://doi.org/10.1007/s11886-014-0504-5.
76. Popescu FD. Support #ContinuousAllergyAwareness twitter campaign by adding a nice #Allergy #Twibbon to your profile photo! X/Twitter. 2016. https://twitter.com/FlorinDanPopesc/status/796739043698450432. Accessed 4 Apr 2024.
77. Bingemann T, Herbert LJ, Young MC, Sicherer SH, Petty CR, Phipatanakul W, Bartnikas LM. Deficits and opportunities in allergists' approaches to food allergy-related bullying. J Allergy Clin Immunol Pract. 2020;8(1):343–5. https://doi.org/10.1016/j.jaip.2019.06.037.

78. Hadjipanayis A, Efstathiou E, Altorjai P, Stiris T, Valiulis A, Koletzko B, Fonseca H. Social media and children: what is the paediatrician's role? Eur J Pediatr. 2019;178(10):1605–12. https://doi.org/10.1007/s00431-019-03458-w.
79. Cooke F, Ramos A, Herbert L. Food allergy-related bullying among children and adolescents. J Pediatr Psychol. 2022;47(3):318–26. https://doi.org/10.1093/jpepsy/jsab099.
80. Gibson-Young L, Martinasek MP, Clutter M, Forrest J. Are students with asthma at increased risk for being a victim of bullying in school or cyberspace? Findings from the 2011 Florida youth risk behavior survey. J Sch Health. 2014;84(7):429–34. https://doi.org/10.1111/josh.12167.
81. D'Amato G, Liccardi G, Cecchi L, Pellegrino F, D'Amato M. Facebook: a new trigger for asthma? Lancet. 2010;376(9754):1740. https://doi.org/10.1016/S0140-6736(10)62135-6.
82. Charles R, Brand PLP, Gilchrist FJ, Wildhaber J, Carroll W. Why are children with asthma bullied? A risk factor analysis. Arch Dis Child. 2022;107(6):612–5. https://doi.org/10.1136/archdischild-2021-321641.
83. Popescu FD. #StopAllergyBullying #Respect #PatientVoices #ContinuousAllergyAwareness. Twitter. 2022. https://twitter.com/FlorinDanPopesc/status/1543942121794699264. Accessed 4 Apr 2024.
84. Chiou H, Voegeli C, Wilhelm E, Kolis J, Brookmeyer K, Prybylski D. The future of Infodemic surveillance as public health surveillance. Emerg Infect Dis. 2022;28(13):S121–8. https://doi.org/10.3201/eid2813.220696.
85. Giachanou A, Zhang X, Barrón-Cedeño A, Koltsova O, Rosso P. Online information disorder: fake news, bots and trolls. Int J Data Sci Anal. 2022;13(4):265–9. https://doi.org/10.1007/s41060-022-00325-0.
86. Muhammed TS, Mathew SK. The disaster of misinformation: a review of research in social media. Int J Data Sci Anal. 2022;13(4):271–85. https://doi.org/10.1007/s41060-022-00311-6.
87. WHO Press release. Infodemics and misinformation negatively affect people's health behaviours, new WHO review finds. 2022. www.who.int/europe/news/item/01-09-2022-infodemics-and-misinformation-negatively-affect-people-s-health-behaviours%2D%2Dnew-who-review-finds. Accessed 4 Apr 2024.
88. Di Sotto S, Viviani M. Health misinformation detection in the social web: an overview and a data science approach. Int J Environ Res Public Health. 2022;19(4):2173. https://doi.org/10.3390/ijerph19042173.
89. Gaeta A, Loia V, Lomasto L, Orciuoli F. A novel approach based on rough set theory for analyzing information disorder. Appl Intell (Dordr). 2022:1–22. https://doi.org/10.1007/s10489-022-04283-9.
90. Doherty TS, Carroll AE. Believing in overcoming cognitive biases. AMA J Ethics. 2020;22(9):E773–8. https://doi.org/10.1001/amajethics.2020.773.
91. Richie M, Josephson SA. Quantifying heuristic bias: anchoring, availability, and representativeness. Teach Learn Med. 2018;30(1):67–75. https://doi.org/10.1080/10401334.2017.1332631.
92. Bergstrom CT. Eight rules to combat medical misinformation. Nat Med. 2022;28(12):2468. https://doi.org/10.1038/s41591-022-02118-1.
93. Aïmeur E, Amri S, Brassard G. Fake news, disinformation and misinformation in social media: a review. Soc Netw Anal Min. 2023;13(1):30. https://doi.org/10.1007/s13278-023-01028-5.
94. Desai AN, Ruidera D, Steinbrink JM, Granwehr B, Lee DH. Misinformation and Disinformation: the potential disadvantages of social media in infectious disease and how to combat them. Clin Infect Dis. 2022;74(Suppl_3):e34–9. https://doi.org/10.1093/cid/ciac109.
95. Ahmed S, Ng SWT, Bee AWT. Understanding the role of fear of missing out and deficient self-regulation in sharing of deepfakes on social media: evidence from eight countries. Front Psychol. 2023;14:1127507. https://doi.org/10.3389/fpsyg.2023.1127507.
96. O'Connor C, Murphy M. Going viral: doctors must tackle fake news in the covid-19 pandemic. BMJ. 2020;369:m1587. https://doi.org/10.1136/bmj.m1587.

97. Stukus DR, Patrick M. How allergists can use social media to counter false information on vaccines. Ann Allergy Asthma Immunol. 2020;125(1):10–1. https://doi.org/10.1016/j.anai.2020.04.015.
98. Garg A, Sohal A, Kalra S, Singh C, Singh I, Grewal J, Kansal R, Malhotra K, Mahajan R, Midha V, Singh A, Sood A, Bawa A. Inflammatory bowel disease and X (formerly twitter) influencers: who are they and what do they say? Cureus. 2023;15(10):e47536. https://doi.org/10.7759/cureus.47536.
99. Díaz-Martín AM, Schmitz A, Yagüe Guillén MJ. Are health e-mavens the new patient influencers? Front Psychol. 2020;11:779. https://doi.org/10.3389/fpsyg.2020.00779.
100. Powell J, Pring T. The impact of social media influencers on health outcomes: systematic review. Soc Sci Med. 2024;340:116472. https://doi.org/10.1016/j.socscimed.2023.116472.

Chapter 19
The Landscape of Digital Health Approaches to Allergy in Australia

Janet M. Davies ⓘ

Contents

Abstract With 14–24% of the population affected, Australia has among the highest rates of allergic diseases globally. However, many patient needs are not adequately addressed across this vast continent with its biogeographically diverse exposures to pollen, insect, and seafood allergen sources. The 2020 Commonwealth Inquiry in Allergy and Anaphylaxis arrived at 24 recommendations to improve education, care, and outcomes for allergy patients nationally. This underpinned a partnership

J. M. Davies (✉)
School of Biomedical Sciences, Centre Immunology and Infection Control and Centre for Environment, Queensland University of Technology, Brisbane, Australia

National Allergy Centre of Excellence, Murdoch Children's Research Institute, Melbourne, VIC, Australia
e-mail: j36.davies@qut.edu.au

© The Author(s), under exclusive license to Springer Nature
Switzerland AG 2025
P. M. Matricardi, S. Dramburg, *Digital Allergology*, Health Informatics,
https://doi.org/10.1007/978-3-031-71021-6_19

299

between the peak professional body; Australasian Society of Clinical Immunology and Allergy, and the patient advocacy foundation; Allergy and Anaphylaxis Australia to form the National Allergy Council, and a collaboration with the Australian Digital Health Agency on projects to increase harmonization, quality, and sharing of allergy notification data. The National Allergy Centre of Excellence was also established to build systems and capabilities that accelerate allergy research. With segregated responsibilities for healthcare across tiers of government, the landscape for digital health systems here is complex with a plethora of stakeholders involved in guiding and governing national standardization, linking and integration of health datasets primarily for safety and quality purposes. Views of the national prevalence of allergies and the scope of allergy research in Australia can be garnered from a National Health Survey, the NACE allergy studies directory, and the Australian and New Zealand Clinical Trials Registry. Australia has been rapid in its adoption of digital approaches including virtual care platforms, transition to electronic medical records, clinical registries of adverse drug reactions (AusCAR, iNAAN), response to biologics for allergic respiratory conditions (e.g., ASAR), mHealth applications to share pollen exposure information, symptom surveys (e.g., AusPollen and AirRater), and manage health (e.g., MASKair, AllergyPal). With these rapidly emerging and sophisticated digital health capabilities, there are an ongoing opportunities and challenges to navigation of the digital health landscape to derive new insights can inform ways to more fully and equitably improve the lives of allergy patients in this country.

19.1 Burden of Allergy in Australia

Australia is an island continent covering 7.7 million km^2 [1]. With a dispersed population of 26.5 million people, 86.5% live in coastal urban centers [2]. While as many as 14% of the Australian population reports having an allergic condition [3], not all individuals affected by allergies can or do access appropriate and timely medical care [4, 5]. Access to allergy care is a challenge, especially for those living in regional, rural, and remote communities [6, 7]. Despite the high burden that allergic disease places on the health system, including high frequency and magnitude of epidemic thunderstorm asthma [8, 9], and the high social, economic, and health impacts that allergies have on patients and their families [10–12], there remain significant unmet needs relating to many aspects of preventing, diagnosing, and treating allergic diseases in this country [6].

The bipartisan Commonwealth Parliamentary Inquiry in Allergy and Anaphylaxis conducted in 2020, arrived at 24 recommendations to improve education, care, and outcomes for allergy patients nationally [6]. However, high-quality, consistently collected, and comprehensive Australian data on population prevalence of allergic conditions has not yet been systematically synthesized and analyzed. The lack of standardized and integrated national allergy data leaves us with a patchy view of the frequency, severity, outcomes, and impacts of allergic diseases at a national population level. With the transition to electronic medical records being adopted in many hospital and health services, in a majority of jurisdictions of Australia, new digital health research opportunities, and initiatives for embedding clinical research with real-time health surveillance, are being enabled. A sophisticated digital health ecosystem is underpinned by a number of initiatives including the drafted National Digital Research Infrastructure Strategy [13] and the Australian Digital Health Agency (ADHA). This chapter will consider allergic diseases, in the context of the national publicly funded health service and the health and medical research landscapes, within the context of emergent capabilities for digital health as it pertains to allergy.

This chapter focuses primarily on aspects of Digital Health related to electronic health records, and the potential for large allergy data analytics and to an extent mobile health applications. Use of digital health approaches within healthcare delivery is aimed at technical and digital transformation for improvement in safety and quality of care [14, 15], with a view to achieving efficiencies in health service systems. However, these safety and quality purposes simultaneously create an additional rich and beneficial secondary opportunity for research to garner insights from large scale, national datasets, and the generation of knowledge to underpin clinical practice improvement. A further implicit goal of digital health capability is to drive personalized medicine, predominantly in the context of pharmacogenomics for cancer therapy [16]. Interestingly, allergy specialists have provided personalized care for many decades with choices of allergen immunotherapy for patients based on individual sensitization profiles [17, 18]. Cybersecurity and privacy legislation govern appropriate secondary use of collections of individual patient health data for the purpose of research [19]. Taking full advantage of digital health opportunities for allergy research at scale requires careful strategic planning and implementation of the necessary digital research infrastructure, including access processes and platforms such as trusted research environments [20], that will help enable safe and secure research use according the "five safes framework" [21, 22] of health service-derived data relating to hospital care for allergy.

Reliance on hospital data sources of allergy patient data records primarily reveals data on allergy patients with severe symptoms who present to emergency departments, are admitted for care, or who are referred to specialist outpatient clinics. This skews data to those with more severe allergies, revealing a subset of patients with allergies in the community (Fig. 19.1), albeit those allergy patients that place the highest burden on healthcare services [23, 24]. There are likely to be many more individuals with allergies who don't access medical care [4, 25], or who are managed through primary healthcare services or private specialist. Health records from primary care are not directly captured and integrated into national datasets in a streamlined manner, obscuring the true scope and scale of allergies in Australia. Moreover, respiratory allergies such as allergic rhinitis (AR) [26] may not be classed as a high priority for hospital care or referral to public clinical immunology services, with the exception of severe asthma and for example thunderstorm asthma [8, 9], which is likely managed in emergency departments or by respiratory physicians [27, 28].

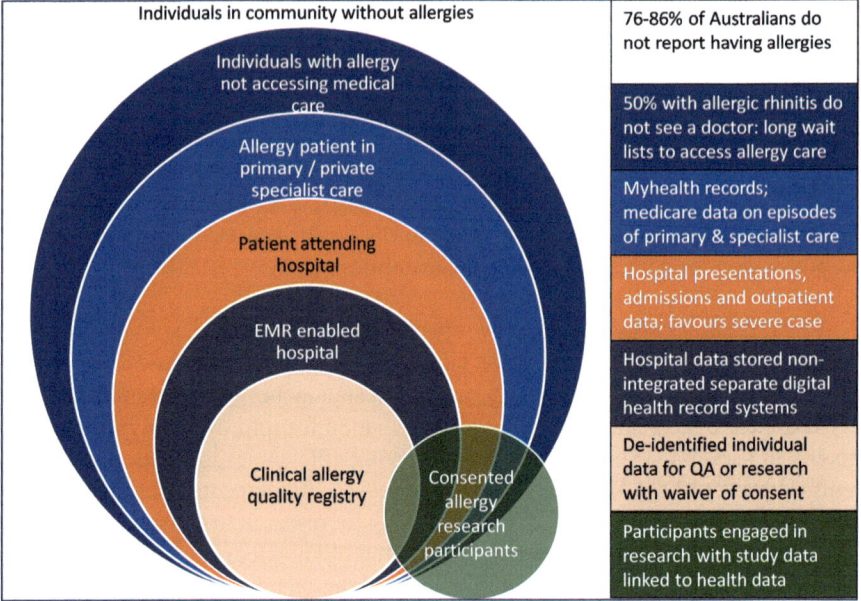

Fig. 19.1 Individuals in Australia stratified by self-reported allergy history, access to care and ways allergy-related data might be sourced and accessed for safety and quality assurance (QA) or research purposes to create new insights through analysis of electronic medical records (EMR) or knowledge generated by research. Numerical information sourced and integrated from [3, 4]

19.2 Australian Health Service Context

Australia has a public health system with distributed responsibility for delivery of care. Funding is granted from the federal government to six state governments in support of a complex healthcare system. State level Departments of Health hold responsibility for delivery of secondary and tertiary public hospital and health service networks, with each state making independent decisions, for instance of suppliers of pathology services and electronic medical record systems, which influences the interoperability of allergy data nationally. In contrast, responsibilities for primary and health community care services, health product regulation including of allergy tests and treatments, resourcing, workforce, medical benefits as well as digital health, health economics, system strategy, research, and digital transformation, rest within seven organizational pillars of the federal Department of Health and Aging [29]. This tiered approach to funding and responsibility for healthcare creates fragmented health data across hospital, allied health (e.g., immunopathology, dietetics, pharmacy), specialists, general practitioner, and other services that manage allergy patients.

In 2016, the Commonwealth ADHA was established, with the purpose of integrating health data nationally for generation of insights from the large collection of medical records [30].

19.3 Sources of Allergy Patient Data

Through Medicare, the national public health resourcing scheme [31], individual Australians can choose to active their personal "MyHealth Record." A patient can self-report an "allergy or adverse reaction," including an open text box for "substance or agent" to indicate the trigger of an allergic reaction within their MyHealth Record [32], which includes unstandardized open text data. Individuals may have a "Shared Health Summary" including diagnoses and medicines prescribed as completed by a patient's primary healthcare provider. A clinician can report an allergy or allergic reaction to a patient MyHealth Record via the digital Fast Reliable Easy Dispensing (FRED) portal [33]. However, current state-based public hospitals, which are overseen by local health district or network boards, do not yet have systems implemented for digitally integrating and viewing patient MyHealth records, including allergy or anaphylaxis history, to support clinical decision-making for patients presenting for hospital care. Accessed on the ADHA website is advice to patients and clinicians on how to add and view medicines, allergies, and adverse reactions [34]. However, while there are over 23 million MyHealth records with data, and there are approximately 460 million clinical documents and 670 million medicine documents within the MyHealth records platform, there are only 498,000 consumer documents [35], indicating individuals are not adding many personal health records, limiting at this stage the breadth and completeness of allergy patient records.

The National Allergy Council [36], formed as a partnership between the peak professional body; Australasian Society of Clinical Immunology and Allergy (ASCIA), and the not-for-profit patient advocacy foundation; Allergy and Anaphylaxis Australia (A&AA), has an active digital health project with the ADHA that aims to improve the scope of data, quality, discoverability, and sharing of allergy patient information with and between health professionals [37]. This project has a focus on educating patients, general practitioners, and nurses on the importance of accurate and complete recording of allergy information, particularly for prevention of anaphylaxis. Notably, serum-specific IgE results can now be uploaded by immunopathologist to a patient's MyHealth record [38], but the process and practice for such uploads are not clear. Moreover, how complete and representative specific IgE data is of allergic sensitization at a population level depends on the rate at which testing is requested, the permissions for data entry specified by the patient as indicated on the pathology request slip, and the process of IgE data entry. Allergy sensitization data will be considered further below, but most routine clinical allergy diagnostics conducted in public or private specialist outpatient clinics rely on skin prick testing, for which the provider needs to be authorized by the Therapeutic Goods Administration (TGA) for special access (Category C) since many allergy skin prick or intradermal test materials are not registered as diagnostic products [39]. Although there are guidelines from ASCIA [40], skin prick test (SPT) testing practices vary from clinic to clinic depending on clinical preferences and availability of products from suppliers, lancet choices, as well as practitioner technique and experience. Methods of interpretation of test outcomes range from a dichotomous positive/negative result to the recommended recording of the average millimeter diameter of the wheel area at 15 min [40, 41]. However, recording and storage of SPT data in clinical records is unstandardized, and furthermore, visibility and sharing of patient level SPT data is restricted to the clinical site for patient privacy reasons. Notably, with separate models of care [42], SPT may be performed across a range of clinical services in Australia; for instance, immunology, gastroenterology, pediatrics, respiratory, as well as ear nose and throat surgery clinics and so on. Importantly, with respect to integration and interoperability of allergy test data from these various clinical sources, these should be digitally recorded and accessible to have value for quality assurance or research purposes.

19.4 Systems for Digital Health Surveillance of Allergy Patients in Australia

Undergirded by a strategy and roadmap, the ADHA aims to align and integrate health data across all tiers of government to improve availability, access, and use of government managed data, but this process is still early stage [43, 44]. The ADHA primarily focuses on systems and use of integrated data for preventative health and health service improvement purposes [45] although researchers and planners are identified stakeholders. The ultimate goal is to create national interoperable health data derived from multiple sources [45], which could encompass allergy data sources summarized in Table 19.1. Clinician awareness, acceptance, and pathways for contributing allergy related data are needed for integration of complete and representative data [36], none of which is straightforward.

The value and benefit of nationally integrating health data can only be realized for improvement of care for allergy by establishing and implementing clear guidelines and frameworks for access and uses; quality assurance and/or research, both of which are under development by the ADHA and the Australian Institute of Health and Welfare (AIHW) [46, 47]. However separately, the Office of National Data Commissioner is developing a scheme for government data access, which will apply to health data, according to the 2022 Commonwealth Data Availability and Transparency Act [48], and the Australian Cybersecurity Strategy and Action Plan [19].

In parallel, the Australian Institute for Digital Health plays an important role in developing the health workforce capability and the clinical application of digital health solutions; for instance, virtual care platforms, digital monitoring devices and mobile apps, to underpin connected patient-centered care. The purpose and scope of the Australian Institute of Digital Health is articulated in its own Blueprint and Action Plan, which identifies academic, medical, and industry researchers as key partners in safe and secure use of health data [49, 50]. While the AIDH may not be directly involved in harmonization and integration of health datasets, it plays a key

Table 19.1 Potential sources of routinely collected data on allergy in Australia

Type of data	Data source	Platform	Custodian	Research access[a]	Identification status[a]
Personal reports of allergy or adverse event	Consumer provided: Shared Health Summary	MyHealth Record	AIHW	Aggregated data; Services Australia	De-identified
Reports of allergy or adverse (drug) event	Clinician entered; GP, ED doctor, or other clinician	FRED	AIHW	Aggregated data; Services Australia	De-identified
Episode of care by GP	Primary Health Network	Medicare	AIHW	Aggregated data: Services Australia	De-identified
Medication prescribed	Medical prescriptions	PBS, other	AIHW	Aggregated data: Services Australia: private companies	De-identified
Prescribed and dispensed, or over the counter medicine related adverse events	Entered by consumer or health professional	DAEN	TGA	Searchable MeDRA terms on dashboard on TGA website	De-identified
Specific IgE results	Pathology laboratory, Shared Health Record	Private or public pathology services	Local site for approved research	To be collated nationally (ADHA)	De-identified data, rarely accessible for research
Hospital presentations	Emergency Department data sets	Local/ integrated EMR	Local site and state Health Department	Local site/ network or State Health Department	De-identified
Hospital Admission	Admitted patient datasets	Local/ integrated EMR	State Health Department	Local site/ network or State Health Department	De-identified
Death codes assigned to anaphylaxis	State death certificate, coroner reports	National Mortality Database	AIHW	Aggregated data: Services Australia	De-identified
Outpatient clinic	Non-admitted patient datasets	Local/ integrated EMR	Local site and State Health Department	Local site/ network or State Health Department	De-identified

ADHA Australian Digital Health Agency; *AIHW* Australian Institute for Health and Welfare; *DAEN* Database of adverse event notifications; *ED* emergency department; *EMR* electronic medical record; *FRED* Fast Reliable Easy Dispensing; *GP* general practitioner; *MeDRA TGA* medical dictionary for regulatory activities; *PBS* Pharmaceutical Benefits Scheme; *TGA* Therapeutic Goods Administration

[a] Unless individual informed consent is obtained

role in implementing systems for applying digital health tools and generation of quality health service data.

Secure research access to and analysis of allergy healthcare data alone, or better still integrated with other national datasets for instance socioeconomic, education, and environmental (e.g., allergen) exposure data [51, 52], that help indicate whole of life, patient centric, social determinants of health [53], are yet to follow and will undoubtedly be a more challenging endeavor.

There are currently few statewide or nationally aggregated or individual level datasets, from which some insights of the scale of allergic disease in Australia is evident. In this chapter, the scope of national digitally enabled allergy research has been examined from three sources: an Allergy Study Directory (ASD) [54], The National Health Survey [3], and the Australian and New Zealand Clinical Trials Registry (ANZCTR) [55].

19.5 Investigator Initiated Registries and Studies of Allergy and Anaphylaxis

As part of the response to Commonwealth Inquiry into Allergies and Anaphylaxis [6], the National Allergy Centre of Excellence (NACE) was established in 2022 to become Australia's peak allergy research body tasked with building tools and capabilities to accelerate allergy research and improve quality of life of Australians living with allergic disease [56]. Among 56 studies listed by NACE ASD by the NACE across drug, food, insect, and respiratory allergies [54], 28 are currently open to recruitment of participants, only 11 (19.6%) indicate using digital health tools such as access to hospital records, online surveys or apps to collect data, and two are identified as registries (Table 19.2). This ASD serves the dual purposes of enabling allergy patients to identify studies they may be eligible to participate in and for researchers to showcase allergy studies that have been completed or that are open for recruitment. That on average less than three of the six states and two territories are involved in listed studies suggests the full scope of allergies across diverse regions may not be fully or equitably represented in the currently listed allergy studies (Table 19.2). This is key given variation in exposure to allergen sources across the continent (Fig. 19.2) [57].

19.5.1 Drug Allergy

The Australasian Registry of Severe Cutaneous Adverse Reactions (AusCAR) is a registry (ANZCTR Registration: ACTRN12619000241134) involving collation of routinely collected adverse drug events, including but not only allergic reactions such as anaphylaxis, from 15 hospital sites, and includes 128 participants, of whom 77 have contributed to the associated biobank [58]. The second registry is the International Network of Antibiotic Allergy Nations (iNAAN) delabeling

Table 19.2 Characteristics of studies listed in the National Allergy Centre of Excellence (NACE) Allergy Study Directory

Allergy Stream	Number aligned studies	Age bracket of study participants (% of studies)				Study design (% of studies)						Average (median; IQR) states	Number with international sites
		Adults	Adults and children	Children	Not specified	Registry	Interventional/ RCT	Observational/ cohort	Survey/ interviews	Other design	Digitally Enabled		
Drug	10	2 (20)	7 (70)	1 (10)		2 (20)	6 (60)	2 (20)			2 (20)	2.6 (1:1–3.0)	2
Food	36	1 (3)	7 (19)	28 (78)			18 (50)	13 (36)	5 (14)	1	5 (17)	2.8 (1:1–3.8)	4
Insect	5		1 (20)		4 (80)		1 (20)			4 (80)	0	2.6 (1:1–2)	1
Respiratory	5		5 (100)					1 (20)	1 (20)	3 (60)	3 (60)	2.8 (1:1–4)	1

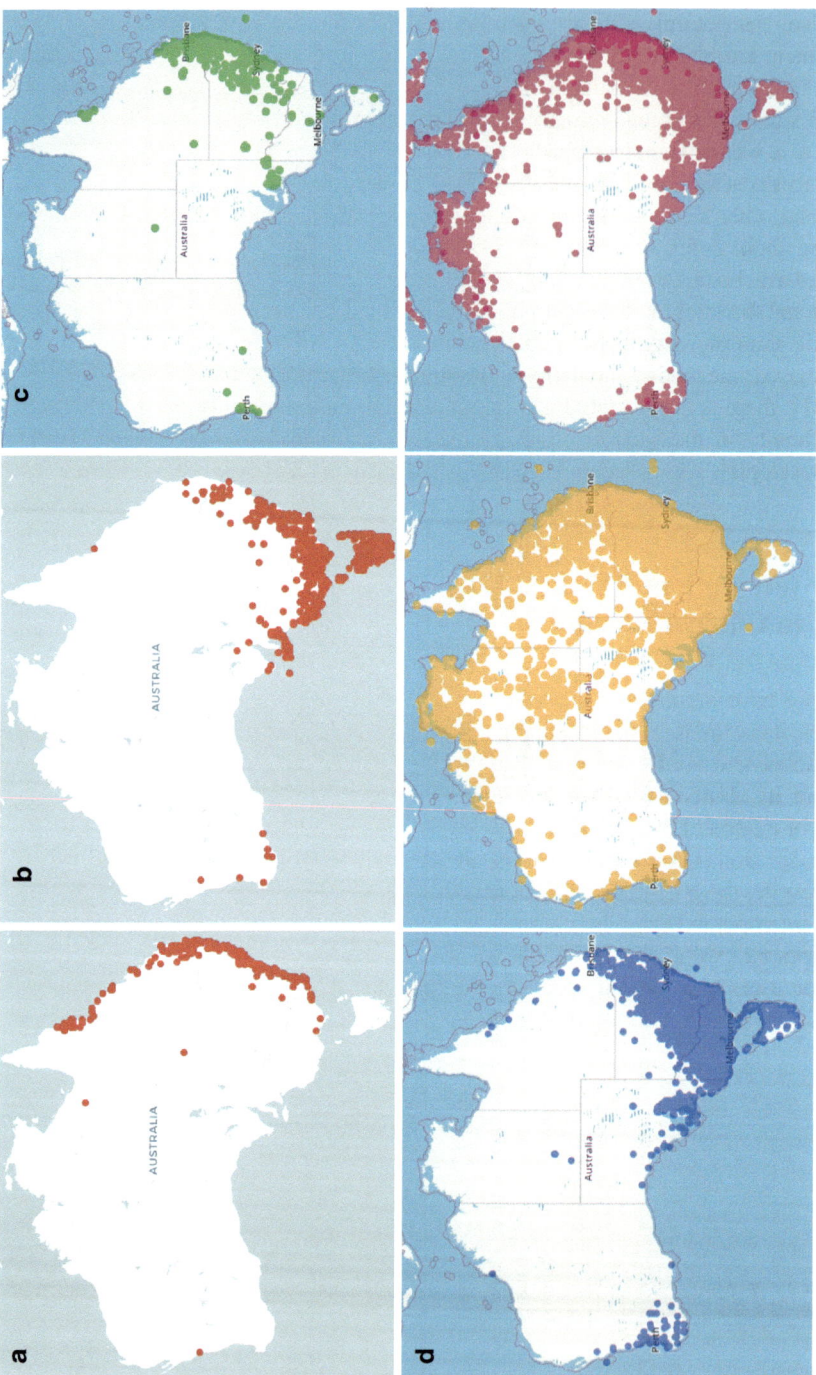

Fig. 19.2 Distribution of examples of clinically relevant environmental allergen sources across the continent of Australia. Insect allergen sources: (**a**) Jack Jumper ant (*Myrmecia pilosula*), (**b**) paralysis tick (*Ixodes holocyclus*), and pollen allergen sources; (**c**) ragweed (*Ambrosia* sp.), and (**d**) ryegrass (*Lolium perenne*, left panel), Bermuda grass (*Cynodon dactylon*, middle panel), and Bahia related grasses (*Paspalum* sp., right panel). Distributions from the Atlas of Living Australia sighting records [57]

study (ANZCTR Registration: ACTRN12623000484640) [59], which incorporates a validated, clinical decision tool digitally integrated for collection at point-of-care oral antibiotic challenge data [60], to assist in adherence to the National Health and Quality Health Service Standard 3; Preventing and Controlling Infections [61]. Although there are nine separate cohort, observational studies or clinical trials related to drug allergy listed within the ASD, these involve different investigators and sites with use of separate protocols and data collection tools, illustrating the challenge for nationally interoperable allergy study and allergy patient data.

Drewett et al. [62] recently analyzed anaphylaxis notification data for the state of Victoria [63], a collection established following a change to that state's Public Health and Welling Being Act in 2018. The Victorian reporting requirements were adapted from national acute management of anaphylaxis guidelines subsequently updated by the Australasian Society for Clinical Immunology and Allergy (ASCIA) [64]. Nationally, the Australian Commission on Safety and Quality in Health Care issued the Acute Anaphylaxis Clinical Care Standard in 2021 [65], which is now in the process of being implemented across other jurisdictions, paves the way for future nationwide analysis of acute anaphylaxis reporting data from hospital and health services.

On a national level, notifications entered by health professionals or consumers on adverse reactions to prescribed or over-the-counter medications are collated nationally by the TGA Database of Adverse Event Notifications (DAEN) [66], which includes data on suspected unverified adverse events inclusive of but not only allergic reactions, coded to the TGA medical dictionary for regulatory activities terms including allergy relevant terms such as pruritus, anaphylaxis, anaphylactoid reaction, allergic respiratory reaction, angioedema, rash, and dyspnea (Table 19.1). However, similar terms such as "swollen tongue" and "tongue oedema" are utilized, suggesting the need to map similar terms to standardized codes. The need for a comprehensive and standardized national integrated registry of drug-induced anaphylaxis has been clearly articulated [67] and is evident by increasing reported rates of anaphylaxis in this country [23, 68, 69].

19.5.2 Food Allergy

Food allergy is an active area of research in Australia with more than half of the studies in the NACE ASD pertaining to food allergy (Table 19.2). As many as 78% involve children and a further 19% involving both pediatric and adult participants, consistent with the high burden of food allergies in Australian children [70, 71]. A number of food allergy studies (17%) are embracing digital tools to enable their studies, for example, digital surveys ($n = 3$) and interviews ($n = 2$).

19.5.3   Insect Allergy

Five studies in the ASD aligned to insect allergy. The nature, prevalence, management, and prevention of allergy to the Australian paralysis tick present across southeastern Australia (Fig. 19.2a), which have been associated with induction of red meat allergy and IgE sensitization to galactose-alpha 1–3-galactose [72, 73] has been communicated to community and health professionals via the efforts of the Tick-Induced Allergies Research and Awareness (TiARA) program [74]. While there are six insect allergy studies or databases listed, some of these appear to overlap in scope but span several eastern states; Tasmania, New South Wales, and Queensland. From a uniquely Australian perspective (Fig. 19.2b), an important insect clinical research program is the delineation of allergens from Jack Jumper ant venom for diagnostic and immunotherapeutic use [75–77].

19.5.4   Respiratory Allergies

Three of five studies listed in the ASD that related to respiratory allergies involved digital health tools, including one discrete choice experiment survey on digital asthma inhaler design [78], a citizen science Grass Gazers project on sources of airborne pollen [79], and an app to track seasonal respiratory allergy symptoms over the grass pollen season as part of the Thunderstorm Asthma in Seasonal AR study [52]. The full scope of digital health research on allergic respiratory disease, often pertaining to or encompassing allergic asthma, may not be captured in the NACE ASD. A significant body of respiratory allergy research would be more visible within the Thoracic Society for Australia and New Zealand community than ASCIA, for instance, the Australasian Severe Asthma Registry for patients with eosinophilic asthma who receive Benralizumab or Dupilumab treatment [80], or mepolizumab [81].

19.6   Insight on Allergy Data Derived the National Health Survey

The Australian Bureau of Statistics recently released data on the latest National Health Survey conducted in 2022 [3], from which insights are generated by the Australian Institute for Health and Welfare (AIHW) [26]. Data was collected by face-to-face interviews with over 13,000 households across urban and rural settings in all states and territories [82]. The AIHW reports on the overall prevalence of asthma extensively with 10.8% of Australians having a diagnosis of asthma. Notably, multimorbidity in asthma was as high as 64.9% [26]. Asthma is the fourth highest common chronic condition with a prevalence of 12.0% in females verses

9.4% in males [26]. Data for AR in adults shows the current rate of 23.8% of Australians [26], with significant increase of 65% since 2004 (Fig. 19.3a), and for children under 14 years the prevalence of AR is 10.4% [83]. Unfortunately, information on AR in adolescents is not reported, even though research shows young people to be particularly vulnerable to AR [84] with significant and complex adverse impact on general health, anxiety, and welling being [4, 85–88].

The National Health Survey data indicates that 14% of Australians reported having an allergy, with 7% of the population overall with reported food allergies, which appeared to vary with age and gender (Fig. 19.3c and d). Data from the HealthNuts studies conducted in state of Victoria show that clinically confirmed food allergy is as high as 11% at 1 year, 3.8% at 4 years, and 4.5% between 10 and 14 years of age [70, 71]. Interestingly, this overall prevalence of 14% having a history of allergy is lower than the reported rate for AR (23.8%), indicating discrepancy in the collection, coding, and analysis of data. It is interesting to note the greater variation between states with respect to AR compared to asthma (Fig. 19.3b), which may be related to biogeographic differences in allergen, particularly pollen, exposure

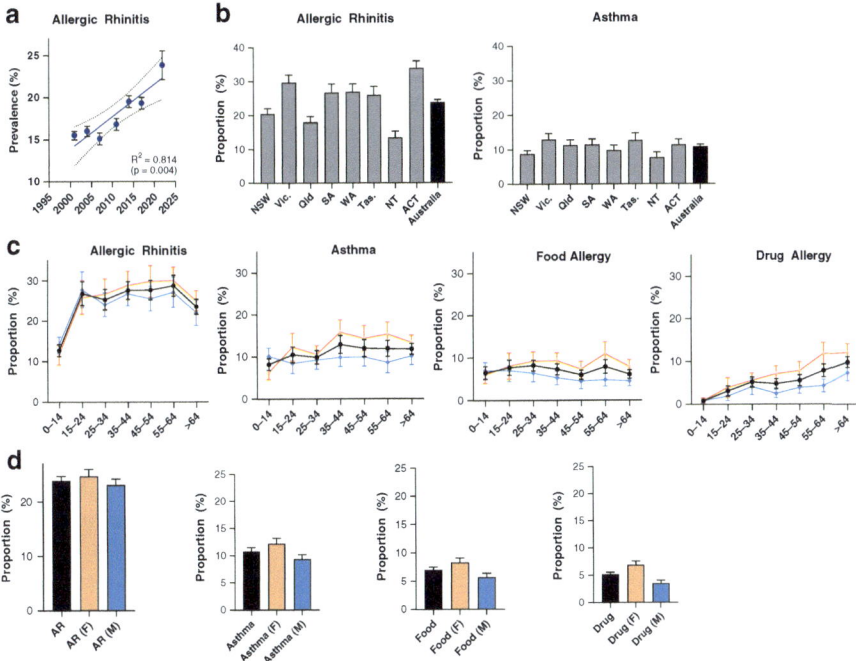

Fig. 19.3 Overview of reported descriptive statistics relevant to allergy from the National Health Surveys of 2022 and earlier. (**a**) Prevalence rate of allergic rhinitis over time, (**b**) population rates for allergic rhinitis and asthma by state (grey bars) and Australia overall (black bar) (data not listed by state for other allergies), (**c**) rates of allergic conditions by age and gender, and (**d**) rates of allergic conditions of the population (black) and for females (F) and males (M). Data derived from [26]. Pearson correlation coefficient and linear regression model for rate of allergic rhinitis over time was analysed

(Fig. 19.3c, d) [51, 89]. Variation in drug and food allergy between states was not reported. With the exception of asthma in children under 14 years of age (Fig. 19.3c and d), the rates of allergies seemed to be higher in females than males for drug, food, and AR, which warrants further interrogation beyond the scope of this chapter.

19.7 Overview of Studies Relating to Allergy in the ANZCTR

The ANZCTR includes metadata about clinical studies conducted in Australia and New Zealand [55]. Of 391 studies approved by a human research ethics committee that are registered with the term allergy mentioned, only 94 contain the word allergy or IgE within in the scientific title, indicating allergy being the central focus of these studies. These, and other trials addressing multiple health conditions, that had included "allergy" or "allergic reaction" as a secondary or safety outcome measure, can generate data that could be useful for informing the extent of allergic reactions (Fig. 19.4d). Of all the registered studies mentioning allergy, 88% involved Australian sites, 11% involved New Zealand sites, and 1% involved other countries. Over 50% of these registered trials where aligned to the study category of treatment, whereas 6% and 20% could be categorized as focusing on diagnosis or prevention, respectively (Fig. 19.4c). Notably, in the ANZCTR over 40% of studies aligned to respiratory allergy compared to 23% for food, 8.5% for drug, and 0.4% for insect allergy, which differed from the composition of studies captured in the NACE ASD with a higher proportion of food allergy studies (Fig. 19.4b). The involvement of various states in studies (Fig. 19.4a) was related to population size [90] (data not shown, spearman $r = 0.952$, $p < 0.005$), but importantly from a biogeographical perspective the majority of studies tended be conducted in southeastern Australia which has a predominantly temperate climate. The studies spanned a wide variety of allergen triggers or organ systems affected by allergy (Fig. 19.4b).

One of six studies including a registry component, that was not captured in the NACE ASD is the Australian Mepolizumab Registry for Chronic Rhinosinusitis with Nasal Polyps (AMR-CRSwNP) (ACTRN12623000692639) [81]. This registry was established to track patient characteristics and effectiveness in a multicenter, observational post-marketing study following the recent approval for Mepolizumab on the PBS in April 2023 [91].

19.8 Sensitization

Comprehensive Australian evidence for population level or individual patient sensitization profiles is guided by the ASCIA position paper [92], but may currently be affected by diversity of allergy diagnostics practices and siloed unstandardized data. Serological testing platforms clinically available in Australia include the high-throughput pathology laboratory ImmunoCAP (ThermoFisher) or Immulite

(Siemens). Allergen extract and/or allergen component arrays; ISAC chip (ThermoFisher), ALEX array (Macro Array Diagnostics, Germany), and Euroline (Euroimmun Germany) are also available. However, testing of specific IgE to molecular allergen components is mostly limited to clinical research settings [93–96] or requests by general practitioner, specialist clinics that do not have capacity for skin prick testing, or for patients for whom SPT is not indicated.

While the state of Victoria, which has individual hospital level pathology services, mostly utilizes the ImmunoCAP platform, other states including Queensland, which has the benefit of an integrated, statewide pathology services and integrated hospital medical records [97], uses a different platform (Siemens Immulite), which has some format and performance differences [98].

Importantly, the relevance of commercially available components to Australian patients who are exposed to locally prevalent and clinically relevant species may limit the utility and adoption of allergen component testing [6, 99]. This unmet need for locally relevant allergen components for clinically appropriate personalized allergy diagnostics extends across aeroallergens; subtropical grass pollen allergen components [95, 100], local stinging insect venom such as paper wasp [101] and Jack jumper ant venom allergy [75, 77], and fish and shellfish allergen components [102, 103].

Medicare rebate structure may restrict the number of specific IgE tests to four allergen sources per episode of care, and the cost to private allergy patients may also present significant economic barriers to adequate allergy diagnostic testing [6, 42]. Long wait times to see a specialist and lack of specialists in regional and rural areas may drive requests for serological testing.

The levels of spIgE that indicate clinically important sensitization appear to be influenced by biogeographical, environmental, and social determinants [104, 105]. Knowledge of biogeographical sensitization patterns in China has been analyzed to guide recommendations of minimum SPT screening panel [106]. There may be locally relevant concentrations of spIgE to particular allergen components, for example, egg Gal d 1 [93], cashew Ana o 3 [107], or peanut Ara h 2 [94], that are associated with clinically relevant symptoms. spIgE concentrations to particular aeroallergens; house dust mite allergens [108] or Phl p 5 allergen of Timothy grass [109] have been associated with asthma elsewhere. In Australia, sensitization to pollen starch granules or Lol p 5 of the same group 5 allergen family from the locally relevant temperate ryegrass pollen source (Fig. 19.2) has been associated with risk of thunderstorm asthma [52, 110–112].

Gradients in sensitization patterns between in urban coastal suburb where atopic children showed higher SPT frequencies to HDM (*Dermatophagoides farinae* and *D. pteronynissinus*) than pollen verses inland rural settings where children showed higher sensitization to pollens extracts including ragweed, ryegrass, and plantain [113]. On a small geographical scale across the Sydney area, which experiences both temperate and subtropical microclimatic zones, variation in aeroallergen sensitization profiles have been found [114]. At a state level, differences in avidity and levels of sensitization to subtropical and temperate grass pollens by SPT and spIgE to pollen extracts, as well as spIgE to pollen allergen components, has been demonstrated [95] with AR patients in the temperate region of Adelaide showing higher spIgE reactivity to ryegrass pollen and Lol p 1 compared to AR patients in subtropical Queensland showing significantly higher spIgE to subtropical Bahia and Bermuda grass pollen, and their allergens Pas n 1 and Cyn d 1, respectively. Sensitive and specific detection of spIgE reactivity with recombinant Pas n 1 and Cyn d 1 on a digitally integrated rapid nanofluidic point of are device has potential to improve access to allergy diagnosis particularly in regional and rural communities where access to care is limited [100].

19.9   Exposure

Exposure to high levels of airborne grass pollen has led to over 10 thunderstorm asthma events in Australia [8]. The AusPollen Partnership established in September 2016 with key university, health, meteorology, and environmental agencies as well as patient and professional bodies, designed and implemented standardized processes for monitoring pollen nationally [115]. During 4 years of the Partnership, the number of sites monitoring pollen in Australia grew from two active sites to 25. The team generated the first continental scale, Southern Hemisphere standardized aerobiology dataset to track shifts in the pollen season loads, providing tens of thousands of people in Brisbane, Sydney, Canberra, and Melbourne with accurate daily grass pollen observations and short-term daily forecasts [51].

In the weeks immediately before and after the major thunderstorm asthma event in Melbourne 2016 [9], women who used the Melbourne Pollen App were more likely to have had a history of hay fever than males [116]. Notably, in that study, 64.7% of males and 59.2% of females reported having no formal diagnosis of hay fever. Our systematic review found that smart phone apps can have a positive effect on asthma control and adherence to prescribed medication use [117]. Mobile phone applications use such as MacVIA [25, 88], or others for symptom surveys including AirRater in Tasmania [118, 119], and crowdsourcing of symptom surveys of allergic rhinitis and asthma patients who access grass pollen information from Melbourne and Canberra [120, 121] have been developed and/or applied here.

Integration of symptom survey data from apps, which may not have been validated as efficacious, and which provide pollen exposure information, has a risk of information bias. Furthermore, approaches to push attention to pollen information apps, which may be funded by sale of data or advertising revenue, or for which pollen forecast information is shared as a "goodie," create further potential biases. Electronic symptom surveys need to balance simplicity of use with the precision of information collected; eyes, nasal and lung symptoms, and they should be independently led and validated to provide a benefit to patients. Unfortunately, a plethora of pollen forecasts can be found online in Australia, many of which may not be informed by or verified by actual pollen concentration data [122].

There is limited spatial coverage of aerobiological monitoring nationally with most sites being disbursed in populated coastal urban centers; the number of sites that monitor pollen in Australia fluctuates with resourcing to sustain pollen monitoring. National collaborative research on understanding Australian aerobiology has been an active endeavor spurred by the Australian Centre for Ecological Synthesis and Analysis working group in 2013 [123–128], extended through the NHMRC AusPollen Partnership [51], further enabled by the University of Tasmania AirRater research [118] [119], and the Victorian thunderstorm asthma pollen surveillance project that established the world's first thunderstorm asthma warning system [129].

Despite implications as a cofactor in thunderstorm asthma [130], there is limited data from few sites on fungal spore aerobiology [131], and airborne fungal spore associations with respiratory illness [132, 133]. This is undoubtedly an important gap in aerobiological monitoring and analysis of environmental health impacts.

Transition to automation of pollen monitoring in Australia commenced in 2021 with the first holographic air monitoring device at the AusPollen Brisbane site with excellent initial experience over the grass pollen monitoring period [134] and in 2022 in Melbourne [135]. However, training and verification of accurate recognition and monitoring of diverse Australian pollen sources is essential for successful transition to real-time monitoring given the well-established knowledge of broad biodiversity of airborne pollen in Australia [125, 126, 136], that has been confirmed by application of environmental DNA metabarcoding studies including innovative use of routinely collected air samples at multiple sites and seasons [89, 137, 138]. This is particularly important given the impact of various types of pollen exposure [125, 139, 140] on allergic respiratory disease in temperate [141, 142] and subtropical regions [143, 144].

19.10   Standardization of Terminology and Sharing of Allergy Data

As well as challenges with access and integration of multiple separate allergy data sources, there does not seem to be an internationally developed and accepted common data model (CDM) for allergic diseases. Thus international or national standards for common allergy data encompassing condition codes, symptoms and diagnostic indicators, and medication labels and doses, or outcome measures have not yet been defined, accepted, and implemented [145]. CDM in the context of food allergy [146], pediatric drug prescription data [147], with some relevance to drug allergy, and by the Observational Medical Outcomes Partnership for respiratory allergies [148], are being addressed. These do not cover all aspects of allergy across drug, food, insect, and respiratory allergen sources or allergic conditions or organs effected. A considerable effort will be required to reach consensus on allergy CDM. For instance, during a project developing CDM for primary care datasets in Australia, less than 10% of structured data extracted could be mapped to standard vocabularies such as Snowmed CT, the rest needed to be mapped manually [149].

The updated National Statement on Ethical Conduct in Human Research, the associated guidelines on Management of Data and Information in Research, and

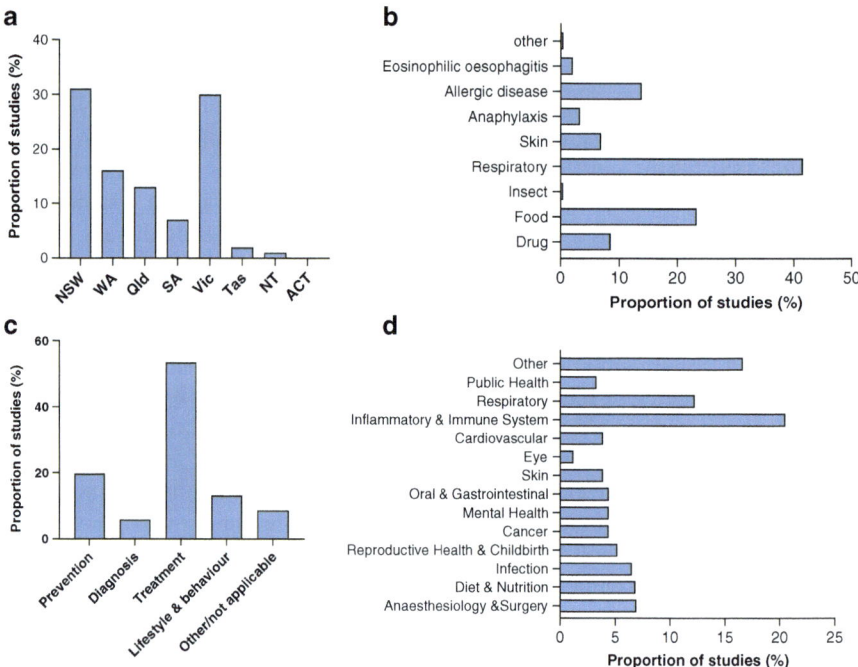

Fig. 19.4 Overview of clinical studies pertaining to allergy entered by investigators into the Australian and New Zealand Clinical Trials Registry Network. (**a**) The proportion of studies by state, (**b**) allergy focus, (**c**) study categories, and (**d**) condition codes. Data derived and anlysed from records identified by search for "allergy" on ANZCTR [55]

Statement on Consumer and Community involvement in Health and Medical Research, require that, without justifiable reasons otherwise (such as respect for Indigenous ownership or unmanageable risks to the privacy of research participants), and to enable equitable access to the benefits of research, investigators should collect and store data generated through research in a way that data can be reused in future projects [150–152]. Reuse of research data derived from publicly funded research is strongly encouraged [150], and adherence to Findable, Accessible, Interoperable, and Reusable (FAIR) principles [153], are advocated but maturity of the application is still emerging [154, 155] (Fig. 19.4).

As many as 76% of studies related to allergy in the ANZCTR [55] indicated that de-identified individual participant data was not available to share, and a further 2% had not decided (Fig. 19.5a). Of those not intending to share participant level data, 113 provided an open text response about the reasons why data would not be shared. These reasons could be coded to an array of themes (Fig. 19.5b), commonly including not having human research ethics approval or plans to share (35%), not having informed participant consent (12%), and privacy and confidentiality concerns (32%). While 18% would publish aggregated data (rather than individual level data), 9% considered there would be no value in sharing data, sometimes because the sample size was small or the study a pilot.

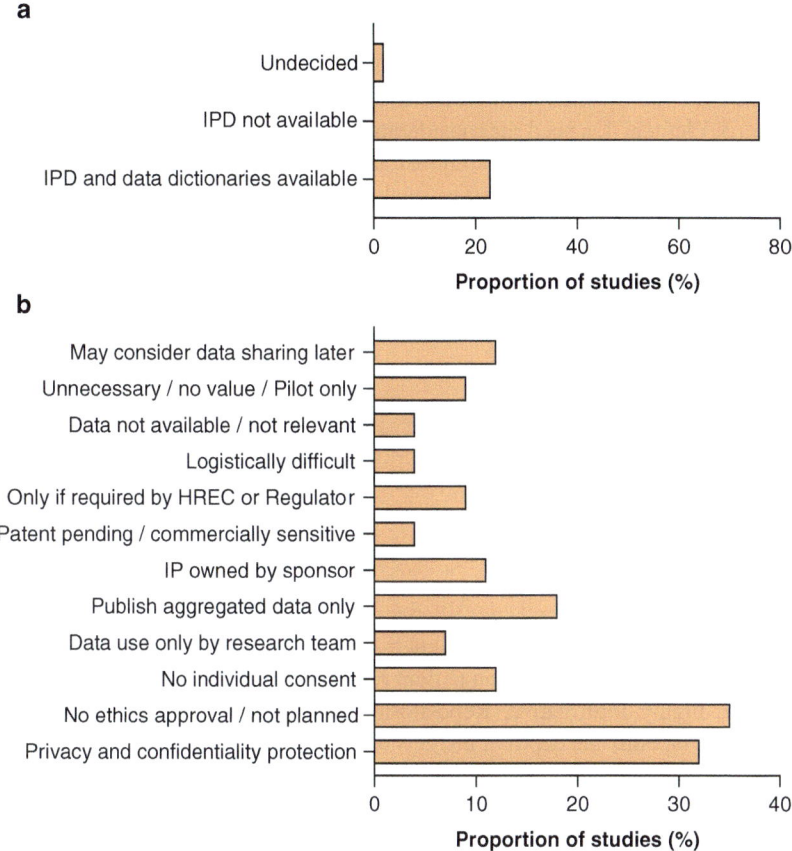

Fig. 19.5 Intent to share and reasons for not sharing data from studies pertaining to allergy entered by investigators into the Australian and New Zealand Clinical Trials Registry Network. a. the proportion of studies for which (de-identified) individual participant data (IPD) and data dictionaries are to be shared for research re-use, and b. proportion of studies giving reasons for not sharing IPD in open text in the 'IPD comments" field. Data derived and thematically analysed from 113 of the 395 human research ethics approved records identified by search for "allergy" on ANZCTR [55]

19.11   Future Directions

The new national mHealth assessment framework articulates requirements for mHealth applications to show efficacy and benefit to patients [156], paving the way for use of apps to support care and safety of allergy patients in future and for symptom surveys [119–121, 157], provision of pollen exposure to benefit respiratory allergy patients [158], and management of medication adherence in real world, regionally relevant practice in Australia [25, 88]. For instance in partnership between Allergy and Anaphylaxis Australia and ASCIA, investigators at the Murdoch

Children's Research Institute have developed the AllergyPal mobile application that digitalizes a child's ASCIA Allergy Action Plan is designed to reliably share allergy information with other health professionals to ensure child safety [159]. Notably, updated National Statement on Responsible Conduct of Research specifies under Section 3, Element 4, a need for consideration of use of large digital health datasets, including routinely collected or administrative electronic medical records collected for purposed other than research (i.e., quality and safety surveillance), mobile apps, biospecimens and derived data, interview, surveys, focus group data, and information generated by analysis of personal information, which will help clarify and enable ethical, safe, secure, and appropriate use of digital health approaches in allergy care and research.

19.12 Challenges and Opportunities for Research Access and Integration of Allergy Health Data

Identifying the right data custodian and seeking approval to access particular fields or sets of individual allergy data remains a challenge, illustrated by the range of separate stored routinely collected allergy data sources (Table 19.1).

Given the unique biodiversity and environmental conditions across the continent, registries of real-world Australian patient responses to biological therapies and AIT would be highly informative. Repositories of integrated allergy patient data to improve the breadth and depth of insights on the scale of allergies across drug, food, insect and respiratory allergen sources, that effect all types of allergy conditions, are needed to garner the complete picture of allergy prevalence, prevention, diagnosis, and treatment nationally.

Navigation of our complex tiered health system with separated responsibilities but overlapping remits of national, state and local organizational stakeholders involved in health care delivery, research systems, cybersecurity, and privacy, particularly pertaining to digital health approaches to research and care for allergy patients is a challenge. Understanding the associated digital health landscape [160] and how the multitude of government agencies described herein influence, enable, and accelerate advancement of digital health capabilities is an active and exciting field of endeavor. With partnership between key stakeholders including ASCIA, NAC, and NACE, Australia is poised to improve the level of evidence on the scale of and inform solutions to the allergy problem nationally. With new insights and rapidly emerging digital health capabilities related to integration and analysis of electronic health records as well as virtual care platforms and mHealth applications, the unmet needs of allergy patients should, in future, be more fully and equitably addressed in this country.

References

1. Australian Bureau of Statistics. National, state and territory population. ABS Website; 2023. https://www.abs.gov.au/statistics/people/population/national-state-and-territory-population/latest-release#cite-window1.
2. The World Bank. Urban population (% of total population): World Bank Group; 2022. https://data.worldbank.org/indicator/SP.URB.TOTL.IN.ZS.
3. Australian Bureau of Statistics. National Health Survey: information on health behaviours, conditions prevalence, and risk factors in Australia 2022. In: The Australian Bureau of Statistics, editor. 2023. https://www.abs.gov.au/statistics/health/health-conditions-and-risks/national-health-survey/latest-release.
4. Katelaris CH, Sacks R, Theron PN. Allergic rhinoconjunctivitis in the Australian population: burden of disease and attitudes to intranasal corticosteroid treatment. Am J Rhinol Allergy. 2013;27:506–9. https://doi.org/10.2500/ajra.2013.27.3965.
5. Cvetkovski B, Kritikos V, Yan K, Bosnic-Anticevich S. Tell me about your hay fever: a qualitative investigation of allergic rhinitis management from the perspective of the patient. NPJ Prim Care Respir Med. 2018;28:3. https://doi.org/10.1038/s41533-018-0071-0.
6. Commonwealth of Australia. Walking the allergy tightrope. In: Standing Committee on Health Aged Care and Sport, editor. Canberra ACT. 2020. https://www.aph.gov.au/Parliamentary_Business/Committees/House/Health_Aged_Care_and_Sport/Allergiesandanaphylaxis/Report.
7. St Clair M, Murtagh D. Barriers to telehealth uptake in rural, regional, remote Australia: what can be done to expand telehealth access in remote areas? IOS Press; 2019.
8. Davies J, Erbas B, Simunovic M, Kouba JAL, Milic A, Fagan D. Literature Review on Thunderstorm Asthma and its implications for Public Health Advice. 2017. https://www2.health.vic.gov.au/about/publications/researchandreports/thunderstorm-asthma-literature-review-may-2107
9. Thien F, Beggs PJ, Csutoros D, Darvall J, Hew M, Davies JM, et al. The Melbourne epidemic thunderstorm asthma event 2016: an investigation of environmental triggers, effect on health services, and patient risk factors. Lancet Planetary Health. 2018;2:e255–e63. https://doi.org/10.1016/S2542-5196(18)30120-7.
10. Borchers-Arriagada N, Jones PJ, Palmer AJ, Bereznicki B, Cooling N, Davies JM, et al. What are the health and socioeconomic impacts of allergic respiratory disease in Tasmania? Aust Health Rev. 2021;45:281–9. https://doi.org/10.1071/AH20200.
11. Deloitte Access Economics Pty Ltd. The Hidden cost of asthma. Asthma Australia and National Asthma Council Australia; 2015. https://asthma.org.au/wp-content/uploads/2022/03/HIdden-cost-of-asthma-final-report-revised-181115-v2-2.pdf.
12. Cook M, Douglass J, Mallon D, Mullins R, Smith J, Wong M. The economic impact of allergic disease in Australia: not to be sneezed at. 2007. https://www.allergy.org.au/images/stories/pospapers/2007_economic_impact_allergies_report_13nov.pdf.
13. Department of Education. National Digital Research Infrastructure Strategy. In: Commonwealth Department of Education, editor. Commonwealth of Australia Department of Education; 2021. https://www.education.gov.au/national-researchinfrastructure/resources/draft-ndri-strategy.
14. Gilbert S, Pimenta A, Stratton-Powell A, Welzel C, Melvin T. Continuous improvement of digital Health applications linked to real-world performance monitoring: safe moving targets? Mayo Clin Proc Digital Health. 2023;1:276–87. https://doi.org/10.1016/j.mcpdig.2023.05.010.
15. Shaw T, Hines D, Kielly-Carroll C. Impact of digital health on the safety and quality of health care. Sydney, Australia: Australian Commission on Safety and Quality in Health Care; 2018. https://www.safetyandquality.gov.au/publications-and-resources/resource-library.

16. Mateo J, Steuten L, Aftimos P, Andre F, Davies M, Garralda E, et al. Delivering precision oncology to patients with cancer. Nat Med. 2022;28:658–65. https://doi.org/10.1038/s41591-022-01717-2.

17. Tripodi S, Frediani T, Lucarelli S, Macri F, Pingitore G, et al. Molecular profiles of IgE to Phleum pratense in children with grass pollen allergy: implications for specific immunotherapy. J Allergy Clin Immunol. 2012;129:834–9. e8. https://doi.org/10.1016/j.jaci.2011.10.045.

18. Incorvaia C, Al-Ahmad M, Ansotegui IJ, Arasi S, Bachert C, Bos C, et al. Personalized medicine for allergy treatment: allergen immunotherapy still a unique and unmatched model. Allergy. 2021;76:1041–52. https://doi.org/10.1111/all.14575.

19. Department of Home Affairs. Australian Cyber Security Strategy. In: Department of Home Affairs, editor. Canberra Australia.: Commonwealth Department of Home Affairs; 2023. https://www.homeaffairs.gov.au/about-us/our-portfolios/cyber-security/strategy/2023-2030-australian-cyber-security-strategy

20. Wood A, Denholm R, Hollings S, Cooper J, Ip S, Walker V, et al. Linked electronic health records for research on a nationwide cohort of more than 54 million people in England: data resource. BMJ. 2021;373:n826. https://doi.org/10.1136/bmj.n826.

21. Australian Institute for Health and Welfare. The five safes framework. Canberra Australia: Australian Institute for Health and Welfare; 2023. https://www.aihw.gov.au/about-our-data/data-governance/the-five-safes-framework.

22. Research Data Scotland. What is the five safes framework? Discover what the five safes framework is and how it's used to keep data secure. Edinburgh Scotland: Research Data Scotland; 2024. https://www.researchdata.scot/our-work/data-explainers/what-is-the-five-safes-framework/.

23. Stiles SL, Sanfilippo FM, Loh R, Said M, Clifford RM, Salter SM. Contemporary trends in anaphylaxis burden and healthcare utilisation in Western Australia: a linked data study. World Allergy Organ J. 2023;16:100818. https://doi.org/10.1016/j.waojou.2023.100818.

24. Hua X, Dalziel K, Brettig T, Dharmage SC, Lowe A, Perrett KP, et al. Out-of-hospital health care costs of childhood food allergy in Australia: a population-based longitudinal study. Pediatr Allergy Immunol. 2022;33:e13883. https://doi.org/10.1111/pai.13883.

25. Bosnic-Anticevich S, Costa E, Menditto E, Lourenco O, Novellino E, Bialek S, et al. ARIA pharmacy 2018 "allergic rhinitis care pathways for community pharmacy": AIRWAYS ICPs initiative (European innovation partnership on active and healthy ageing, DG CONNECT and DG Sante) POLLAR (impact of air POLLution on asthma and rhinitis) GARD demonstration project. Allergy. 2019;74:1219–36. https://doi.org/10.1111/all.13701.

26. The Australian Institute of Health and Welfare. Australia's Health 2022: data insights. In: The Australian Institute of Health and Welfare, editor. Canberra Australia: The Australian Institute of Health and Welfare; 2022. https://www.aihw.gov.au/reports/australias-health/australias-health-2022-in-brief/summary.

27. Davies JM. Pollen allergens. In: Nriagu J, editor. Encyclopedia of environmental health. The Netherlands: Elsevier; 2019. https://doi.org/10.1016/B978-0-12-409548-9.11537-4.

28. Erbas B, Jazayeri M, Lambert KA, Katelaris CH, Prendergast LA, Tham R, et al. Outdoor pollen is a trigger of child and adolescent asthma emergency department presentations: a systematic review and meta-analysis. Allergy. 2018;73:1632–41. https://doi.org/10.1111/all.13407.

29. Commonwealth Department of Health and Aged Care. Corporate plan. Canberra Australia: Commonwealth Department of Health and Aged Care; 2023. https://www.health.gov.au/sites/default/files/2023-12/corporate-plan-2023-24.pdf.

30. Commonwealth Department of Health and Aged Care. Australian Digital Health Agency: Connecting Australia to a healthier future. Canberra Australia. Australian Government Australian Digital Health Agency; 2024. https://www.digitalhealth.gov.au/

31. The National Museum of Australia. Defining moments: Medicare 1984: the introduction to Medicare Canberra ACT. Australia: The National Museum of Australia; 2023. https://www.nma.gov.au/defining-moments/resources/medicare.

32. Australian Digital Health Agency. My health record; allergies, medicines, adverse reactions. Canberra Australia: Australian Digital Health Agency; 2024. https://www.digitalhealth.gov.au/initiatives-and-programs/my-health-record/whats-inside/allergies-medicines-adverse-reactions.
33. Australian Digital Health Agency. FRED dispense fact sheet: uploading an allergy as an event summary. 2022. https://www.digitalhealth.gov.au/media/1739
34. Australian Digital Health Agency. Allergies, medicines, adverse reactions. Canberra Australia: Australian Digital Health Agency; 2024. https://www.digitalhealth.gov.au/initiatives-and-programs/my-health-record/whats-inside/allergies-medicines-adverse-reactions.
35. Australian Digital Health Agency. My health record THE BIG picture. Canberra Australia: Australian Digital Health Agency; 2024. https://www.digitalhealth.gov.au/initiatives-and-programs/my-health-record/statistics.
36. National Allergy Council. National allergy strategy. National Allergy Council; 2022. https://nationalallergycouncil.org.au/images/doc/NAS_Document_Final_WEB.pdf.
37. Australian Digital Health Agency, National Allergy Council. Digital Health (My Health Record) project National Allergy Council; 2023. https://nationalallergycouncil.org.au/projects/digital-health.
38. National Allergy Council. National Allergy Council position statement: changes to pathology test results. In: Agency ADH, editor. Canberra ACT Australia: Australian Digital Health Agency; 2023. https://nationalallergycouncil.org.au/digital-health-project-position-statement.
39. Therapeutic Goods Administration. Authorised Prescriber Scheme. In: Commonwealth Department of Health and Aged Care, editor. Canberra Australia.: Therapeutic Goods Adminsitration; 2022. https://www.tga.gov.au/resources/resource/guidance/authorised-prescriber-scheme.
40. Australasian Society for Clinical Immunology and Allergy. Skin prick testing guide for diagnosis of allergic disease. 2020. http://www.allergy.org.au.
41. van der Valk JP, Gerth van Wijk R, Hoorn E, Groenendijk L, Groenendijk IM, de Jong NW. Measurement and interpretation of skin prick test results. Clin Transl Allergy. 2015;6:8. https://doi.org/10.1186/s13601-016-0092-0.
42. National Allergy Council. Shared care for allergy project overview. National Allergy Council; 2023. https://nationalallergycouncil.org.au/images/doc/scm/Shared_Care_Project_Overview_for_participants_April_2023_V2.pdf.
43. Australian Digital Health Agency. National Digital Health Strategy Delivery Roadmap 2023–2028. Sydney Australia: Australian Digital Health Agency; 2023. https://www.digitalhealth.gov.au/sites/default/files/documents/national-digital-health-strategy-roadmap-2023-2028.pdf.
44. Australian Digital Health Agency. National Digital Health Strategy 2023–2028. Sydney Australia: Australian Digitial Health Agency; 2023. https://www.digitalhealth.gov.au/sites/default/files/documents/national-digital-health-strategy-2023-2028.pdf.
45. Australian Digital Health Agency. Connecting Australian Healthcare: NATIONAL HEALTHCARE INTEROPERABILITY PLAN 2023–2028. 2023. https://www.digitalhealth.gov.au/sites/default/files/documents/national-healthcare-interoperability-plan-2023-2028.pdf.
46. Commonwealth Department of Health. Framework to guide the secondary use of My Health Record system data. In: Commonwealth Department of Health, editor. Canberra Australia: Commonwealth Department of Health; 2018. https://www.health.gov.au/sites/default/files/documents/2021/12/framework-to-guide-the-secondary-use-of-my-health-record-system-data.pdf.
47. Australian Institute for Health and Welfare. DATA GOVERNANCE FRAMEWORK 2021. In: Australian Institute for Health and Welfare, editor: Australian Institute for Health and Welfare; 2021. https://www.aihw.gov.au/getmedia/c3e00f60-c40d-4989-ad22-de1be3ab5380/data-governance-framework-2021.pdf.aspx.

48. Commonwealth Office of the National Data Commissioner. Introducing the DATA Scheme: a scheme for sharing Australian Government data Commonwealth Office of the National Data Commissioner; 2022. https://www.datacommissioner.gov.au/the-data-scheme.

49. Commonwealth Department of Health and Aged Care. Digital Health Blueprint 2023–2033. In: Commonwealth Department of Health and Aged Care, editor. Canberra Australia; 2023. https://www.health.gov.au/sites/default/files/2024-01/the-digital-health-blueprint-and-action-plan-2023-2033_0.pdf.

50. Commonwealth Department of Health and Aged Care. Action Plan for the Digital Health Blueprint 2023–2033. In: Commonwealth Department of Health and Aged Care, editor. Canberra Australia; 2023. https://www.health.gov.au/sites/default/files/2023-12/the_action_plan_for_the_digital_health_blueprint_2023-2033.pdf.

51. Davies JM, Smith BA, Milic A, Campbell B, Van Haeften S, Burton P, et al. The AusPollen partnership project: allergenic airborne grass pollen seasonality and magnitude across temperate and subtropical eastern Australia, 2016-2020. Environ Res. 2022;214:113762. https://doi.org/10.1016/j.envres.2022.113762.

52. Douglass JA, Lodge C, Chan S, Doherty A, Tan JA, Jin C, et al. Thunderstorm asthma in seasonal allergic rhinitis: the TAISAR study. J Allergy Clin Immunol. 2021;149:1607. https://doi.org/10.1016/j.jaci.2021.10.028.

53. Delpierre C, Lefevre T. Precision and personalized medicine: what their current definition says and silences about the model of health they promote. Implication for the development of personalized health. Front Sociol. 2023;8:1112159. https://doi.org/10.3389/fsoc.2023.1112159.

54. The National Allergy Centre of Excellence. Allergy Studies Directory. 2022. https://www.nace.org.au/allergy-studies-directory/.

55. National Health and Medical Research Council. Australian and New Zealand clinical trials registry: National Health and Medical Research Council; 2024. https://www.anzctr.org.au/Support/AboutUs.aspx.

56. The National Allergy Centre of Excellence. Research to transform the lives of Australians living with allergic disease: Murdoch Childrens' Research Insititute; 2022. https://www.nace.org.au/.

57. National Research Infrastructure Australia, Commonwealth Scientific and Industrial Research Organisation. Atlas of Living Australia. Canberra Australia. Commonwealth Scientific and Industrial Research Organisation; 2024.

58. James F, Goh MSY, Mouhtouris E, Vogrin S, Chua KYL, Holmes NE, et al. Study protocol: Australasian registry of severe cutaneous adverse reactions (AUS-SCAR). BMJ Open. 2022;12:e055906. https://doi.org/10.1136/bmjopen-2021-055906.

59. Centre for Antibiotic Allergy and Research. National Antibiotic Allergy Network; 2018. https://antibioticallergy.org.au/naan#.

60. Trubiano JA, Vogrin S, Chua KYL, Bourke J, Yun J, Douglas A, et al. Development and validation of a penicillin allergy clinical decision rule. JAMA Intern Med. 2020;180:745–52. https://doi.org/10.1001/jamainternmed.2020.0403.

61. Australian Commission on Safety and Quality in Health Care. National Safety and Quality Health Service Standards Sydney Australia: Australian Commission on Safety and Quality in Health Care; 2021. https://www.safetyandquality.gov.au/sites/default/files/2021-05/national_safety_and_quality_health_service_nsqhs_standards_second_edition_-_updated_may_2021.pdf.

62. Drewett GP, Encena J, Gregory J, Franklin L, Trubiano JA. Anaphylaxis in Victoria: presentations to emergency departments, with a focus on drug- and antimicrobial-related cases. Med J Aust. 2022;216:520–4. https://doi.org/10.5694/mja2.51459.

63. Victorian Department of Health. Anaphylaxis notifications guidance for Victorian hospitals. Melbourne Australia: Victorian Department of Health; 2019. https://www.health.vic.gov.au/publications/anaphylaxis-notifications-guidance-for-victorian-hospitals.

64. Australasian Society for Clinical Immunology and Allergy. ASCIA guidelines—acute management of anaphylaxis. Sydney Australia: Australasian Society for

Clinical Immunology and Allergy; 2023. https://www.allergy.org.au/hp/papers/acute-management-of-anaphylaxis-guidelines.

65. Australian Commission on Safety and Quality in Health Care. Acute Anaphylaxis Clinical Care Standard. Canberra Australia: Australian Commission on Safety and Quality in Health Care; 2021. https://www.safetyandquality.gov.au/sites/default/files/2021-11/Acute-Anaphylaxis-Clinical-Care-Standard-2021.pdf.

66. Therapeutic Goods Administration. Database of Adverse Event Notifications (DAEN)—medicines: Department of Health and Aged Care; 2023. https://www.tga.gov.au/safety/safety/safety-monitoring-daen-database-adverse-event-notifications/database-adverse-event-notifications-daen.

67. Lucas M, Vale S. Drug-induced anaphylaxis in Australia: we need a national drug allergy registry. Med J Aust. 2022;216:515–6. https://doi.org/10.5694/mja2.51527.

68. Salter SM, Marriott RJ, Murray K, Stiles SL, Bailey P, Mullins RJ, et al. Increasing anaphylaxis events in Western Australia identified using four linked administrative datasets. World Allergy Organ J. 2020;13:100480. https://doi.org/10.1016/j.waojou.2020.100480.

69. Mullins RJ, Camargo CA. Latitude, sunlight, vitamin D, and childhood food allergy/anaphylaxis. Curr Allergy Asthma Rep. 2012;12:64–71. https://doi.org/10.1007/s11882-011-0230-7.

70. Sasaki M, Koplin JJ, Dharmage SC, Field MJ, Sawyer SM, McWilliam V, et al. Prevalence of clinic-defined food allergy in early adolescence: the SchoolNuts study. J Allergy Clin Immunol. 2018;141:391–8. e4. https://doi.org/10.1016/j.jaci.2017.05.041.

71. Peters RL, Koplin JJ, Gurrin LC, Dharmage SC, Wake M, Ponsonby AL, et al. The prevalence of food allergy and other allergic diseases in early childhood in a population-based study: HealthNuts age 4-year follow-up. J Allergy Clin Immunol. 2017;140:145–53. e8. https://doi.org/10.1016/j.jaci.2017.02.019.

72. van Nunen SA, O'Connor KS, Clarke LR, Boyle RX, Fernando SL. An association between tick bite reactions and red meat allergy in humans. Med J Aust. 2009;190:510–1. https://doi.org/10.5694/j.1326-5377.2009.tb02533.x.

73. van Nunen S. Tick-induced allergies: mammalian meat allergy and tick anaphylaxis. Med J Aust. 2018;208:316–21. https://doi.org/10.5694/mja17.00591.

74. Tick Induced Allergies Research and Awareness. Allergy and anaphylaxis Australia webinar: mammalian meat allergy. 2022. https://www.tiara.org.au/news.

75. Wanandy T, Dwyer HE, McLean L, Davies NW, Nichols D, Gueven N, et al. Factors influencing the quality of *Myrmecia pilosula* (Jack jumper) ant venom for use in in vitro and in vivo diagnoses of allergen sensitization and in allergen immunotherapy. Clin Exp Allergy. 2017;47:1478–90. https://doi.org/10.1111/cea.12987.

76. Wanandy T, Le TA, Lau WY, Wiese MD, Heddle RJ, Brown SGA. The development of Jack jumper ant venom immunotherapy: our 25 years' experience. Intern Med J. 2023;53:1716–21. https://doi.org/10.1111/imj.16217.

77. Wanandy T, Wilson R, Gell D, Rose HE, Gueven N, Davies NW, et al. Towards complete identification of allergens in Jack jumper (*Myrmecia pilosula*) ant venom and their clinical relevance: an immunoproteomic approach. Clin Exp Allergy. 2018;48:1222–34. https://doi.org/10.1111/cea.13224.

78. The University of Auckland Medical and Health Science. Digital inhaler preferences in health providers and in patients with asthma: A discrete choice experiment. 2021. https://www.auckland.ac.nz/en/fmhs/research/research-study-recruitment/research-study-recruitment-a-l-fmhs/digital-inhaler-preferences.html.

79. Van Haften S, Milic A, Addison-Smith B, Butcher C, Davies JM. Grass gazers: using citizen science as a tool to facilitate practical and online science learning for secondary school students during the COVID-19 lockdown. Ecol Evol. 2020;11(8):3488–500. https://doi.org/10.1002/ece3.6948.

80. The Thoracic Society of Australia and New Zealand. Australian Severe Asthma Registry. The Thoracic Society of Australia and New Zealand. https://thoracic.org.au/wp-content/uploads/2024/01/ASAR2022.png.

81. University of Newcastle College of Health Medicine and Wellbeing. Australian Mepolizumab registry for chronic rhinosinusitis with nasal polyps. Newcastle Australia: University of Newcastle College of Health Medicine and Wellbeing; 2024. https://treatabletraits.org.au/australian-mepolizumab-registry-for-chronic-rhinosinusitis-with-nasal-polyps/.

82. Australian Bureau of Statistics. National Health Survey methodology. In: Australian Bureau of Statistics, editor. Canberra Australia; 2023. https://www.abs.gov.au/methodologies/national-health-survey-methodology/2022.

83. Australian Institute for Health and Welfare. Australia's children: in brief. Canberra Australia: Australian Institute for Health and Welfare; 2022. https://www.aihw.gov.au/reports/children-youth/australias-children/contents/about.10.25816/5ebca4d0fa7dd.

84. Wise SK, Damask C, Roland LT, Ebert C, Levy JM, Lin SD, et al. International consensus statement on allergy and rhinology: allergic rhinitis-2023. Int Forum Allergy Rh. 2023;13:293–859. https://doi.org/10.1002/alr.23090.

85. Garcia-Sanchez D, Darssan D, Lawler SP, Warren CM, De Klerk-Braasch A, Osborne NJ. Asthma and anxiety development in Australian children and adolescents. Pediatr Allergy Immunol. 2023;34:e13941. https://doi.org/10.1111/pai.13941.

86. Blaiss MS, Hammerby E, Robinson S, Kennedy-Martin T, Buchs S. The burden of allergic rhinitis and allergic rhinoconjunctivitis on adolescents: a literature review. Ann Allergy Asthma Immunol. 2018;121:43–52. e3. https://doi.org/10.1016/j.anai.2018.03.028.

87. Owens L, Laing IA, Zhang G, Turner S, Le Souef PN. Prevalence of allergic sensitization, hay fever, eczema, and asthma in a longitudinal birth cohort. J Asthma Allergy. 2018;11:173–80. https://doi.org/10.2147/JAA.S170285.

88. Bosnic-Anticevich S, Smith P, Abramson M, Hespe CM, Johnson M, Stosic R, et al. Impact of allergic rhinitis on the day-to-day lives of children: insights from an Australian cross-sectional study. BMJ Open. 2020;10:e038870. https://doi.org/10.1136/bmjopen-2020-038870.

89. Van Haeften S, Campbell BC, Milic A, Addison-Smith E, Al Kouba J, Huete A, et al. Environmental DNA analysis of airborne poaceae (grass) pollen reveals taxonomic diversity across seasons and climate zones. Environ Res. 2023;247:117983. https://doi.org/10.1016/j.envres.2023.117983.

90. Australian Bureau of Statistics. National, state and territory population. Australian Bureau of Statistics; 2023. https://www.abs.gov.au/statistics/people/population/national-state-and-territory-population/latest-release#states-and-territories.

91. Australasian Society of Clinical Immunology and Allergy. Nucala® (mepolizumab) PBS listed for CRSwNP—April 2023. Sydney Australia: Australasian Society of Clinical Immunology and Allergy; 2023. https://www.allergy.org.au/about-ascia/info-updates/nucala-mepolizumab-pbs-listed-for-crswnp.

92. Australasian Society for Clinical Immunology and Allergy. ASCIA position paper: laboratory investigation of allergic diseases. Sydney Australia: Australasian Society of Clinical Immunology and Allergy; 2020. https://www.allergy.org.au/images/stories/pospapers/ASCIA_HP_Allergy_Testing_Laboratory_2020.pdf.

93. Dang TD, Peters RL, Koplin JJ, Dharmage SC, Gurrin LC, Ponsonby AL, et al. Egg allergen specific IgE diversity predicts resolution of egg allergy in the population cohort HealthNuts. Allergy. 2019;74:318–26. https://doi.org/10.1111/all.13572.

94. Dang TD, Tang M, Choo S, Licciardi PV, Koplin JJ, Martin PE, et al. Increasing the accuracy of peanut allergy diagnosis by using Ara h 2. J Allergy Clin Immunol. 2012;129:1056–63. https://doi.org/10.1016/j.jaci.2012.01.056.

95. Kailaivasan TH, Timbrell VL, Solley G, Smith WB, McLean-Tooke A, van Nunen S, et al. Biogeographical variation in specific IgE recognition of temperate and subtropical grass pollen allergens in allergic rhinitis patients. Clin Transl Immunol. 2020;9:e01103. https://doi.org/10.1002/cti2.1103.

96. Timbrell VL, Riebelt L, Simmonds C, Solley G, Smith WB, McLean-Tooke A, et al. An immunodiagnostic assay for quantitation of specific IgE to the major pollen allergen component, Pas n 1, of the subtropical Bahia grass. Int Arch Allergy Immunol. 2014;165:219–28. https://doi.org/10.1159/000369341.

97. Digital Strategy and Transformation Branch. Digital Health 2031 A digital vision for Queensland's health system. In: eHealth Queensland, editor.: State of Queensland (Queensland Health); 2022. https://www.health.qld.gov.au/__data/assets/pdf_file/0020/1153910/QH_Digital_Health_2031.pdf.

98. Park KH, Lee J, Sim DW, Lee SC. Comparison of Singleplex specific IgE detection immunoassays: ImmunoCAP Phadia 250 and Immulite 2000 3gAllergy. Ann Lab Med. 2018;38:23–31. https://doi.org/10.3343/alm.2018.38.1.23.

99. Dramburg S, Hilger C, Santos AF, de Las Vecillas L, Aalberse RC, Acevedo N, et al. EAACI molecular Allergology user's guide 2.0. Pediatr Allergy Immunol. 2023;34(Suppl 28):e13854. https://doi.org/10.1111/pai.13854.

100. Davies JM, Pralong C, Tickner J, Timbrell V, Rodger A, Bogaard PVD, et al. Nanofluidic point-of-care IgE test for subtropical grass pollen for rapid diagnosis of allergic rhinitis. Ann Allergy Asthma Immunol. 2023;132:497. https://doi.org/10.1016/j.anai.2023.11.025.

101. Australasian Society for Clinical Immunology and Allergy. Allergic reactions to bites and stings. Sydney Australia: Australasian Society for Clinical Immunology and Allergy; 2019. https://www.allergy.org.au/images/pcc/ASCIA_PCC_Allergic_Reactions_Bites_Stings_2019.pdf.

102. Nugraha R, Kamath SD, Johnston E, Zenger KR, Rolland JM, O'Hehir RE, et al. Rapid and comprehensive discovery of unreported shellfish allergens using large-scale transcriptomic and proteomic resources. J Allergy Clin Immunol. 2018;141:1501–4. e8. https://doi.org/10.1016/j.jaci.2017.11.028.

103. Ruethers T, Taki AC, Johnston EB, Nugraha R, Le TTK, Kalic T, et al. Seafood allergy: a comprehensive review of fish and shellfish allergens. Mol Immunol. 2018;100:28–57. https://doi.org/10.1016/j.molimm.2018.04.008.

104. Minami T, Fukutomi Y, Inada R, Tsuda M, Sekiya K, Miyazaki M, et al. Regional differences in the prevalence of sensitization to environmental allergens: analysis on IgE antibody testing conducted at major clinical testing laboratories throughout Japan from 2002 to 2011. Allergol Int. 2019;68:440–9. https://doi.org/10.1016/j.alit.2019.03.008.

105. Tanaka J, Fukutomi Y, Shiraishi Y, Kitahara A, Oguma T, Hamada Y, et al. Prevalence of inhaled allergen-specific IgE antibody positivity in the healthy Japanese population. Allergol Int. 2022;71:117–24. https://doi.org/10.1016/j.alit.2021.08.009.

106. Lou H, Ma S, Zhao Y, Cao F, He F, Liu Z, et al. Sensitization patterns and minimum screening panels for aeroallergens in self-reported allergic rhinitis in China. Sci Rep. 2017;7:9286. https://doi.org/10.1038/s41598-017-10111-9.

107. Brettig T, Koplin JJ, Dang T, Lange L, McWilliam V, Sato S, et al. Cashew allergy diagnosis: a two-step algorithm leads to fewer oral food challenges. J Allergy Clin Immunol Pract. 2022;10:1652–4. e2. https://doi.org/10.1016/j.jaip.2021.12.042.

108. Muddaluru V, Valenta R, Vrtala S, Schlederer T, Hindley J, Hickey P, et al. Comparison of house dust mite sensitization profiles in allergic adults from Canada, Europe, South Africa and USA. Allergy. 2021;76:2177–88. https://doi.org/10.1111/all.14749.

109. Hatzler L, Panetta V, Lau S, Wagner P, Bergmann RL, Illi S, et al. Molecular spreading and predictive value of preclinical IgE response to Phleum pratense in children with hay fever. J Allergy Clin Immunol. 2012;130:894–901. e5. https://doi.org/10.1016/j.jaci.2012.05.053.

110. Bellomo R, Gigliotti P, Treloar A, Holmes P, Suphioglu C, Singh MB, et al. Two consecutive thunderstorm associated epidemics of asthma in the city of Melbourne. The possible role of rye grass pollen. Med J Aust. 1992;156:834–7.

111. Hew M, Lee J, Varese N, Aui PM, McKenzie CI, Wines BD, et al. Epidemic thunderstorm asthma susceptibility from sensitization to ryegrass (Lolium perenne) pollen and major allergen Lol p 5. Allergy. 2020;75:2369. https://doi.org/10.1111/all.14319.

112. Davies JM, Thien F, Hew M. Thunderstorm asthma: controlling (deadly) grass pollen allergy. BMJ. 2018;360:k432. https://doi.org/10.1136/bmj.k432.

113. Britton WJ, Woolcock AJ, Peat JK, Sedgwick CJ, Lloyd DM, Leeder SR. Prevalence of bronchial hyperresponsiveness in children: the relationship between asthma and skin reactivity to allergens in two communities. Int J Epidemiol. 1986;15:202–9.

114. Kam AW, Tong WW, Christensen JM, Katelaris CH, Rimmer J, Harvey RJ. Microgeographic factors and patterns of aeroallergen sensitisation. Med J Aust. 2016;205:310–5. https://doi.org/10.5694/mja16.00264.

115. National Health and Medical Research Council. Airborne pollen and respiratory allergies: case study. In: Commonwealth Ministry of Health, editor. Canberra Australia,: National Health and Medical Research Council; 2023. https://www.nhmrc.gov.au/about-us/resources/impact-case-studies/airborne-pollen-and-respiratory-allergies-case-study.

116. AlQuran A, Batra M, Harry Susanto N, Holland AE, Davies JM, Erbas B, et al. Community response to the impact of thunderstorm asthma using smart technology. Allergy Rhinol (Providence). 2021;12:21526567211010728. https://doi.org/10.1177/21526567211010728.

117. Alquran A, Lambert KA, Farouque A, Holland A, Davies J, Lampugnani ER, et al. Smartphone applications for encouraging asthma self-management in adolescents: a systematic review. Int J Environ Res Public Health. 2018;15:15. https://doi.org/10.3390/ijerph15112403.

118. Jones PJ, Koolhof IS, Wheeler AJ, Williamson GJ, Lucani C, Campbell SL, et al. Can smartphone data identify the local environmental drivers of respiratory disease? Environ Res. 2020;182:109118. https://doi.org/10.1016/j.envres.2020.109118.

119. Jones PJ, Koolhof IS, Wheeler AJ, Williamson GJ, Lucani C, Campbell SL, et al. Characterising non-linear associations between airborne pollen counts and respiratory symptoms from the AirRater smartphone app in Tasmania, Australia: a case time series approach. Environ Res. 2021;200:111484. https://doi.org/10.1016/j.envres.2021.111484.

120. Silver JD, Spriggs K, Haberle S, Katelaris CH, Newbigin EJ, Lampugnani ER. Crowd-sourced allergic rhinitis symptom data: the influence of environmental and demographic factors. Sci Total Environ. 2020;705:135147. https://doi.org/10.1016/j.scitotenv.2019.135147.

121. Silver JD, Spriggs K, Haberle SG, Katelaris CH, Newbigin EJ, Lampugnani ER. Using crowd-sourced allergic rhinitis symptom data to improve grass pollen forecasts and predict individual symptoms. Sci Total Environ. 2020;720:137351. https://doi.org/10.1016/j.scitotenv.2020.137351.

122. Emmerson K, Addison-Smith B, Milic A, Davies AM. The performance of short-term curated daily airborne grass pollen forecasts in diverse biogeographical regions during the AusPollen Partnership project 2016–2020. Atmos Environ X. 2022;15:100183. https://www.sciencedirect.com/science/article/pii/S2590162122000375.

123. Medek DE, Beggs PJ, Erbas B, Jaggard AK, Campbell BC, Vicendese D, et al. Regional and seasonal variation in airborne grass pollen levels between cities of Australia and New Zealand. Aerobiologia. 2016;32:289–302. https://doi.org/10.1007/s10453-015-9399-x.

124. Beggs PJ, Katelaris CH, Medek D, Johnston FH, Burton PK, Campbell B, et al. Differences in grass pollen allergen exposure across Australia. Aust N Z J Public Health. 2015;39:51–5. https://doi.org/10.1111/1753-6405.12325.

125. Haberle SG, Bowman DMJS, Newnham RM, Johnston FH, Beggs PJ, Buters J, et al. The macroecology of airborne pollen in Australian and New Zealand urban areas. PLoSOne. 2014;9:e97925. https://doi.org/10.1371/journal.pone.0097925.

126. Stevenson J, Haberle S, Johnston F, Bowman DM. Seasonal distribution of pollen in the atmosphere of Darwin, tropical Australia: preliminary results. Grana. 2007;46:34–42.

127. Johnston FH, Hanigan IC, Bowman DM. Pollen loads and allergic rhinitis in Darwin, Australia: a potential health outcome of the grass-fire cycle. EcoHealth. 2009;6:99–108. https://doi.org/10.1007/s10393-009-0225-1.

128. Davies JM, Beggs PJ, Medek DE, Newnham RM, Erbas B, Thibaudon M, et al. Trans-disciplinary research in synthesis of grass pollen aerobiology and its importance for respiratory health in Australasia. Sci Total Environ. 2015;534:85–96. https://doi.org/10.1016/j.scitotenv.2015.04.001.

129. Bannister T, Ebert E, Silver J, Newbigin E, Lampugnani E, Csutoros D, et al. A pilot forecasting system for epidemic thunderstorm asthma in South-Eastern Australia. Bull Am Meteorol Soc. 2020:1–54. https://doi.org/10.1175/BAMS-D-19-0140.1.

130. Thien F, Davies JM, Hew M, Douglass JA, O'Hehir RE. Thunderstorm asthma: an overview of mechanisms and management strategies. Expert Rev Clin Immunol. 2020;16:1005–17. https://doi.org/10.1080/1744666X.2021.1826310.
131. Rutherford S, Owen JAK, Simpson RW. Survey of airspora in Brisbane, Queensland, Australia. Grana. 2009;36:114–21. https://doi.org/10.1080/00173139709362597.
132. Tham R, Vicendese D, Dharmage SC, Hyndman RJ, Newbigin E, Lewis E, et al. Associations between outdoor fungal spores and childhood and adolescent asthma hospitalizations. J Allergy Clin Immunol. 2017;139:1140–7. e4. https://doi.org/10.1016/j.jaci.2016.06.046.
133. Tham R, Katelaris CH, Vicendese D, Dharmage SC, Lowe AJ, Bowatte G, et al. The role of outdoor fungi on asthma hospital admissions in children and adolescents: a 5-year time stratified case-crossover analysis. Environ Res. 2017;154:42–9. https://doi.org/10.1016/j.envres.2016.12.016.
134. Addison-Smith E, Milic A, Armitage C, Davies JM. First trial of automated pollen monitoring in an Australian subtropical region 26th Clean Air and Environment Conference; 2022 CONFERENCE PROCEEDINGS; 20221; Adelaide: Clean Air Society of Australia and New Zealand.
135. Air Health Labs. Commercial services: access cutting-edge air quality data and technology. 2024. https://www.airhealthlab.com/index.php/what-we-do/commercial-services.
136. Katelaris C, Baldo BA, Howden ME, Matthews PA, Walls RS. Investigation of the involvement of *Echium plantagineum* (Paterson's curse) in seasonal allergy. IgE antibodies to Echium and other weed pollens. Allergy. 1982;37:21–8.
137. Campbell BC, Al Kouba J, Timbrell V, Noor MJ, Massel K, Gilding EK, et al. Tracking seasonal changes in diversity of pollen allergen exposure: targeted metabarcoding of a subtropical aerobiome. Sci Total Environ. 2020;747:141–89. https://doi.org/10.1016/j.scitotenv.2020.141189.
138. Campbell BC, Van Haeften S, Massel K, Milic A, Al Kouba J, Addison-Smith B, et al. Metabarcoding airborne pollen from subtropical and temperate eastern Australia over multiple years reveals pollen aerobiome diversity and complexity. Sci Total Environ. 2023;862:160585. https://doi.org/10.1016/j.scitotenv.2022.160585.
139. Lambert KA, Katelaris C, Burton P, Cowie C, Lodge C, Garden FL, et al. Tree pollen exposure is associated with reduced lung function in children. Clin Exp Allergy. 2020;50:1176–83. https://doi.org/10.1111/cea.13711.
140. Tegart LJ, Schiro G, Dickinson JL, Green BJ, Barberan A, Marthick JR, et al. Decrypting seasonal patterns of key pollen taxa in cool temperate Australia: a multi-barcode metabarcoding analysis. Environ Res. 2024;243:117808. https://doi.org/10.1016/j.envres.2023.117808.
141. Erbas B, Dharmage SC, Tang ML, Akram M, Allen KJ, Vicendese D, et al. Do human rhinovirus infections and food allergy modify grass pollen-induced asthma hospital admissions in children? J Allergy Clin Immunol. 2015;136:1118–20. e2. https://doi.org/10.1016/j.jaci.2015.04.030.
142. Erbas B, Akram M, Dharmage SC, Tham R, Dennekamp M, Newbigin E, et al. The role of seasonal grass pollen on childhood asthma emergency department presentations. Clin Exp Allergy. 2012;42:799–805.
143. Simunovic M, Boyle J, Erbas B, Baker P, Davies JM. Airborne grass pollen and thunderstorms influence emergency department asthma presentations in a subtropical climate. Environ Res. 2023;236:116754. https://doi.org/10.1016/j.envres.2023.116754.
144. Simunovic M, Dwarakanath D, Addison-Smith B, Susanto NH, Erbas B, Baker P, et al. Grass pollen as a trigger of emergency department presentations and hospital admissions for respiratory conditions in the subtropics: a systematic review. Environ Res. 2020;182:109125. https://doi.org/10.1016/j.envres.2020.109125.
145. Gupta RS, Sehgal S, Wlodarski M, Bilaver LA, Wehbe FH, Spergel JM, et al. Accelerating food allergy research: need for a data commons. J Allergy Clin Immunol Pract. 2023;11:1063–7. https://doi.org/10.1016/j.jaip.2023.02.003.

146. Sehgal S, Gupta RS, Wlodarski M, Bilaver LA, Wehbe FH, Spergel JM, et al. Development of food allergy data dictionary: toward a food allergy data commons. J Allergy Clin Immunol Pract. 2022;10:1614–21. e1. https://doi.org/10.1016/j.jaip.2022.02.024.
147. Brauer R, Wong ICK, Man KK, Pratt NL, Park RW, Cho SY, et al. Application of a common data model (CDM) to rank the paediatric user and prescription prevalence of 15 different drug classes in South Korea, Hong Kong, Taiwan, Japan and Australia: an observational, descriptive study. BMJ Open. 2020;10:e032426. https://doi.org/10.1136/bmjopen-2019-032426.
148. Observational health data sciences and informatics. Allergic rhinitis search terms. 2024. https://athena.ohdsi.org/search-terms/terms?query=allergic+rhinitis&bo&page=1.
149. Ward R, Hallinan CM, Ormiston-Smith D, Chidgey C, Boyle D. The OMOP common data model in Australian primary care data: building a quality research ready harmonised dataset. Research Square. 2023;19(4):e0301557. https://doi.org/10.21203/rs.3.rs-2618841/v1.
150. National Health and Medical Research Council, Australian Research Council, Universities Australia. Management of Data and Information in research: a guide supporting the Australian code for the responsible conduct of research. National Health and Medical Research Council; 2019. https://www.nhmrc.gov.au/sites/default/files/documents/attachments/Management-of-Data-and-Information-in-Research.pdf.
151. National Health and Medical Research Council. National Statement on Ethical Conduct in Human Research 2023. In: National Health and Medical Research Council, editor. Canberra Australia: National Health and Medical Research Council; 2023. https://www.nhmrc.gov.au/about-us/publications/national-statement-ethical-conduct-human-research-2023.
152. National Health and Medical Research Council, Consumers Health Forum of Australia. Statement on consumer and community involvement in health and medical research. Canberra Australia: National Health and Medical Research Council; 2016. www.nhmrc.gov.au/guidelines/publications/s01.
153. Wilkinson MD, Dumontier M, Sansone SA, Santos LOBD, Prieto M, Batista D, et al. Evaluating FAIR maturity through a scalable, automated, community-governed framework. Sci Data. 2019;6:174. https://doi.org/10.1038/s41597-019-0248-6.
154. Jacobsen A, Azevedo RD, Juty N, Batista D, Coles S, Cornet R, et al. FAIR principles: interpretations and implementation considerations. Data Intelligence. 2020;2:10–29. https://doi.org/10.1162/dint_r_00024.
155. Santos LOBD, Burger K, Kaliyaperumal R, Wilkinson MD. FAIR data point: a FAIR-oriented approach for metadata publication. Data Intelligence. 2023;5:163–83. https://doi.org/10.1162/dint_a_00160.
156. Australian Digital Health Agency. Assessment framework for mHealth apps: summary. In: commonwealth Department of Health and Aged Care, editor. Sydney Australia: Australian Digital Health Agency; 2022. https://www.digitalhealth.gov.au/about-us/strategies-and-plans/assessment-framework-for-mhealth-apps.
157. Medek DE, Kljakovic M, Fox I, Pretty DG, Prebble M. Hay fever in a changing climate: linking an internet-based diary with environmental data. EcoHealth. 2012;9:440–7. https://doi.org/10.1007/s10393-012-0787-1.
158. Medek D, Suminovic M, Erbas B, Katelaris C, Lampugnani ER, Huete A, et al. Enabling self-management of pollen allergies a pre-season questionnaire evaluating the perceived benefit of providing local pollen information. Aerobiologia. 2019;35:777–82. https://doi.org/10.1007/s10453-019-09602-1.
159. Allergy & Anaphylaxis Australia, Australasian society for clinical immunology and allergy. AllergyPal; 2023. https://allergyfacts.org.au/resources/apps/allergy-pal
160. Australian Research Data Commons. Health Studies Australian National Data Assets (HeSANDA) development priorities: research community consultation report. Canberra Australia: Australian Research Data Commons; 2021. https://ardc.edu.au/wp-content/uploads/2022/05/HeSANDA-Development-Priorities.pdf.

Chapter 20
Digital Allergology and Allergen-Immunotherapy in Germany

Ludger Klimek, Uso Walter, Sven Becker, Ingrid Casper, Roya Kianfar, Stefani Röseler, Astrid Schareina, Holger Wrede, and Stephanie Dramburg

Contents

L. Klimek (✉) · I. Casper · R. Kianfar
Center for Rhinology and Allergology Wiesbaden, Wiesbaden, Germany
e-mail: Ludger.Klimek@allergiezentrum.org; Ingrid.Casper@allergiezentrum.org; Roya.
Kianfar@allergiezentrum.org

U. Walter
ENT joint practice Duisburg, Duisburg, Germany

S. Becker
Department of Otolaryngology, University of Tübingen, Tübingen, Germany
e-mail: Sven.Becker@med.uni-tuebingen.de

S. Röseler
Clinic for Pneumology, Allergology, Sleep and Respiratory Medicine, Augustinerinnen
Hospital, Cologne, Germany
e-mail: sroeseler@ukaachen.de

A. Schareina
Joint Practice for internal medicine and allergology, Cologne, Germany
e-mail: a.schareina@praxisschareina-lind.de

H. Wrede
ENT and Allergy Center Herford, Herford, Germany

S. Dramburg
Department of Pediatric Respiratory Medicine, Immunology and Critical Care Medicine,
Charité–Universitätsmedizin Berlin, a corporate member of Freie Universität Berlin and
Humboldt–Universität zu Berlin, Berlin, Germany
e-mail: stephanie.dramburg@charite.de

© The Author(s), under exclusive license to Springer Nature   329
Switzerland AG 2025
P. M. Matricardi, S. Dramburg, *Digital Allergology*, Health Informatics,
https://doi.org/10.1007/978-3-031-71021-6_20

Abstract The rapid adoption of telemedicine and remote ambulatory healthcare during the COVID-19 pandemic has accelerated the use of digital health applications in allergology. This chapter explores the implementation and potential of digital technologies in allergen-specific immunotherapy (AIT) in Germany and highlights the advantages and challenges they present. In addition, it provides an overview of eHealth and its various terms, such as digital health, mHealth, and healthtech, and their role in the convergence of the internet and medicine in Germany. The potential cost savings and benefits of mobile applications in healthcare are explored, along with the concept of blended care. The chapter also emphasizes the need to leverage the positive experiences and lessons learned from the pandemic to improve patient care in the future.

20.1   Introduction

Digital health applications have received a major boost from the COVID19 pandemic—particularly the various forms of telemedicine. In allergology, many aspects of remote ambulatory healthcare were rapidly implemented, while professional societies and medical associations produced guidance documents to support patient triage and remote treatment pathways [1–6]. In the field of allergy and clinical immunology, published reports and individual examples encouraged the use of digital technologies to support safe telemedicine care [7–9]. Although many health professionals appreciated the support provided by new digital technologies and the state of emergency led to reimbursement for remote care in several countries, widespread implementation has been lacking [10, 11]. An example of COVID-19-independent early adoption in the reimbursement system is provided by the German Ministry of Health, which regulated mandatory reimbursement of health apps (so-called DiGA—Digitale Gesundheitsanwendungen) by statutory health insurers once the app(s) have undergone a standardized evaluation process [12].

The special effects of the pandemic for telemedicine have now ceased—but there is still a need for telemedicine follow-up visits, follow-up care, and medium-term treatments [13].

The experience and positive lessons learned in the pandemic must be used to improve everyday patient care in the future [14]. Healthcare professionals can benefit from digital support for routine activities, especially repetitive actions and data-based decision support [15, 16]. In particular, medium- to long-term treatments with repetitive applications and follow-up appointments, such as allergen-specific immunotherapy (AIT) [17], are an excellent application area for digital and/or remote support.

This chapter summarizes different concepts of digital allergology for AIT in Germany and highlights both advantages and challenges for their implementation, referring to our previous publications on the subject [18].

20.2 An Overview of the Topic of Digital Health

Health apps, the Apple Watch, electronic patient files and artificial intelligence in hospitals, or video consultations with a doctor from the comfort of your own couch: digitization has become an indispensable part of healthcare [10].

More and more people are using their smartphones and tablets for fitness or health applications. Health or fitness apps in conjunction with wearables are particularly popular. Thus, these apps, sensors and data-based monitoring help to significantly improve preventive healthcare.

According to the Mobile Health Market Report (mHealth), sales of mobile eHealth offerings will reach a global volume of USD 115 billion by 2025 [19].

Driven by the consumer sector and the general mobility trend, the market for eHealth offerings is also growing rapidly in Germany.

20.3 Digital Health Is the Term Used to Describe Digitization in Medicine

Digital health, eHealth, mHealth, and healthtech serve as collective terms for the convergence of the Internet and medicine. We prefer the term digital health as an expression of digitization in medicine and referring to the electronic processing of communication, information, and data acquisition for medical care, documentation, and other tasks in healthcare.

Today, technology companies such as Google, Apple, or IBM are mingling at the forefront of medical research.

20.4 eHealth as an Innovative Force for Medicine

eHealth is now understood not just as a technical development, but rather as a mindset that looks away from individual healthcare to a networked, global mindset. Communication and information technologies will help improve healthcare worldwide in the future.

The fact that the concept of eHealth seems to encompass a great deal more is also shown by the large number of related terms such as *digital health*, new *health*, *healthtech, online health, health 2.0, cybermedicine, cyberdoc, and consumer health informatics*. Here it becomes clear that the term touches on a variety of topics. Mobile Health or mHealth is the area that focuses on the use of mobile devices in the healthcare sector. Mobile health is currently the growth driver on the market—the focus here is primarily on consumer-oriented fitness and health offerings.

eHealth Breaks Down into Five Major Levels:

1. **The Consumer Level**
   At the consumer level are all offerings such as web-based information portals for patients, apps, measurement and assistance systems, or digital fitness tools.
2. **The Professional Level**
   The professional level comprises the digital offerings (healthtech) financed by the traditional players in the primary healthcare market, i.e., doctors, hospitals, or insurance companies. These include, in particular, offerings from telemedicine, such as IT-supported expert consults or remote monitoring of patients' vital signs.
3. **The Macro Level**
   In the future, the macro level is to network the various digital offerings with each other. This is the greatest challenge, but it is also where the greatest potential for innovation lies dormant. First, network infrastructures must be provided, the protection and security of patient data must be ensured, and finally, the cross-sector flow of information between patients, physicians, hospitals, and payers must be regulated. A first step in this direction is the introduction of the electronic health card (eGK) in Germany [20].
4. **The Level of Artificial Intelligence**
   Thanks to artificial intelligence (AI), machines are competing with doctors, especially in diagnosis. This development can no longer be stopped.
5. **Programmable Level**
   Genomes can be read today. Experts are trying to use technology to rewrite genes and have them installed. DNA tests provide important findings for preventive medicine, allow insights into the basic structure of people, and are to become standard.

20.5   eHealth Is Being Held Back by Data Protection in Germany

A study conducted by the EU Commission last year shows that Germany still has a lot of catching up to do in the area of eHealth applications [21].

Most medical practices now have a computer with an Internet connection in their consulting rooms, but there is still a lack of electronic data capture and data exchange. This affects the areas of EHR (electronic health record): The systematic recording of an individual's or population's health data in electronic health records; *HIE (Health information exchange):* The electronic exchange of health information between different healthcare organizations (hospitals, doctors' offices, insurance companies, pharmacies); *Telehealth:* The care of patients from a distance (doctor to patient) or telemedicine applications for consultations with colleagues as well as telemedicine applications for training purposes (doctor to doctor) in the form of web conferencing or e-learning; and *PHR (Personal health record):* A personalized health record in which patients are provided with their health data digitally.

In the areas mentioned, the German healthcare system is currently not well positioned and an interoperable and digitized healthcare system still seems a long way off. Regulatory problems are primarily responsible for this and can only be remedied by means of a political framework and appropriate legislation. Too many decision-makers are expressing concerns about data protection law and slowing down development.

20.6 Cost Savings Are Possible Especially Through Mobile Applications

In addition to improving the quality of medical care, mobile applications in particular promise to reduce medical costs. If a routine examination does not have to be performed by a doctor in every case, but is automated using a smartphone and appropriate equipment, this is safer for the patient and cheaper for the entire healthcare system.

20.7 Development in the eHealth Market Starts with the Consumer

The fact that eHealth applications have recently enjoyed increasing popularity is primarily due to impetus from the consumer sector. Digitization of the healthcare sector is currently taking place bottom-up: consumers are setting the direction [22]. The main reason for this is increased health awareness. Fitness and wellness offerings are also becoming increasingly popular [23, 24]. Over 100,000 different apps from the health and fitness sector are now available on iOS and Android. In recent months, activity trackers have also conquered the German market. As smart companions, usually worn on the wrist in the form of a bracelet, they record movements and convert these into steps, distance covered, and calories burned.

Fitness apps evaluate the data in the form of tables and statistics and provide an overall impression of physical fitness. Fitness apps and wearables form the interface between leisure and health offerings and are currently the growth engine on the eHealth market [22–24].

20.8   Blended Care: Personal Healthcare and Digital Support

Blended care describes the combination of in-person healthcare visits with distance or online training sessions [25, 26]. This allows continuous access to therapy and care without overstretching the capacity of healthcare systems. In allergy care, blended care approaches have been shown to increase adherence to mobile symptom monitoring for seasonal allergic rhinitis to over 80% over several weeks [27]. As the use of monitoring apps decreases significantly faster when not accompanied or prescribed by a healthcare professional [28], this might indicate that blended care concepts could also be a valuable tool in allergy care. In particular, the prospective recording of symptoms in combination with exposure data creates a broad database for clinicians to evaluate the clinical relevance of sensitization, but also the efficacy of treatment and possible side effects.

20.9   eHealth for AIT Management

Once a diagnostic workup has led to the prescription of AIT, adherence to therapy is an essential aspect regarding efficacy outcomes. While subcutaneous use of AIT (SCIT) is subject to some control and motivation by healthcare professionals due to regular injection visits, adherence to sublingual immunotherapy (SLIT) depends primarily on the intrinsic motivation and coordination of the patients (or caregivers) themselves [29]. Because this challenge applies not only to AIT but to most chronic diseases that require continuous medication adherence, several digital support strategies have been proposed. From relatively simple reminder systems [30] to more complex models with feedback on efficacy [31, 32] and the use of artificial intelligence [33], a variety of tools have been developed and some have been evaluated in clinical trials with varying results [34]. A challenge for digital assistive technologies is that one tool is not suitable for all patients, but the choice of support should ideally be based on individual needs and preferences. During the SARS-CoV-2 pandemic, video consultations gained importance, especially for patients who needed regular checkups and follow-up [35]. In allergy care, intermittent remote video visits have been described as a viable tool to assess treatment efficacy, potential side effects, and the need for prescription renewal without having to be there in person [18]. Telehealth technologies such as video consultations and electronic prescription renewals allow healthcare professionals to maintain close contact with their patients to review individual needs and ensure optimal disease and treatment management. Finally, patient-reported outcomes provide a valuable basis for stratifying patients and deciding whether to continue or stop treatment, as efficacy can be assessed in conjunction with individual burden [36]. Direct feedback of these results in the form of intuitive summaries for patients may also increase intrinsic motivation as success can be directly monitored.

20.10   Big Data Enables New Therapy Concepts in Medicine

In the future, more and more people will be collecting data about their state of health alongside medical institutions. It is the consumers and patients themselves who are driving the Big Data development by measuring biosignals with their smartphones and corresponding sensors, for example. Self-tracking is the name of this trend from the USA. Quantified self is the movement behind it.

It is all about self-measurement and self-optimization. In addition to medical data, more and more paramedical data is also being generated. The lifelong recording and consolidation of personal data in an electronic health record could open new perspectives for research. New drugs and therapy concepts could be developed by combining and evaluating the data. However, political and social discussions make it difficult to use this data.

The comprehensive networking of all things (IoT—Internet of Things), processes, and infrastructures is unleashing enormous growth impulses on the one hand, but on the other hand it must be integrated into a new image of society. While physicians, health insurers, and the pharmaceutical industry rejoice, others fear for data protection and warn of permanent surveillance.

20.11   Data-Based Therapy Prescription

According to current guidelines and standard clinical practice, the decision to prescribe AIT is based on a thorough history and diagnostic in vitro and/or in vivo tests such as determination of serum IgE antibodies, skin prick tests, or specific provocation tests [37]. Once diagnosed, the clinical significance of the findings must be established before symptomatic medication or the only causal treatment to date— AIT—is prescribed. Therapeutic decision-making requires a thorough evaluation of symptom severity and duration combined with an assessment of allergen exposure and information on the use of symptomatic over-the-counter medications. Assessment of disease control under symptomatic treatment is particularly useful for consideration of AIT [38]. Although the preventive potential of early immunotherapy is widely discussed, patients with mild and intermittent symptoms in particular may benefit adequately from symptomatic therapy; previous recommendations have mainly targeted patients in whom this treatment has proven inadequate [37]. The diagnostic process and the assessment of disease control are associated with several challenges that can be overcome with the help of digital health technologies [39].

20.12 Digital Decision Support for Early Identification of Patients Who May Benefit from AIT

Several years may elapse between the first onset of potential allergy symptoms and diagnostic workup, in part because patients self-medicate with over-the-counter medications based on assumptions and Internet searches [40]. Because underdiagnosed and undertreated allergic rhinitis represents a significant burden not only on quality of life but also on the economy, it is desirable to improve access for patients with symptoms to proper diagnostic workup [41]. Potential solutions may include widely available symptom assessment apps [42, 43], digital diaries that highlight a potential link between symptoms and exposure [28, 43], and clinical decision support systems for primary care physicians and specialists [44, 45]. Examples of validated symptom and exposure monitoring apps include: MASK-Air [28, 38, 39, 46], Hay Fever Diary/Pollen App [47], and AllergyMonitor [43]. While mobile application systems give a (mostly probabilistic) assessment of a possible pre-diagnosis, encouraging patients to seek medical attention rather than self-treatment [36], symptom diaries enable the precise and prospective recording of symptoms in preparation for a medical visit [28, 42, 45, 47]. At the primary point of contact between patients and health professionals, usually in primary care settings, general practitioners and pediatricians can be supported by clinical decision support systems (CDSS) on diagnostic procedures and referrals [48, 49]. Finally, pharmacists are an important point of contact for patients who do not see a physician. Decision support systems have been proposed to assist pharmacists in selecting patients and recommending appropriate over-the-counter medications or referring them to a physician for diagnosis and possible prescription of AIT [50, 51].

20.13 Digital Assistive Technologies for AIT Prescribing in Polysensitized Patients

In areas with a high prevalence of polysensitization and overlapping pollen seasons, prescribing AIT can be challenging even for specialists. Retrospective clinical histories and multiple positive results in SPT or IgE to allergen extracts complicate the identification of the triggering allergen and thus the prescription of AIT. For this scenario, a clinical decision support system is currently under investigation to assist in the diagnostic workup of polysensitized patients, considering the clinical history, skin prick test, molecular IgE results, and finally eDiary results cross-referenced with local pollen data [46]. Initial evaluations among allergists and non-allergists suggest a positive effect on diagnosis and AIT prescription rates [52]. Importantly, none of the previously mentioned technologies aims to replace a healthcare professional. The common goal is to enable informed, shared decision-making and improve access to specialized medical care in a timely manner.

References

1. Conway R, Kelly DM, Mullane P, Ni Bhuachalla C, O'Connor L, Buckley C, et al. Epidemiology of COVID-19 and public health restrictions during the first wave of the pandemic in Ireland in 2020. J Public Health (Oxf). 2021;43(4):714–22.
2. Eberly LA, Kallan MJ, Julien HM, Haynes N, Khatana SAM, Nathan AS, et al. Patient characteristics associated with telemedicine access for primary and specialty ambulatory care during the COVID-19 pandemic. JAMA Netw Open. 2020;3(12):e2031640-e.
3. Shaker MS, Oppenheimer J, Grayson M, Stukus D, Hartog N, Hsieh EW, et al. COVID-19: pandemic contingency planning for the allergy and immunology clinic. J Allergy Clin Immunol Pract. 2020;8(5):1477–88. e5
4. Pfaar O, Klimek L, Jutel M, Akdis CA, Bousquet J, Breiteneder H, et al. COVID-19 pandemic: practical considerations on the organization of an allergy clinic—an EAACI/ARIA position paper. Allergy. 2021;76(3):648–76.
5. Brough HA, Kalayci O, Sediva A, Untersmayr E, Munblit D, Rodriguez del Rio P, et al. Managing childhood allergies and immunodeficiencies during respiratory virus epidemics–the 2020 COVID-19 pandemic: a statement from the EAACI-section on pediatrics. Pediatr Allergy Immunol. 2020;31(5):442–8.
6. Klimek L, Pfaar O, Hamelmann E, Kleine-Tebbe J, Taube C, Wagenmann M, et al. COVID-19 vaccination and allergen immunotherapy (AIT)–a position paper of the German Society for Applied Allergology (AeDA) and the German Society for Allergology and Clinical Immunology (DGAKI). Allergologie Select. 2021;5:251.
7. Malipiero G, Heffler E, Pelaia C, Puggioni F, Racca F, Ferri S, et al. Allergy clinics in times of the SARS-CoV-2 pandemic: an integrated model. Clin Transl Allergy. 2020;10(1):1–9.
8. Malipiero G, Paoletti G, Puggioni F, Racca F, Ferri S, Marsala A, et al. An academic allergy unit during COVID-19 pandemic in Italy. J Allergy Clin Immunol. 2020;146(1):227.
9. Persaud YK, Portnoy JM. Ten rules for implementation of a telemedicine program to care for patients with asthma. J Allergy Clin Immunol Pract. 2021;9(1):13–21.
10. Dramburg S, Matricardi PM, Casper I, Klimek L. Use of telemedicine by practising allergists before and during the SARS-CoV-2 pandemic: a survey among members of the Association of German Allergists (AeDA). Allergo J Int. 2021;30(6):193–7.
11. Armstrong CM, Wilck NR, Murphy J, Herout J, Cone WJ, Johnson AK, et al. Results and lessons learned when implementing virtual health resource centers to increase virtual care adoption during the COVID-19 pandemic. J Technol Behav Sci. 2021;7:1–19.
12. Geier AS. Digital health applications (DiGA) on the road to success—the perspective of the German Digital Healthcare Association. Bundesgesundheitsblatt-Gesundheitsforschung-Gesundheitsschutz. 2021:1–4.
13. Walker MJ, Meggetto O, Gao J, Espino-Hernández G, Jembere N, Bravo CA, et al. Measuring the impact of the COVID-19 pandemic on organized cancer screening and diagnostic follow-up care in Ontario, Canada: a provincial, population-based study. Prev Med. 2021;151:106586.
14. Frick NR, Möllmann HL, Mirbabaie M, Stieglitz S. Driving digital transformation during a pandemic: case study of virtual collaboration in a German Hospital. JMIR Med Inform. 2021;9(2):e25183.
15. Miller S, Gilbert S, Virani V, Wicks P. Patients' utilization and perception of an artificial intelligence–based symptom assessment and advice technology in a British primary care waiting room: exploratory pilot study. JMIR Hum Factors. 2020;7(3):e19713.
16. Montazeri M, Multmeier J, Novorol C, Upadhyay S, Wicks P, Gilbert S. Optimization of patient flow in urgent care centers using a digital tool for recording patient symptoms and history: simulation study. JMIR Format Res. 2021;5(5):e26402.
17. Pfaar O, Bousquet J, Durham SR, Kleine-Tebbe J, Larché M, Roberts G, et al. One hundred and ten years of allergen immunotherapy: a journey from empiric observation to evidence. Allergy. 2022;77(2):454–68.

18. Dramburg S, Walter U, Becker S, Casper I, Röseler S, Schareina A, et al. Telemedicine in allergology: practical aspects: a position paper of the Association of German Allergists (AeDA). Allergo J Int. 2021;30(4):119–29.
19. Intelligence M. MHEALTH MARKET SIZE & SHARE ANALYSIS—GROWTH TRENDS & FORECASTS (2023–2028) Hyderabad, Telangana, India. https://www.mordorintelligence.com; 2023. https://www.mordorintelligence.com/industry-reports/mobile-health-market?gclid=EAIaIQobChMI5-GH0cC4gAMVr41oCR0_vAC-EAAYASAAEgLcTfD_BwE.
20. Gesetz für sichere digitale Kommunikation und Anwendungen im Gesundheitswesen sowie zur Änderung weiterer Gesetze Vom 21. Dezember 2015, Jahrgang 2015 Teil I Nr. 54. 2015.
21. The European eHealth initiative—objectives and solutions. European Mathematical Information Service. 2022. https://cs.emis.de/LNI/Proceedings/Proceedings91/GI-Proceedings-91-2.pdf.
22. Zöllner JP, Noda AH, McCoy J, Schulz J, Tsalouchidou P-E, Langenbruch L, et al. Use of health-related apps and telehealth in adults with epilepsy in Germany: a multicenter cohort study. Telemed J E Health. 2022;29(4):540–50.
23. Balakrishnan P, Owen E, Eberl M, Friedrich B, Etter T. A retrospective real-world observational pilot analysis of Waya: a self-monitoring fitness app in Germany. Cardiovasc Endocrinol Metab. 2022;11(3):e0266.
24. Davergne T, Meidinger P, Dechartres A, Gossec L. The effectiveness of digital apps providing personalized exercise videos: systematic review with meta-analysis. J Med Internet Res. 2023;25:e45207.
25. Wu MS, Chen S-Y, Wickham RE, O'Neil-Hart S, Chen C, Lungu A. Outcomes of a blended care coaching program for clients presenting with moderate levels of anxiety and depression: pragmatic retrospective study. JMIR Mental Health. 2021;8(10):e32100.
26. Witlox M, Garnefski N, Kraaij V, De Waal MW, Smit F, Bohlmeijer E, et al. Blended acceptance and commitment therapy versus face-to-face cognitive behavioral therapy for older adults with anxiety symptoms in primary care: pragmatic single-blind cluster randomized trial. J Med Internet Res. 2021;23(3):e24366.
27. Di Fraia M, Tripodi S, Arasi S, Dramburg S, Castelli S, Villalta D, et al. Adherence to prescribed e-diary recording by patients with seasonal allergic rhinitis: observational study. J Med Internet Res. 2020;22(3):e16642.
28. Bédard A, Basagana X, Anto JM, Garcia-Aymerich J, Devillier P, Arnavielhe S, et al. Mobile technology offers novel insights into the control and treatment of allergic rhinitis: the MASK study. J Allergy Clin Immunol. 2019;144(1):135–43. e6
29. Pitsios C, Dietis N. Ways to increase adherence to allergen immunotherapy. Curr Med Res Opin. 2019;35(6):1027–31.
30. Prabhakaran L, Wei YC. Effectiveness of the eCARE programme: a short message service for asthma monitoring. BMJ Health Care Inform. 2019;26(1):e100007.
31. Mosnaim GS, Stempel DA, Gonzalez C, Adams B, BenIsrael-Olive N, Gondalia R, et al. The impact of patient self-monitoring via electronic medication monitor and Mobile app plus remote clinician feedback on adherence to inhaled corticosteroids: a randomized controlled trial. J Allergy Clin Immunol Pract. 2021;9(4):1586–94.
32. Pizzulli A, Perna S, Florack J, Pizzulli A, Giordani P, Tripodi S, et al. The impact of telemonitoring on adherence to nasal corticosteroid treatment in children with seasonal allergic rhinoconjunctivitis. Clin Exp Allergy. 2014;44(10):1246–54.
33. Babel A, Taneja R, Mondello Malvestiti F, Monaco A, Donde S. Artificial Intelligence solutions to increase medication adherence in patients with non-communicable diseases. Front Digit Health. 2021;3:669869.
34. Matricardi PM, Dramburg S, Alvarez-Perea A, Antolín-Amérigo D, Apfelbacher C, Atanaskovic-Markovic M, et al. The role of mobile health technologies in allergy care: an EAACI position paper. Allergy. 2020;75(2):259–72.
35. Portnoy JM, Pandya A, Waller M, Elliott T. Telemedicine and emerging technologies for health care in allergy/immunology. J Allergy Clin Immunol. 2020;145(2):445–54.

36. Gilbert S, Mehl A, Baluch A, Cawley C, Challiner J, Fraser H, et al. How accurate are digital symptom assessment apps for suggesting conditions and urgency advice? A clinical vignettes comparison to GPs. BMJ Open. 2020;10(12):e040269.
37. Alvaro-Lozano M, Akdis CA, Akdis M, Alviani C, Angier E, Arasi S, et al. Allergen immunotherapy in children user's guide. Pediatr Allergy Immunol. 2020;31:1–101.
38. Sousa-Pinto B, Schünemann HJ, Sá-Sousa A, Vieira RJ, Amaral R, Anto JM, et al. Consistent trajectories of rhinitis control and treatment in 16,177 weeks: the MASK-air® longitudinal study. Allergy. 2023;78(4):968–83.
39. Bousquet J, Jutel M, Pfaar O, Fonseca JA, Agache I, Czarlewski W, et al. The role of mobile health technologies in stratifying patients for AIT and its cessation: the ARIA-EAACI perspective. J Allergy Clin Immunol Pract. 2021;9(5):1805–12.
40. Cvetkovski B, Kritikos V, Yan K, Bosnic-Anticevich S. Tell me about your hay fever: a qualitative investigation of allergic rhinitis management from the perspective of the patient. NPJ Primary Care Respirat Med. 2018;28(1):3.
41. Maurer M, Zuberbier T. Undertreatment of rhinitis symptoms in Europe: findings from a cross-sectional questionnaire survey. Allergy. 2007;62(9):1057–63.
42. Alvarez-Perea A, Dimov V, Popescu FD, Zubeldia JM. The applications of eHealth technologies in the management of asthma and allergic diseases. Clin Transl Allergy. 2021;11(7):e12061.
43. Tripodi S, Giannone A, Sfika I, Pelosi S, Dramburg S, Bianchi A, et al. Digital technologies for an improved management of respiratory allergic diseases: 10 years of clinical studies using an online platform for patients and physicians. Ital J Pediatr. 2020;46:1–11.
44. Dramburg S, Marchante Fernández M, Potapova E, Matricardi PM. The potential of clinical decision support systems for prevention, diagnosis, and monitoring of allergic diseases. Front Immunol. 2020;11:2116.
45. Pereira AM, Jácome C, Almeida R, Fonseca JA. How the smartphone is changing allergy diagnostics. Curr Allergy Asthma Rep. 2018;18:1–10.
46. Bédard A, Antó JM, Fonseca JA, Arnavielhe S, Bachert C, Bedbrook A, et al. Correlation between work impairment, scores of rhinitis severity and asthma using the MASK-air® app. Allergy. 2020;75(7):1672–88.
47. Bastl K, Bastl M, Bergmann K-C, Berger M, Berger U. Translating the burden of pollen allergy into numbers using electronically generated symptom data from the patient's hayfever diary in Austria and Germany: 10-year observational study. J Med Internet Res. 2020;22(2):e16767.
48. Flokstra-de Blok BM, van der Molen T, Christoffers WA, Kocks JW, Oei RL, Oude Elberink JN, et al. Development of an allergy management support system in primary care. J Asthma Allergy. 2017;10:57–65.
49. Flokstra-de Blok BM, Brakel TM, Wubs M, Skidmore B, Kocks JW, Oude Elberink JN, et al. The feasibility of an allergy management support system (AMSS) for IgE-mediated allergy in primary care. Clin Transl Allergy. 2018;8(1):18.
50. Cvetkovski B, Cheong L, Tan R, Kritikos V, Rimmer J, Bousquet J, et al. Qualitative exploration of pharmacists' feedback following the implementation of an "allergic rhinitis clinical management pathway (AR-CMaP)" in Australian community pharmacies. Pharmacy. 2020;8(2):90.
51. Lourenço O, Bosnic-Anticevich S, Costa E, Fonseca JA, Menditto E, Cvetkovski B, et al. Managing allergic rhinitis in the pharmacy: an ARIA guide for implementation in practice. Pharmacy. 2020;8(2):85.
52. Arasi S, Castelli S, Di Fraia M, Villalta D, Tripodi S, Perna S, et al. @ IT2020: an innovative algorithm for allergen immunotherapy prescription in seasonal allergic rhinitis. Clin Exp Allergy. 2021;51(6):821–8.

Chapter 21
Digital Allergology in Spain

Darío Antolín-Amérigo, Alberto Álvarez-Perea, Teresa Garriga-Baraut, and Irene García-Gutiérrez

Contents

D. Antolín-Amérigo (✉)
Allergy Department, Ramón y Cajal University Hospital. Ramón y Cajal Research Institute (IRYCIS), Madrid, Spain

Universidad de Alcalá, Alcalá de Henares, Madrid, Spain

A. Álvarez-Perea
Allergy Service, Hospital General Universitario Gregorio Marañón; Gregorio Marañón Health Research Institute, Madrid, Spain
e-mail: alberto@alvarezeperea.com

T. Garriga-Baraut
Pediatric Allergy Unit, Vall d'Hebron University Hospital, Barcelona, Spain
e-mail: teresa.garriga@vallhebron.cat

I. García-Gutiérrez
Allergy Department. Hospital Universitario Marqués de Valdecilla, Marqués de Valdecilla Research Institute (IDIVAL), Santander, Spain

Universidad de Alcalá, Alcalá de Henares, Madrid, Spain

© The Author(s), under exclusive license to Springer Nature Switzerland AG 2025
P. M. Matricardi, S. Dramburg, *Digital Allergology*, Health Informatics, https://doi.org/10.1007/978-3-031-71021-6_21

Abstract The National Health System of Spain (SNS) provides different structures and public services for the protection of health throughout the State, offering universal access to its services, which are financed through taxes. The opportunities in the field of Digital Health, and specifically in Digital Allergology are diverse and will be revised in this chapter. The SNS has large databases whose exploitation allows the generation of numerous indicators accounting for the current health situation. The development of a Digital Health Strategy (DHS) in Spain requires a prior review of the framework for digital transformation of the public administration as a whole and the need to adopt measures to address the problems of the manifest health system as a challenge. The new Spanish Strategy for Science, Technology, and Innovation, 2021–2027 constitutes a very good opportunity to achieve innovative operative goals. In this chapter, the reader will gain knowledge on reimbursement structures, mobile health developments, telemedicine and the utilization of digital health tools in the Spanish healthcare system.

21.1   Current State of Digitization in the Spanish Healthcare System

The Spanish Constitution, in its Article 43, recognizes for all people the right to health protection [1]. Its implementing regulations specify this right from a comprehensive perspective including health surveillance, promotion and maintenance, preventive, diagnostic, therapeutic and rehabilitative activities, all of which constitute the service portfolio of the Spanish National Health System (SNS, from *Sistema Nacional de Salud* in Spanish).

The SNS provides different structures and public services for the protection of health throughout the State, offering universal access to its services, which are financed through taxes. The baseline provision of healthcare, or first level of care, is organized via professional primary care teams (medicine and nursing), who are responsible for the population of a certain area. Primary care staff focuses on the promotion and preservation of health, treating prevalent problems, and ensuring continuous follow-ups. In this way, equity in access to services is reinforced, minimizing geographical barriers and increasing personal autonomy [2].

The second level (specialist care) has more complex and costly diagnostic and treatment resources, which have to be concentrated in order to be efficient. These services are accessible only by referral from primary healthcare professionals or by other specialists.

Electronic medical record systems have clearly advanced in terms of their availability and accessibility from different digital devices. Still, they are not yet perceived as an essential asset for the relationship between professionals and patients. The decision support systems that have been adopted to date consist fundamentally of generic aids with little development of tools based on massive data management.

Decision support systems are not developed enough, but there is a recent trend on delabeling drug hypersensitivities in a nationwide movement called PROA [3].

The diversification of contact channels, which can facilitate patient access to services and appointment management has exponentially increased during the pandemics, providing sometimes more agile and appropriate medical advice when in-person consultations may pose a risk. There is also room for improvements in the information provided to the patient and reference persons on the evolution of their process: quality healthcare requires health information to be provided in a timely manner, taking advantage of the different available communication options.

The introduction of portable digital devices aimed at improving the management and control of diseases, especially those with a chronic course. For instance, insulin pumps and continuous glucose monitors, electronic peak-flow meters or smart-watch pulsioxymeters provide the patient with greater autonomy and quality of life allowing them to interact with health services in a more flexible way and in a passive manner. Its use needs a decided impulse, always supported by its systematic evaluation and follow-up, so that its incorporation into clinical practice is based on a correct cost/effectiveness ratio.

It is also necessary to review the situation of the SNS Health Information System, defined in Chapter V of Law 16/2003, of May 28, on cohesion and quality of the SNS, which must guarantee standardization, comparability, transparency, and accessibility within the legal framework for the protection of personal data [2].

The SNS has large databases whose exploitation allows the generation of numerous indicators accounting for the health situation, system resources, activity, clinical or cost-effectivity results, including the opinion and expectations of the population/patients. This information system, which constitutes one of the backbones of the SNS, is based on specific records and statistics, existing both at state level and in the Autonomous Communities. The national and regional health databases are subject to a significant degree of standardization.

However, there are still underdeveloped aspects, related to the socioeconomic, cultural, and environmental determinants of health, or the physical, social, and family environment that play a relevant role in the health status of the population. Other issue to be improved is a progress in the analysis of health results, information that would enrich the knowledge and, consequently, would facilitate the prioritization of health policies.

Because of the health crisis caused by COVID-19, the need for shared information in real time has become more evident, both for epidemiological surveillance and to orchestrate the response of care and assistance to the population. This need was also important for patients suffering from allergic diseases, in need of continuous or acute care [4]. The pandemic has promoted systems for the registration and exploitation of health information, monitoring and control of the care capacity, including the effective allocation of the available resources. The information systems must support all the activities of the SNS, from health surveillance to personalized medicine seeking the best option for each patient.

Finally, one of the fundamental challenges facing the health system and related entities is the massive storage of data for advanced analysis thereof. It is necessary to establish a National Health Data Space, including data from the SNS and other repositories of health agencies or non-health-related public administrations. Also, information from the academic field or the Internet of Things (IoT) may be included. This comprehensive database will then give ground to digital exploitation methodologies, such as massive data analysis ("big data") or artificial intelligence (AI) tools, machine learning (ML), or natural language processing (NLP) [2].

21.2   Digital Cross-Linking of Different Stakeholders in the Healthcare System

Undertaking the development of a Digital Health Strategy (DHS) in Spain requires a prior review of the framework for the digital transformation of the public administration as a whole.

There is a need to adopt measures to address the problems of the health system as a challenge: establishing the new foundations of a system that requires the systematic incorporation of novel digital technologies, prevention of disease and disability, clinical practice, planning, management and decision-making [5].

It is necessary to align the approach and objectives of this Strategy with the lines of action established in the Digital Spain 2025 [6] Strategy plan, of the Ministry of Economic Affairs and Artificial Intelligence [7], as well as with the National Artificial Intelligence Strategy, the Industrial Policy Strategy for Spain 2030 and the Personalized Medicine Strategy (both in preparation). Likewise, the DHS must take advantage of the synergies that may derive from the national research plans, within the framework of the new Spanish Strategy for Science, Technology and Innovation, 2021–2027 [2], as well as the European programs.

The Spanish DHS 2025 [6] is built around 10 axes, to achieve the following objectives: (1) 100% coverage of the population with Internet access of more than 100Mbps; (2) 80% of people with basic digital skills; (3) 20,000 specialists in cybersecurity, AI and data; (4) 50% of public services available through apps, and (5) 25% of companies using AI and "big data". Specifically, it envisages a project to drive the digital transformation of the healthcare sector through innovation, research, care and patient empowerment, with the ultimate goal of increasing the quality of life of the population.

This transformation of the SNS is proposed as the result of a coordinated, interoperable, integrated and multidimensional development that generates applications for the entire biohealth ecosystem. In addition, it establishes that it will work with all ministerial departments. The Recovery, Transformation, and Resilience Plan [8] also includes as one of its projects the "Renewal and expansion of the capabilities of the SNS": technological modernization, renewal of equipment and digital transformation; digitalization and accessibility of patients to their own medical data; and the development of new diagnostic and therapeutic techniques (e.g., for the diagnosis and treatment of allergies).

Likewise, the Spanish Strategy for Science, Technology and Innovation 2021–2027 [2] includes precision medicine and new diagnostic and therapeutic techniques (for example, for the diagnosis and treatment of Allergy) among its contents.

The AI Strategy establishes seven strategic objectives or results to be achieved with its application: scientific excellence and innovation in AI, the projection of Spanish language, the creation of qualified employment, the transformation of the productive factory, the creation of confidence in the use of AI, the incorporation of humanistic values to AI and the development of an inclusive and sustainable AI.

The DHS is therefore aimed at a public health system based on the right to health protection recognized in the Spanish Constitution and on the responsibility of public administrations; focused on people, processes, data and innovation oriented to 5P healthcare (population, preventive, predictive, personalized and participatory).

Its guiding principles are: (1) to promote the values of the SNS; (2) to increase patient autonomy and professional development, and (3) to prioritize innovative actions for positive health outcomes (Fig. 21.1).

DHS action plan (Fig. 21.1):

The Strategy must be considered as a living and dynamic working instrument, which will be reviewed periodically within the Digital Health Commission and, when appropriate, in the Interterritorial Council of the SNS.

21.3   Access to Digital Health and Reimbursement Structures

The Spanish public healthcare system is funded through taxes and primarily operates through its own resources. Management is controlled by public authorities. Besides, there is involvement of the private sector in certain contracted activities.

Approximately 26.7% of the total healthcare expenditure in Spain is attributed to private healthcare. This activity may be funded through out of the pocket fees, but it is mostly covered by private insurance policies. The number of Spaniards with private health insurance was estimated to be 10.3 million in 2022 [9].

Allergology is a recognized specialty in Spain, with fully defined aims and competencies [10]. In 2018, the SNS had a ratio of 2.3 allergists per 100,000 inhabitants. The number showed significant variation across autonomous communities, ranging from 0 allergists in the Balearic Islands, 0.49 in Asturias, and 0.77 in Andalusia to 2.31 in Castilla La Mancha and 2.45 in Madrid. On average, there was a 41% variability among communities [11].

Private allergy practice is present in hospitals, specialty centers and independent clinics all over the country.

Over the past decade, certain regions have taken steps to increase the utilization of telehealth to enhance accessibility, particularly for patients dealing with chronic conditions. Among the medical specialties implementing telemedicine extensively nationwide, dermatology stands out as one of the leaders. Galicia, the Basque Country, Cataluña, and Andalusia have been at the forefront of teledermatology

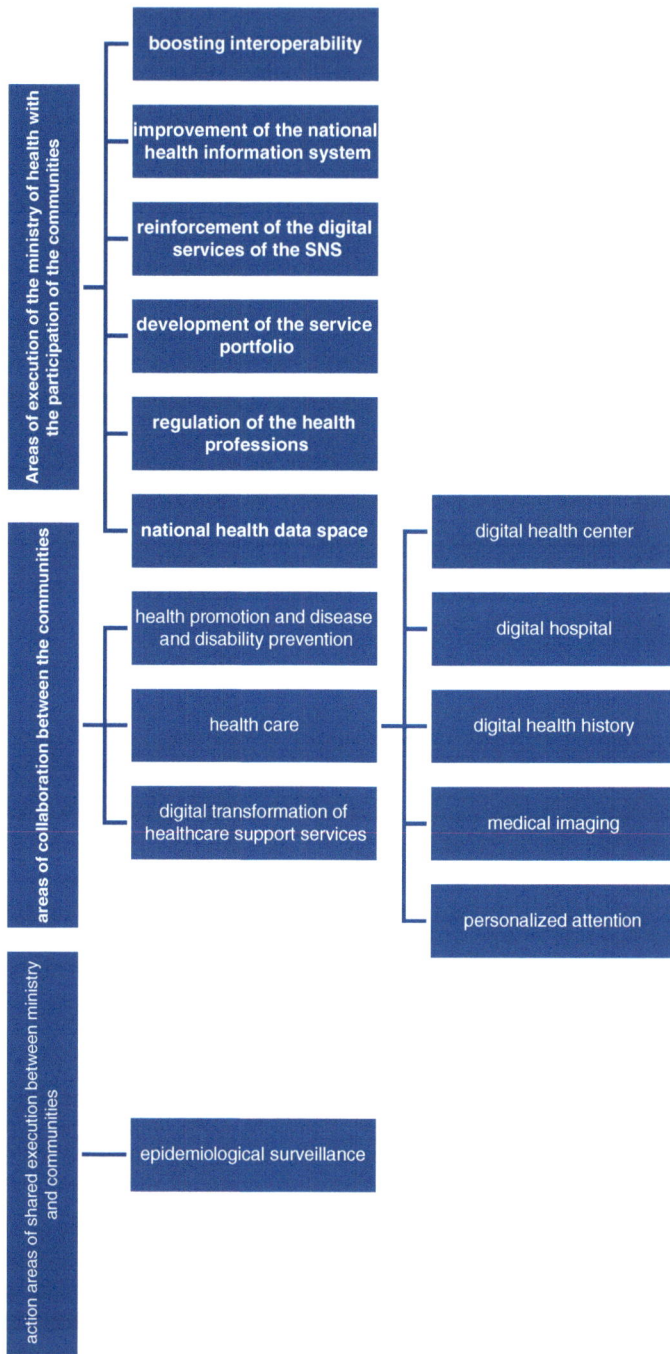

Fig. 21.1 Digital Health Strategy action plan in Spain

services. Additionally, Galicia was a pioneer in conducting teleconsultations for pneumology as well [12].

The outbreak of the COVID-19 pandemic further accelerated the adoption of remote consultations and telemedicine, aiming to minimize patients' physical visits to healthcare centers. As a result, phone triage became a widespread practice for all patients in need of primary care consultations or specialized follow-up appointments. During the initial 12 months of the pandemic, approximately 72% of the population in Spain stated that they had experienced a medical consultation either through online means or over the telephone, encompassing both public and private healthcare services. Additionally, various remote communication systems, such as video conferencing or synchronous messaging, were implemented to facilitate seamless communication across different levels of care [13].

The access to digital health services has been added in the last few years to the conditions of many private insurance policies, most frequently telemedicine, including teleconsultation (telephone and video platforms), appointment managing and online access to health records. It has been perceived by the insurers as a mean to improve access, but also as a potential reduction in cost [14].

Unfortunately, no specific initiatives aimed at digitalizing Allergology have been established in either the public or private healthcare sectors up to this point.

21.4 Digital Health Tools for Allergic Patients

The Spanish Government has developed a strategic plan for the implementation of eHealth interventions in the national health care system. Data from the national Health Care Barometer-prior to the COVID-19 pandemic-show a frankly positive assessment of select digital services by the population, such as online appointments (rating 8.4/10), access to clinical reports (7.9/10), electronic prescriptions (8.8/10) or telephone consultations with the doctor (8.1/10). However, the availability of these tools, including telemedicine, has been limited until the outbreak of the pandemic.

Telemedicine received a tremendous boost in acceptance and utilization during COVID-19 [15]. The most heavily affected countries, such as Spain, saw their allergy practices being converted to telemedicine within days [16]. In many cases, the radical change in practice had to happen without much of the needed preparation or advanced planning [17]. Despite this almost overnight transformation, there are reports that allergic patients' satisfaction with telemedicine during the pandemic was high. A survey conducted in a Spanish allergy unit, demonstrated that half of the patients who underwent a telephone consultation during the first peak of the pandemic would welcome this practice also after the resolution of the epidemiological emergency [18].

An often-underestimated tool for the delivery of health-related guidance is social media platform. Social media has become a popular source of health information for the general population and, particularly, for the patients with asthma and allergic diseases. A survey conducted by the Spanish Government in 2015 revealed that 37.6% of the respondents searched social media for health-related information [19]. A study, based on a survey among caretakers of food-allergic patients attending a Spanish pediatric allergy unit, described that over two thirds of them used social media and 25% gathered information related to their disease. The most popular food allergy-related use of social media was receiving food allergen information, followed by medical information and socializing with other patients [20].

Moreover, patients show a significant level of engagement during the annual meetings of the major professional organizations. It has been described that, during the period from 2013 to 2016, up to 12.3% of the users of the official hashtags of the SEAIC annual congresses were patients [21].

Nevertheless, the main limitation for the use of social media for patients is reliability. There is no standardized method to measure the characteristics of information available in social networks [22]. And there are no specific studies assessing the quality of information about allergic diseases available on social media in Spanish. Studies in English have shown that quality is mostly low [23–25]. In line with these findings, only 14.7% of Spaniards consider social media as a trustworthy source for health-related information, according to a survey published in 2016 by the National Observatory of Telecommunications [19].

In the field of mobile health, an open-label randomized controlled trial demonstrated that an epinephrine autoinjector smart case, attached to a mobile app, reduced anxiety in patients with anaphylaxis. In addition, it improved the patient's perception of the management of an acute episode of anaphylaxis [26]. Unfortunately, it is not commercially available, so there is no actual use of this tool by Spanish patients.

The plans for the Spanish Digital Health strategy include research and development funds to be invested in the transformation of the National Healthcare System, including implementation in clinical practice and patient empowerment. We still don't know how this will affect the progress of Digital Allergology in Spain, but growth seems the most likely scenario when we are practically starting from scratch [6].

21.5   Telemedicine and Remote Care: Revolutionizing Healthcare in Spain

Telemedicine and remote care have emerged as revolutionary forces in the healthcare sector, transforming the way medical services are delivered and accessed in various specialties, including Allergology. With the advancements in technology and the growing demand for efficient healthcare, telemedicine has become an essential tool for allergists and patients alike. The specialty of Allergology has witnessed significant advancements in telemedicine in recent years. Telemedicine in Allergology in Spain involves the use of telecommunications and digital technologies to provide virtual consultations, monitor patients remotely, offer allergy advice, and facilitate follow-up care. This approach has proven to be particularly beneficial for Spanish allergic patients who often require ongoing management and support [27].

Telemedicine in Spain has proven particularly effective in managing asthma and allergic rhinitis, one of the most common allergic conditions. Patients can consult with allergists through video calls, receive personalized treatment plans, and learn about environmental control measures to mitigate allergen exposure. Moreover, patients can use connected devices to monitor their lung function and share the data with healthcare providers. This allows for early detection of asthma exacerbations and timely intervention.

Telemedicine and remote care have had a profound impact on allergy care in Spain, bringing specialized allergy care within reach of patients across the country. However, in certain cases, face-to-face consultations are still required for comprehensive diagnosis and treatment. Integrating telemedicine with traditional healthcare practices is essential to ensure continuity of care, comprehensive allergy diagnostics and treatment, and to ensure the best disease control. Building trust through virtual consultations may require extra effort on the part of healthcare professionals [28].

One interesting study about telemedicine performed in Spain was the COMETA consensus describing that a total of 96% of participants continue using telemedicine after the COVID19 pandemic. Landline telephones, videoconference platforms, email addresses and mobile phones were provided by health service providers for, respectively, 100%, 73.3%, 73.3%, and 38.7% of the participants. However, 48% of participants declared to still use their private email address and 33.3% their private telephone line for work purposes. Likewise, according to the results obtained, there is a wide interest in implementing telemedicine in Spain in daily clinical practice, but it is necessary to work on the limitations [29].

Table 21.1 describes the main benefits of telemedicine in the specialty of Allergology in Spain, which resulted in more effective disease management and enhanced patient education. However, while telemedicine brings numerous advantages and holds immense promise to the specialty of Allergology, several challenges and considerations have been encountered during its implementation in Spain, as described in Table 21.2 [30, 31].

21.6 Telemedicine and its Impact on Spanish Healthcare

In Spain, the adoption of telemedicine in the field of the allergology has steadily increased, offering a wide range of medical services including virtual consultations, remote patient monitoring, digital diagnostics (such as prickFILM or GEMAST, among others), and online prescriptions [28]. The Spanish healthcare system has embraced telemedicine to address long waiting times, improve accessibility in rural areas, and enhance the overall patient experience. Telemedicine has had a profound impact on the Spanish healthcare system. It has helped alleviate the burden on

Table 21.1 Main benefits of telemedicine in the specialty of Allergology in Spain

Improved accessibility	Telemedicine has made specialized care more accessible to patients residing in remote or rural areas of Spain. It reduces the need for patients to travel long distances to consult with allergists, leading to better compliance with treatment plans, improving healthcare equity while saving time and money
Remote monitoring	Allergists can remotely monitor patients' allergic reactions and responses to treatment. This continuous monitoring allows for early intervention and adjustments to treatment plans as needed
Cost-effectiveness	Telemedicine in Allergology can help reduce healthcare costs for both patients and the healthcare system. It minimizes the need for physical consultations and emergency visits, optimizing resource allocation and saving time and travel expenses
Enhanced allergy education	Telemedicine platforms offer opportunities for allergists to educate patients about allergies, triggers, and preventive measures. This empowers patients to better manage their allergies and make informed lifestyle choices, fostering a more proactive approach to allergy care
Better disease management	Regular virtual check-ups and monitoring enable allergists to track patients' progress and make necessary adjustments to treatment plans, leading to improved allergy management. This facilitates more effective management of chronic allergic conditions and reduces the need for frequent hospital visits
Rapid response during emergencies	In cases of severe allergic reactions, telemedicine can serve as an immediate means of communication, providing patients with potentially life-saving advice before emergency services arrive
Flexibility and convenience	Telemedicine offers flexibility to both patients and healthcare professionals, making healthcare more efficient and saving time and travel expenses
Timely medical advice	Telemedicine has enabled real-time communication between patients and healthcare providers. This timely access to medical advice allows for early diagnosis and intervention, leading to better treatment outcomes, reducing hospitalization rates, and leading to improved quality of life

Table 21.2 Challenges and considerations of telemedicine in the specialty of Allergology in Spain

Technological barriers (Digital gap)	Some elderly or economically disadvantaged patients may lack access to the necessary technology or face challenges related to digital literacy, hindering their participation in telemedicine services
Allergic testing limitations	Certain allergic tests, such as skin prick tests or patch tests, require in-person evaluation and are not yet fully replicable in remote settings
Privacy and data security	Protecting patient data and ensuring the confidentiality of medical information are critical considerations in telemedicine implementation. Cybersecurity measures must be robust to protect sensitive medical information from unauthorized access
Establishing trust	Establishing a strong doctor-patient relationship is vital in Allergology
Medical licensure and regulations	Telemedicine may involve crossing regional or national borders, which can complicate medical licensure and regulatory compliance

overcrowded hospitals and clinics, making it easier for patients to access medical advice and specialized care. The remote care model has also improved the coordination between primary care providers and specialists, leading to more efficient healthcare delivery. Furthermore, telemedicine has demonstrated its usefulness during public health crises, such as the COVID-19 pandemic [32]. It enabled health-care providers to continue delivering essential services while minimizing the risk of infection and reducing the strain on healthcare facilities.

Finally, to address and improve the legal and healthcare gaps that currently exist in telemedicine applied to allergology, the Pediatric Allergy Committee of the Spanish Society of Allergy is actively working on the development of what will be the first Spanish Telemedicine Guide for the management of pediatric and adolescent patients with asthma and allergies.

21.7 Mobile Health Developments: Revolutionizing Healthcare at Patients' Fingertips

Mobile health, commonly known as mHealth, has emerged as a transformative force in the healthcare industry, leveraging the power of mobile technology to enhance medical services and improve overall health outcomes. These devices have become an indispensable part of modern life, offering a variety of healthcare-related applications and services [33]. With the widespread adoption of smartphones and other portable devices, mHealth has enabled individuals to access healthcare resources, monitor their health, and receive medical guidance. And, as it could not be otherwise, mHealth applications specific to Allergology have gained big popularity also in Spain. Moreover, it is well documented that the developments in mHealth have had a profound impact on patient care and healthcare delivery, as described in Fig. 21.2 [34, 35].

However, it is important to highlight the importance of understanding the mHealth regulatory framework, because, as technology continues to evolve, clear and comprehensive regulatory guidelines are necessary to ensure the safety and effectiveness of mobile health applications. Despite these challenges, the future of mHealth looks promising. Advancements in AI, wearable technology, and 5G connectivity are set to further enhance mHealth capabilities. The integration of mHealth with other emerging technologies, such as remote procedures and smart health devices, holds immense potential for revolutionizing healthcare on a global scale [27]. Table 21.3 describes some Spanish useful apps for allergic patients. All of them have been developed in Spain and offer features like symptom trackers, allergy diaries, and/or medication reminders. Moreover, patients can record allergy triggers, monitor their daily symptoms, and share the data with allergists for better-informed decision-making [36, 37].

mHealth developments have ushered in a new era of healthcare, empowering individuals to actively engage in their well-being and access medical services with unprecedented ease. From health tracking to telemedicine, mHealth applications have reshaped patient care, making it more personalized, efficient, and accessible. Mobile applications developed in Spain cater to individuals with allergies, offering valuable tools for allergy management, pollen monitoring, allergen identification in products, and safe dining experiences. By leveraging technology, these apps

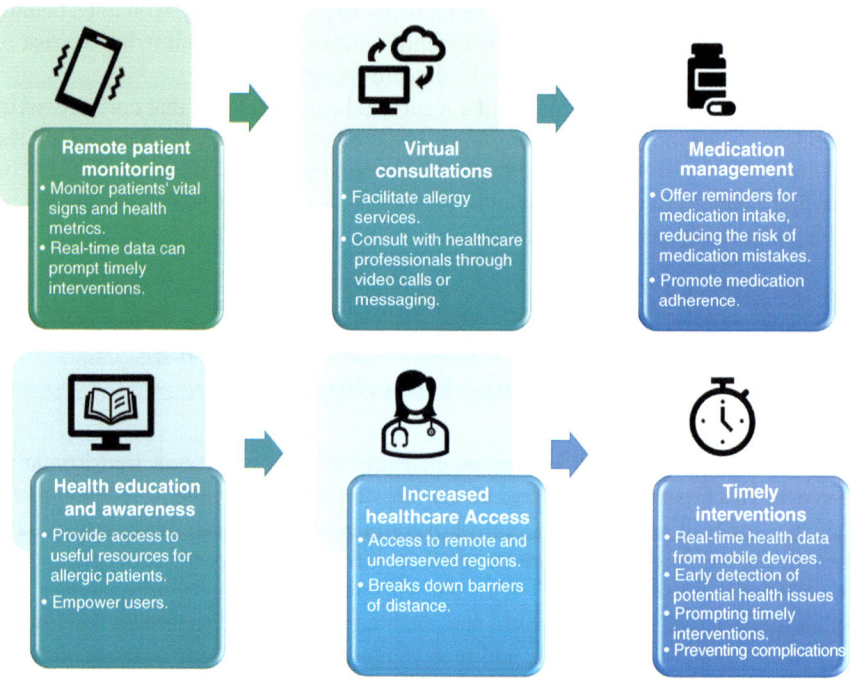

Fig. 21.2 Mobile Health applications benefits

empower allergy sufferers in Spain to take better control of their conditions and improve their quality of life.

21.8   Conclusions

Although decision support systems are not developed enough, there is a recent trend on delabeling drug hypersensitivities in a nationwide movement called PROA.

The Spanish DHS 2025 which is built around ten axes, aims to achieve the requirements for digital transformation of the provision of healthcare, promoting the implementation, formation of healthcare professionals and patients.

Mobile applications developed in Spain cater to individuals with allergies, offering valuable tools for allergy management, pollen monitoring, allergen identification in products, and safe dining experiences. By leveraging technology, these apps empower allergy sufferers in Spain to take better control of their conditions and improve their quality of life.

In Spain, the adoption of telemedicine in the field of the allergology has steadily increased, offering a wide range of medical services including virtual consultations, remote patient monitoring, digital diagnostics, and online prescriptions.

Table 21.3 Spanish useful apps for allergic patients developed in Spain

App name	Logo	Useful information
Polen Control		It is a free application that allows to check environmental pollen levels. It also enables users to track their allergies daily by entering information about their current condition, symptoms, and medications.
Pollen		Designed by the Austrian Pollen Alert Service and the Spanish Aerobiology Network (REA). It allows us to check allergy risk results and record symptoms in a diary, all personalized by allergen type.
Niveles de polen		It is an application to quickly check the pollen levels in an area. It gathers data from 85 measurement stations spread throughout Spain, nine in Portugal, and another one in the Principality of Andorra.
Polen REA		It provides information about the pollen content in the atmosphere through a weekly update and it offers maps of Spain that reflect the pollen levels of the most important plants.
Polen Salud Madrid		In the Community of Madrid checks the status of pollen collectors near mobile patient's device's location, visualizing it on a map in graphic format. This app also emits notifications of alerts for high levels of pollen.
Alerta Polen		Is a comprehensive platform that provides real-time information about allergenic pollen levels in different regions of Spain. The app uses data from official pollen monitoring stations to deliver allergy forecasts and alerts.
Plant·tes		Citizens contribute to creating a map of the phenological state of plants (presence of closed/opened flowers and/or fruits). Knowing the state of the plant allows to interpret if it is in the phase of pollen emission or not.
Anapphylaxis		It is a medical device which includes a smart case and an app. It provides information on the storage conditions, effectiveness, and physical proximity of your adrenaline auto-injector.
EPI-TRAK		It works by using the GPS of the smartphone to monitor alarms and a screen pops remembering your adrenaline pen.
Alimentium - Restalergia		Technological platform of scientific knowledge on nutritional composition and allergens of food products, food safety, global management and compliance with current legislation.
Allergeneat		An innovative mobile app designed to assist users with food allergies and intolerances. It helps users identify allergens in packaged food products by scanning their barcodes.
ControlASMApp		An interactive resource designed for use in the physician's daily clinical practice to better track the evolution of patients with asthma. It allows monitoring of clinical data, activities, and evaluated parameters at each visit.
OITcontrol		App that guides and monitors your oral immunotherapy treatment with food. It allows close communication with your doctor, informing you of intakes, incidents and home reactions in real time. With OITcontrol you will have all the information about your oral immunotherapy treatment always at hand.
Itk diary card		Application in which the user will enter daily the number of symptoms and the medication taken related to their allergic pathology
GEMAST		In order to facilitate its identification and diagnosis and thus improve the quality of life of patients, the Spanish Group of Advanced Systemic Mastocytosis (GEMAST), belonging to the Spanish Society of Hematology and Hemotherapy (SEHH), with the collaboration of Novartis has developed the application for mobile devices to help in the identification and diagnosis of Systemic Mastocytosis.
EASI-SCORAD		The EASI SCORAD is a tool used to measure the extent and severity of Atopic Dermatitis. With this APP, you can calculate the EASI SCORAD easily and accurately
MyHAE		App for Hereditary Angioedema patients which includes: 1) HAE Crisis Diary; 2) Custom reports; 3) Treatment Planning; 4) Calendar reminders; 5) Evolution over time
UrticariApp		App developed by AAUC - Association of Chronic Urticaria Affected patients to monitor chronic urticaria. It allows calibrating the affectation through images and graphs that facilitate the introduction of data. The application stabilized in 2016 and is an example of Apps developed by patient associations.

The future of Digital Allergology in Spain is bright, but requires a profound involvement of the different stakeholders and that the innovation units of hospitals, Allergology Societies, healthcare professionals and patients associations would join efforts, forces, and ideas to embrace the challenges of this particular but useful provision of care.

Telemedicine and remote care have ushered in a new era of healthcare accessibility and efficiency in Spain. By leveraging technology, the Spanish healthcare system has empowered patients with better access to medical services, while healthcare providers have gained the ability to reach a broader patient base and improve overall healthcare outcomes. While challenges persist, the positive impact of telemedicine on Spanish healthcare is undeniable, making it a pivotal component of the country's healthcare landscape. As technology continues to advance, telemedicine is poised to play an even more significant role in the future, ensuring a healthier and more connected population in Spain.

References

1. España Ministerio de Educación Cultura y Deporte. The Spanish Constitution (English). 1978:1–54. http://www.boe.es/legislacion/documentos/ConstitucionINGLES.pdf.
2. Ministerio de ciencia e innovación. Spanish Science, Technology andInnovation Strategy 2021–27. 2021. https://cpage.mpr.gob.es.
3. Paño-Pardo JR, Moreno Rodilla E, Cobo Sacristan S, Cubero Saldaña JL, Periañez Párraga L, Del Pozo León JL, Retamar-Gentil P, Rodríguez Oviedo A, Torres Jaén MJ, Vidal-Cortes P, Colás SC. Management of patients with suspected or confirmed antibiotic allergy: executive summary of guidelines from the Spanish Society of Infectious Diseases and Clinical Microbiology (SEIMC), the Spanish Society of Allergy and Clinical Immunology (SEAIC), the Spanish Society of Hospital Pharmacy (SEFH) and the Spanish Society of Intensive Medicine and Coronary Care Units (SEMICYUC). J Investig Allergol Clin Immunol. 2023;33(2):95–101. https://doi.org/10.18176/jiaci.0859.
4. Izquierdo-Domínguez A, Rojas-Lechuga MJ, Alobid I. Management of Allergic Diseases during COVID-19 outbreak. Curr Allergy Asthma Rep. 2021;21(2):8.
5. Secretaria General de Salud Digital I e I para el S. Estrategia de salud digital. Sistema nacional de salud. Minist Sanidad Gob España. 2021. https://www.sanidad.gob.es/ciudadanos/pdf/Estrategia_de_Salud_Digital_del_SNS.pdf.
6. Sistema Nacional de Salud. Estrategia de Salud Digital. 1st ed. Gobierno de España; 2021. p. 62. https://avancedigital.mineco.gob.es/programas-avance-digital/Documents/EspanaDigital_2025_TransicionDigital.pdf.
7. Sistema Nacional de Salud. Estrategia Nacional de Inteligencia Artificial. Ministerio de Asuntos Económicos y Transformación Digital. 2020. https://portal.mineco.gob.es/RecursosArticulo/mineco/ministerio/ficheros/201202_ENIA_V1_0.pdf
8. https://www.lamoncloa.gob.es/presidente/actividades/Documents/2020/07102020_PlanRecuperacion.pdf.
9. Instituto para el Desarrollo e Integración de la Sanidad. Sanidad Privada, Aportando Valor. 1st ed. Madrid: Fundación IDIS; 2023.
10. Sastre J, Valero Santiago A, Montoro Lacomba J, Quirce S, Vidal Pan C, Dávila González I, et al. SEAIC specialty forum: analysis of the current situation of allergology in Spain and outlook for the future. J Investig Allergol Clin Immunol. 2021;31(2):120–31.
11. Barber Pérez P, González López-Valcárcel B. Estimación de la Oferta y Demanda de Médicos Especialistas. España 2018–2030. Vol. 1. 2019. p. 168.
12. Vivo Ocaña A, Bermejo P, Tárraga López PJ. Baja implantación de la teledermatología. J Negativae No Posit Results. 2020;5(3):259–94.
13. OECD/European Observatory on Health Systems and Policies. Spain: country health profile 2021, state of health in the EU. 1st ed. Brussels: OECD Publishing; 2021. p. 1–22.
14. Sigmados. Healthcare system survey. Fundación IDIS; 2023.
15. Thomas I, Siew LQC, Rutkowski K. Synchronous telemedicine in allergy: lessons learned and transformation of care during the COVID-19 pandemic. J Allergy Clin Immunol Pract. 2021;9(1):170–176.e1.
16. González-Pérez R, Sánchez-Machín I, Poza-Guedes P, Matheu V, Álava-Cruz C, Mederos LE. Pertinence of telehealth in a rush conversion to virtual allergy practice during the COVID-19 outbreak. J Investig Allergol Clin Immunol. 2021;31(1):71–80.
17. Amorim P, Brito D, Castelo-Branco M, Fàbrega C, Gomes Da Costa F, Martins H, et al. Telehealth opportunities in the COVID-19 pandemic early days: what happened, did not happen, should have happened, and must happen in the near future? Telemed e-Health. 2021;27(10):1194–9.
18. Bermejo Becerro A, Skrabski F, Pérez Pallisé M, Rodríguez Hermida S, Zubeldia Ortuño J, Alvarez-Perea A. Patient's perceived quality and satisfaction of teleconsultation Services in an Allergy Department during COVID-19 pandemic era. J Allergy Clin Immunol. 2021;147(Suppl 2):AB112.

19. ONTSI. Los Ciudadanos ante la e-Sanidad. Opiniones y expectativas de los ciudadanos sobre el uso y aplicación de las TIC en el ámbito sanitario. 2016.

20. Alvarez-Perea A, Cabrera-Freitag P, Fuentes-Aparicio V, Infante S, Zapatero L, Zubeldia JM. Social media as a tool for the management of food allergy in children. J Investig Allergol Clin Immunol. 2018;28(4):233–40.

21. Alvarez-Perea A, Ojeda P, Zubeldia JM. Trends in twitter use during the annual meeting of the Spanish Society of Allergology and Clinical Immunology (2013-2016). J Allergy Clin Immunol Pract. 2018;6(1):310–2.

22. Gabarron E, Fernandez-Luque L, Armayones M, Lau AY. Identifying measures used for assessing quality of YouTube videos with patient health information: a review of current literature. Interact J Med Res. 2013;2(1):e6.

23. Dimov V, Eidelman F. Utilizing social networks, blogging and YouTube in allergy and immunology practices. Expert Rev Clin Immunol. 2015;11(10):1065–8.

24. Reddy K, Kearns M, Alvarez-Arango S, Carrillo-Martin I, Cuervo-Pardo N, Cuervo-Pardo L, et al. YouTube and food allergy: an appraisal of the educational quality of information. Pediatr Allergy Immunol. 2018;29(4):410–6.

25. Rosenzweig D, Nickels AS. #asthma #inhaler: evaluation of visual social media depictions of inhalers and spacers. J Allergy Clin Immunol Pract. 2017;5(6):1787–8.

26. Sala-Cunill A, Luengo O, Curran A, Moreno N, Labrador-Horrillo M, Guilarte M, et al. Digital technology for anaphylaxis management impact on patient behaviour: a randomized clinical trial. Allergy Eur J Allergy Clin Immunol. 2021;76(5):1507–16.

27. Alvarez-Perea A, Dimov V, Popescu F-D, Zubeldia JM. The applications of eHealth technologies in the management of asthma and allergic diseases. Clin Transl Allergy. 2021;11(7):e12061.

28. Jácome C, Pereira AM, Amaral R, Alves-Correia M, Almeida R, Mendes S, et al. The use of remote care during the coronavirus disease 2019 pandemic: a perspective of Portuguese and Spanish physicians. Eur Ann Allergy Clin Immunol. 2022;54(1):25–9.

29. Molina Paris J, Almonacid Sánchez C, Blanco-Aparicio M, Domínguez-Ortega J, Giner Donaire J, Sánchez Marcos N, et al. Current expert opinion and attitudes to optimize telemedicine and achieve control in patients with asthma in post-pandemic era: the COMETA consensus. Aten Primaria. 2022;54(12):102492.

30. Martínez Rivera C, Crespo-Lessmann A, Arismendi E, Muñoz-Esquerre M, Aguilar X, Ausín P, et al. Challenges for asthma units in response to COVID-19: a qualitative group dynamics analysis. J Asthma. 2022;59(6):1195–202.

31. Vidal-Aliaball J, Acosta-Roja R, Pastor Hernández N, Sanchez Luque U, Morrison D, Narejos Pérez S, et al. Telemedicine in the face of the COVID-19 pandemic. Aten Primaria. 2020;52(6):418–22.

32. Fernández-de-Alba I, Brigido C, García-Gutierrez I, Antolín-Amérigo D, Sánchez-García S. COVID-19 and allergy: allergists' workload during the pandemic. J Investig Allergol Clin Immunol. 2021;31(2):187–90.

33. Matricardi PM, Dramburg S, Alvarez-Perea A, Antolín-Amérigo D, Apfelbacher C, Atanaskovic-Markovic M, et al. The role of mobile health technologies in allergy care: an EAACI position paper. Allergy. 2020;75(2):259–72.

34. Alvarez-Perea A, Sánchez-García S, Muñoz Cano R, Antolín-Amérigo D, Tsilochristou O, Stukus DR. Impact of "eHealth" in allergic diseases and allergic patients. J Investig Allergol Clin Immunol. 2019;29:94.

35. Knibb RC, Alviani C, Garriga-Baraut T, Mortz CG, Vazquez-Ortiz M, Angier E, et al. The effectiveness of interventions to improve self-management for adolescents and young adults with allergic conditions: a systematic review. Allergy. 2020;75(8):1881–98.

36. Nievas Soriano BJ, Uribe-Toril J, Ruiz-Real JL, Parrón-Carreño T. Pediatric apps: what are they for? A scoping review. Eur J Pediatr. 2022;181(4):1321–7.

37. Mayoral K, Garin O, Caballero-Rabasco MA, Praena-Crespo M, Bercedo A, Hernandez G, et al. Smartphone app for monitoring asthma in children and adolescents. Qual life Res. 2021;30(11):3127–44.

Index

© The Author(s), under exclusive license to Springer Nature Switzerland AG 2025
P. M. Matricardi, S. Dramburg, *Digital Allergology*, Health Informatics, https://doi.org/10.1007/978-3-031-71021-6